Lumbar Spinal Imaging in Radicular Pain and Related Conditions

Jan T. Wilmink

Lumbar Spinal Imaging in Radicular Pain and Related Conditions

Understanding Diagnostic Images in a Clinical Context

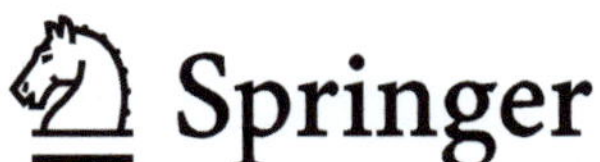 Springer

Prof. Dr. Jan T. Wilmink
University Hospital Maastricht
Dept. Radiology
6202 AZ Maastricht
Netherlands
jtwilmink@hotmail.com

Additional material to this book can be downloaded from http://extras.springer.com

ISBN: 978-3-642-43238-5   ISBN: 978-3-540-93830-9 (eBook)

DOI: 10.1007/978-3-540-93830-9

Springer Heidelberg Dordrecht London New York

© Springer-Verlag Berlin Heidelberg 2010
Softcover re-print of the Hardcover 1st edition 2010

This work is subject to copyright. All rights are reserved, whether the whole or part of the material is concerned, specifically the rights of translation, reprinting, reuse of illustrations, recitation, broadcasting, reproduction on microfilm or in any other way, and storage in data banks. Duplication of this publication or parts thereof is permitted only under the provisions of the German Copyright Law of September 9, 1965, in its current version, and permission for use must always be obtained from Springer. Violations are liable to prosecution under the German Copyright Law.

The use of general descriptive names, registered names, trademarks, etc. in this publication does not imply, even in the absence of a specific statement, that such names are exempt from the relevant protective laws and regulations and therefore free for general use.

Product liability: The publishers cannot guarantee the accuracy of any information about dosage and application contained in this book. In every individual case the user must check such information by consulting the relevant literature.

Cover design: eStudio Calamar, Figueres/Berlin

Printed on acid-free paper

Springer is part of Springer Science+Business Media (www.springer.com)

Many years ago as a young neurologist I found myself, more or less by chance, with a temporary appointment in the neuroradiological staff of the University Hospital Groningen. As it turned out, this "temporary" excursion proved to be more permanent than I had anticipated, and some thirty years later, I look back on a career in neuroradiology, which has centred importantly on spinal imaging.

An encounter of crucial importance for me was with Lourens Penning, then professor of neuroradiology and head of the department in Groningen. Lourens was a gifted and driven researcher and an accomplished illustrator, as well as being strongly interested in spinal morphometry and biomechanics. He imparted to me an understanding of the principles of spinal imaging, especially functional imaging, as well as of clinical research. Our co-operation was a fruitful one, as numerous joint references in this book attest.

I have been privileged to experience an era of almost bewildering change in the field of medical imaging. At the time of my arrival on the scene in 1976, the mainstays of cerebral diagnosis were still pneumoencephalography, the notorious air study, together with cerebral angiography, with subsidiary roles for brain isotope scanning and echoencephalography. In the spine, diagnosticians still relied heavily on plain X-ray films, with contrast myelography available to image the soft contents of the spinal canal and isotope studies to study CSF flow patterns and detect vertebral lesions.

Computed tomography (CT scanning) of the brain had recently been introduced, but was not generally available. Spinal CT would not become feasible until the advent of large-bore body scanners and high-resolution algorithms. When this did occur in the late-1970s, techniques such as epidural venography and peridurography, which had been introduced as attempted substitutes for myelography, quickly disappeared from the scene. Myelography was relegated to second place, but remained of value, usually in combination with CT.

The advent of magnetic resonance imaging (MRI) provided another great advance in imaging technology and image resolution. MRI has become the prime modality for diagnostic imaging of the brain and spine, and has proven to be superior in many ways to CT. To neurologists and neurosurgeons trained in the last twenty years, it seems almost incredible that neurological diagnosis could previously be achieved without access to these sophisticated imaging modalities. Yet this was actually the case, and while it is undoubtedly true that modern imaging has made life much easier for present-day diagnosticians and patients, it is also a fact that the application of this technology by itself has not provided answers to many important questions which still confront us.

This is also true in the diagnosis of lumbosacral radicular pain and related conditions such as neurogenic claudication. Whereas it is now possible to detect and classify even the smallest disc herniation and measure accurately the dimensions of the spinal canal, fundamental questions are still unanswered.

Much is still unclear about the pathogenesis of sciatica, but it has now become obvious that there is more involved than simply "rupture of the intervertebral disc with involvement of the spinal canal" as Mixter and Barr described in their historic article in 1934. Inflammatory components have proved to play an important role. In neurogenic claudication presenting in patients with lumbar spinal stenosis, vascular factors appear to be at work beside compression of the cauda equina within the narrowed canal. Functional spinal imaging in different postures has, however, helped us to explain the posture-dependency of this complaint

Lumbar disc herniations are frequently encountered by chance in individuals who are not suffering and who will not suffer from symptoms attributable to these herniations. The prevalence of these incidentally-found herniations in the healthy population is generally estimated at around 30%, though even higher percentages have been reported! It is still not fully clear in which ways these asymptomatic herniations and these individuals differ from morphologically similar herniations in patients who do present with radicular symptoms.

Radicular pain episodes tend to be self-limiting, and the presence of a herniated disc causing radicular pain is not a mandatory indication for surgical therapy, as the majority of these pain syndromes will show spontaneous remission. On the other hand, the complaints can be persistent in a small minority of these and it would obviously be useful to be able to select such cases for early surgical therapy, thereby saving these patients an extended period of fruitless conservative therapy.

This book represents an attempt to formulate the beginning of an answer to some of these questions. As a consequence of my neurological and neuroradiological background, I have chosen to focus on the assessment of the state of the nerve root. For this reason, much attention is devoted to technical aspects and interpretation of MR myelographic imaging.

Chapter 1 on the nature of radicular pain presents an overview of the evolution of this concept, from a simple mechanical compression model to a complex phenomenon with humoral and auto-immune inflammatory components, and featuring besides pain by direct involvement of the nerve root, pain originating in spinal musculoskeletal structures, which is referred via a central mechanism to the lower extremities

In Chapter 2, lumbar spinal imaging techniques are reviewed, briefly discussing methods formerly used and focusing on MRI with special attention to MR myelography.

Chapter 3 deals with normal topographic and sectional spinal anatomy, with a section devoted to functional imaging, describing the effects of postural changes on normal spinal structures and dimensions.

Chapter 4 is devoted to pathologic anatomy and the way in which symptomatic nerve root compression can come about. In this chapter as well as the next, case illustrations are captioned with a brief summary of the presenting clinical symptoms of the patients illustrated.

Chapter 5 describes pre- and post-operative imaging, and attention is devoted to features which may help to predict the natural evolution of radicular complaints in an individual patient. In the same chapter, the presentation of various adverse post-operative events is reviewed.

Maastricht, The Netherlands   Prof. Dr. Jan T. Wilmink

Acknowledgements

I consider myself fortunate to have encountered so many gifted clinicians and teachers during my general medical and post-graduate neurological and radiological training, many of whom were especially interested in spinal diagnosis and therapy. I have tried to pass on their teaching to my students and trainees, who have also played a vital part in my own ongoing post-graduate training.
The most important message is probably always to keep in view the patient behind the image.

I thank the medical, technical and administrative staff of the radiology department of the University Hospital Maastricht, my home since 1989. In particular, my thanks go to Ine Kengen from the secretarial staff, whose help in the preparation of the manuscript and whose Photoshop expertise proved literally invaluable. Many thanks go to Geertjan van Zonneveld from the Audiovisual Department of the University Hospital Maastricht, as well as Hans Rensema and Rogier Trompert from the Anatomy Department of the University of Maastricht for providing many illustrations and producing much of the artwork in this book. Many other illustrations in the book are by Lourens Penning, and taken from joint publications and personal communications.
To Ute Heilmann, Meike Stoeck and their associates at Springer, whose professionalism and co-operative attitude made working together on this project a real pleasure. Paul Hofman and Linda Jacobi, my neuroradiological associates and successors, helped me greatly by their enthusiastic interest, advice and suggestions, and also provided a critical review of the text and illustrations. I thank them most warmly.
Finally, Jelleke, to whom this book is dedicated, for reasons that require no explanation.

Contents

The Nature of Radicular Pain and Related Conditions

1

1.1 Introduction

Sciatica, or pain in the distribution of the sciatic nerve due to a condition afflicting the nerve itself, is a fairly common occurrence with a yearly incidence of 1–5% (Frymoyer 1988). Clinical descriptions of sciatica go back to the times of Hippocrates and Cotugno, and the etiology of this affliction has puzzled medical practitioners for equally long. Much is still unclear.

In the course of the twentieth century, surgical techniques and insights improved to a degree in which sciatica was transformed from a symptom related to a "rheumatic" condition causing inflammation of the sciatic nerve to a symptom which could be relieved by an operation. In 1934, Mixter and Barr published their report on "Rupture of the intervertebral disc with the involvement of the spinal canal". The "dynasty of the disc" had begun!

Material extruded from the ruptured disc was thought to compress the adjacent nerve root and thereby produce radicular pain: pain apparently arising in the area of sensory supply of a spinal nerve root but caused by activation of afferent pain fibres within the spinal nerve or nerve root. It becames clear, however, that compression of a nerve root by a herniated disc or by another cause is not the only factor potentially involved in the production of sciatica. Garfin et al. (1991), reporting on four patients with radicular pain, saw no change in the radiological severity of nerve root compression after spontaneous remission of the complaints. Karppinen et al. (2001) were unable to correlate degree of disc displacement, nerve compression, or nerve root contrast enhancement with subjective symptoms. Beattie et al. (2000) have pointed out that although the presence of a herniated disc causing severe nerve root compression is strongly associated with distal leg pain, there can be considerable variations in radicular symptoms between people with similar MRI findings. They also found that radicular symptoms can occur without nerve root compression by a herniated disc or another cause: out of 256 patients in their study with no MRI signs of nerve root compression, 58% reported having unilateral and 23% bilateral lower extremity symptoms. In a study by Modic et al. (1995), out of 25 patients with acute radicular pain, MRI revealed normal findings in five.

On the other hand, disc herniations are frequently asymptomatic: Boos et al. (1995) reported finding herniations in 96% of 46 patients with low back pain or sciatica but also in 76% of a similar group of asymptomatic individuals matched for age, sex, and risk factors. This is a considerably higher percentage than in previous reports.

Surgical therapy for radicular compression has been reported to yield unsatisfactory results in up to one-third of operated patients (Loupasis et al. 1999).

Nerve roots that are compressed by a herniated disc causing sciatica often present an inflammatory aspect compared with normal adjacent nerve roots (Lindahl and Rexed 1951; Haddox 1992).

A large and growing body of experimental data, therefore, support the concept of radicular pain as being the result of compression of a nerve root which has undergone intrinsic changes, due to compression as well as an inflammatory process (Saal 1995; Modic and Ross 2007). This will be discussed in more detail below.

1.2 Radicular Pain: Nomenclature and Pathogenesis

For detailed reviews the reader is referred to recent, articles dealing with pathogenesis as well as other aspects of radicular pain syndromes (Stafford et al.

J. T. Wilmink, *Lumbar Spinal Imaging in Radicular Pain and Related Conditions*
DOI: 10.1007/978-3-540-93830-9_1, © Springer-Verlag Berlin Heidelberg 2010

2007; Mulleman et al. 2006) and a review of terminology by Van Akkerveeken (1993).

Sciatica has been defined above as pain in the distribution of the sciatic nerve due to pathology of the nerve itself. The term sciatica (Latin *ischialgia*) is composed from two Greek words meaning "pain in the buttock or upper thigh". Hippocrates called the symptom "hip pain", but Cotugno in 1764 first made the distinction between diseases of the hip and diseases of the sciatic nerve, the latter also known as "neuralgia ischiadica", "sciatic neuralgia"and "ischias". In the nineteenth century, Lasegue and others described tests to differentiate the "hip syndrome" from "true sciatica", the latter was considered to be caused by untreated diabetes mellitus and alcoholism.

Pain in the presence of a normal nervous system (somatic pain) can only occur through stimulation of nociceptors. Pain as a result of direct stimulation of nerve root fibres may occur in the presence of neural injury or disease, and is called "de-afferentation pain" (Van Akkerveeken 1993).

In the context of degenerative spinal disease the term "radicular pain" is a more precise and specific term than "sciatica", and should be preferred. Many and varying radicular symptoms are reported: pain can be severe and sometimes disabling, with often a sharp and burning component, sometimes cramping and vise-like, frequently accompanied by paresthesia, sometimes with sensory loss and motor weakness.

Radicular pain is defined as pain arising in a limb or the trunk by pathological processes involving the nerve root itself. Some have speculated that in disc-related radicular pain there is no stimulation of the radicular nerve root fibres themselves, but rather of the receptors of the nervi nervorum which innervate the root sleeve containing the nerve root (Verbiest 1973, 1975). This would imply that the symptom which we refer to as radicular pain is in fact a form of "referred pain". Referred pain originates in musculoskeletal structures such as ligaments, muscles and joint capsules and intervertebral discs, (as well as – apparently – dural root sleeves), and is "referred" to an extremity by a central reflex mechanism, sometimes mimicking a radicular distribution and then described as "pseudoradicular" pain. In this view much "radicular pain" is then in fact "pseudoradicular".

Van Akkerveeken (1993) concluded that radicular pain can be produced in two ways:

1. Radicular *de-afferentation pain* caused by traumatic or other pathologic changes of the nerve root fibres, such as compression of the root by a herniated disc. The pain is experienced in the segmental area of the nerve root involved, manifests itself days to months after the neural injury and differs from somatic pain in being characterised by feelings of constant burning and unpleasant dysesthesia accompanied by paroxysmal lancinating pain and sometimes hyperpathia, or pain caused by non-noxious stimuli. In another review (Patel 2002) the pain is described as dull and aching, with occasional sharp or shooting exacerbations, sometimes aggravated by coughing, sneezing, bending or prolonged sitting. At physical examination the irradiating pain can be provoked or exacerbated by various tests aimed at applying tension to the inflamed and irritated nerve root. The best known of these is the straight-leg-raising (SLR) test in which the leg is lifted with extended knee in order to stretch the sciatic nerve. The sciatic stretching effect can be reinforced by simultaneously flexing the cervical spine and/or applying dorsiflexion in the ankle joint. Occasionally the pain can be induced lifting the contralateral leg (crossed-SLR test), or even by bilateral compression of the jugular veins in the neck; this manoeuvre increases intracranial and intraspinal CSF pressure and presumably expands the dural sac and displaces the nerve root against the herniation.

2. Radicular *referred pain* due to stimulation of receptors in the nerve root sleeve, also due to compression by a herniated disc. The main difference between this type of pain and de-afferentation pain appears to lie in its distribution, which does not correspond with the segmental area of the nerve root involved. This may explain the fact that the pattern of pain distribution in L5 (referred) radicular pain does not differ significantly from that occurring when the S1 root sleeve is compressed (Van Akkerveeken 1993). Referred pain can originate in musculoskeletal spinal and paraspinal structures, and is described as having a deep localisation and a dull, aching or boring nature, sometimes irradiating over a considerable distance but difficult to localise exactly, with the area of pain irradiation varying within a group but constant per individual. There may be associated signs such as muscle spasm and local tenderness which can be elicited at physical examination, with deep palpation of gluteal and

paraspinal muscles or manipulation of hip or sacroiliac joints causing irradiating pain. With the patient supine, straight-leg-raising can induce referred pain from musculoskeletal structures in the low back region which deceptively resembles radicular pain due to increased root tension caused by the same manoeuvre.There may be autonomic signs as well, but usually no signs of neurologic deficit (Inman and Saunders 1944; Hockaday and Whitty 1967). Kellgren (1938) elicited referred pain from spinal muscles by injecting hypertonic saline, while Mooney and Robertson (1976) provoked back and leg pain by saline injection into lumbar facet joints. The pain, which occasionally irradiated as far as the foot, was relieved by a subsequent intrafacet injection of lidocaine while depressed tendon reflexes which were also noted in some cases, returned to normal. It was reported by Ohnmeiss et al. (1997) that this type of referred pain can originate in a degenerated and disrupted disc, and irradiate to the lower extremity without a lumbosacral nerve root being compressed or otherwise involved. Milette et al. (1995) reported that such referred pain could be reduced or abolished by intradiscal injection of lidocaine.

As mentioned, by the nineteenth century sciatica was generally considered to be the result of inflammation of the sciatic nerve, as the result of some unspecified rheumatic condition.

Mixter and Barr (1934) established the concept of nerve root compression by material extruded from a ruptured disc as a surgically treatable cause of sciatica. Initially it was thought that the irradiating pain associated with a herniated disc was the sole result of mechanical compression of the root by the displaced disc material, but it was argued by others that compression of peripheral nerves such as the ulnar or peroneal nerve is associated not with pain but rather with loss of function and paresthesia (Cavanaugh 1995). Rydevik et al. (1984) pointed out the role of compression-related changes in nerve root microcirculation leading to ischemia and formation of intraneural oedema, with the latter, in combination with demyelination, being critical factors in pain production.

Smyth and Wright (1958) noted that compressed lumbosacral nerve roots are much more sensitive to mechanical stimulation than uncompressed roots. In a series of experiments nylon loops were placed during operation around nerve roots previously compressed by a disc herniation which had just been excised. Gentle traction on these loops caused severe sciatica similar in nature but more intense than the pain which had been present before the operation, with limitation of straight-leg-raising. Traction on a nylon loop passed around adjacent uncompressed nerve roots caused much less sciatic pain. Traction on a nylon loop passed through the dura mater adjacent to the nerve root, caused no discomfort in most patients, as was also the case with nylon loops passed through the flaval ligaments, the interspinous ligaments or, in a single case, the annulus fibrosus. It was concluded that prolonged irritation made a nerve root hypersensitive, and that merely touching such a nerve root is then sufficient to cause severe sciatica.

Similar findings of hyperaesthesia of compressed nerve roots stimulated by light touch during operation under local anaesthesia, were reported by Murphey (1968, 1973), later also by Greenbarg et al. (1988). It was noted that the root sleeve of such a nerve root was frequently hyperaemic, and the hyperaesthesia could be abolished by the application of a local anaesthetic. Murphey also reported that hypersensitivity of a nerve root compressed by a herniated disc could be accompanied by hypersensitivity of the adjacent annulus and the posterior longitudinal ligament over the herniation. Kuslich et al. (1991) found that a patient's sciatica could be reproduced by mechanical or electrical stimulation of a compressed or stretched nerve root, while normal nerve roots were completely insensitive to such stimuli. Stimulation of the annulus fibrosus reproduced previous complaints of low back pain in about two-thirds of the patients.

As mentioned earlier, histological evidence of inflammation can be found in nerve roots inspected during laminectomy (Lindahl and Rexed 1951). McCarron et al. (1987) injected homogenised autologous nucleus pulposus material into the epidural space of dogs, and observed an intense inflammatory reaction involving the dura and nerve roots, with no such reaction in a control group injected with saline. A macrophage reaction also featuring neovascularisation was found by Ito et al. (1996) in postoperative histological examination of extruded disc material, and this reaction was considered to represent a process of "absorption" of the extrusion. The radiological expression of this reaction appears to be the finding of MRI contrast enhancement around an extruded disc fragment located in the epidural space (See chapter 5). Contrast enhancement can also be seen in compressed and irritated nerve roots, sometimes visible from the site of compression to the insertion of the root in the conus medullaris, and considered to be due to breakdown of the normally present blood–nerve barrier (Jinkins 1993; see also Chap. 5).

Application of nucleus pulposus material in rats also reduces blood flow in the dorsal root ganglion and increases endoneural fluid pressure within the root (Yabuki et al. 1998), and morphologic and functional changes in nerve roots of dogs can reportedly be produced by merely making an incision in the adjacent annulus fibrosus (Kayama et al. 1996). In human studies herniated nucleus pulposus material has proved to contain high levels of phospholipase A2 (PLA2), an enzyme involved in the inflammatory process (Saal et al. 1990). PLA2, which is also found in normal discs, is present at higher levels in sequestrated, as opposed to contained, disc material (Piperno et al. 1997) and acts on the cell membrane to release arachidonic acid, and this substance is a precursor of inflammatory mediators (leukotrines and thromboxanes) which are present at high levels in disc material removed at operation in patients with radicular pain (Nygaard et al. 1997).

Human PLA2 provokes an inflammatory reaction in mice (Franson et al. 1992), and when injected into the epidural space of rats causes demyelination of the nerve roots with weakness and sensory changes in the posterior limbs (Chen et al. 1997).

In addition several cytokines have been demonstrated in disc material of patients with radicular syndromes. Tumour necrosis factor α (TNFα) is the most important in connection with inflammatory properties of nucleus pulposus, but interleukins and prostaglandins are also mentioned (Takahashi et al. 1996).

Involvement of an auto-immune component in acute as well as chronic radicular pain has been reported, with antibodies being formed against glycosphingolipids in the central and peripheral nervous system (Brisby et al. 2002), and markers of glial cell and nerve cell damage present or elevated within the CSF (Brisby et al. 1999).

Animal experiments performed in rats by Myers and Olmarker (1988) showed that exposure of the nerve root to nucleus pulposus material, or chronic nerve root displacement separately do not alter mechanical or thermal stimulation thresholds. In rats exposed to nerve root displacement as well as application of nucleus pulposus material to the root however, there was a significant and lengthy reduction in threshold for thermal stimuli, accompanied by histologic changes indicating cellular injury. Later studies by Kawakami et al. (2003) and Hou et al. (2003) provided similar findings.

In their review, Stafford et al. (2007) conclude that radicular pain in sciatic nerve roots arises from a complex interaction of inflammatory, immune and pressure-related elements. Pressure alone does not cause pain in the compressed roots but the inflammatory process seems to be exacerbated by the effects of nerve root pressure (see also Boos et al. 1995).

1.3 Neurogenic Claudication

In this condition the dural sac and the cauda equina within it are compressed due to some form of stenosis, or narrowing of the spinal canal. The symptoms of this condition may differ from the radicular pain which is associated with compression and inflammation of a single nerve root by a herniated disc, and which has been described above. Common symptoms in neurogenic claudication are irradiating low back pain, also numbness or tingling of the legs (Goh et al. 2004). Complaints are related to posture and sometimes exercise, and the irradiating pain, usually bilateral, may have paresthetic qualities and feelings of numbness, coldness, sometimes burning or cramping, with often a "sensory march" of the symptoms proximally to distally in the legs. These symptoms commence and progress during certain activities (walking erect, standing still: "dysbasia et dysstasia"), and when the activity is discontinued there is rapid relief. If the activity is continued, muscular weakness may set in and eventually collapse (Wilson 1969). Neurologic examination at rest usually reveals no clear motor, sensory or reflex deficits, but one report (Johnsson et al. 1987) mentions bilateral neurogenic EMG changes and high thresholds to vibration and temperature changes in the legs at neurophysiologic testing, most frequently in patients with spinal stenosis and a complete myelographic block. The straight-leg-raising test is usually normal, as well as other tests evoking nerve root tension.

Neurogenic claudication in most cases first manifests itself in older patients than disc-related radicular pain does, its clinical course is slowly progressive and less acute and episodic, patients tend to wait longer before seeking medical help and are generally managed by conservative measures over a longer period of time before operative therapy is sought (Paine 1976).

Patients with unilateral or bilateral entrapment of a single nerve root in a narrowed lateral recess (see Chap. 4) may experience monoradicular pain, and sometimes neurologic deficit in the area of the affected root, similar to that caused by a lumbar disc herniation, with the difference that the nerve root compression is more frequently posture-dependent (Penning and Wilmink 1987). This is sometimes referred to as "root claudication" (Patel 2002).

The pathogenesis of neurogenic claudication is associated with lumbar spinal stenosis or narrowing of the spinal canal, through developmental or degenerative causes, with compression of the dural sac and the cauda equina fibres within it, at one or more disc levels (see Chap. 4). However, it has been noted that anatomically identical changes in a single motion segment may produce either no clinical symptoms at all, or persistent radicular pain, or neurogenic claudication (Findlay 2000). In addition to the components of nerve root compression and inflammation mentioned above, an ischemic factor due to venous congestion is probably of significance in explaining the clinical features of neurogenic claudication. Venous congestion is especially severe when compression occurs at multiple levels: single-level compression of a porcine cauda equina model has little effect on function, but when applied at two levels causes a marked reduction by 64% in blood flow, as well as reduction of protein transport and nerve root conduction (Olmarker and Rydevik 1992). Compression of only 10 mmHg can lead to impaired supply of nutrition to the root (Olmarker et al. 1990). In addition, epidural pressure in patients with stenosis is increased compared to normals, and the pressure further increases during walking, and is reduced when walking with flexed lumbar spine (Takahashi et al. 1995). This is consistent with functional imaging studies indicating that sagittal movement of the spine from lordosis to kyphosis increases intraspinal dimensions, while increasing lordosis has the opposite effect (Penning and Wilmink 1981). In a stenotic spinal canal the effect of increasing lumbar lordosis will then be to reduce intraspinal dimensions beyond a critical degree and to set in motion the process of cauda equina compression and ischemia described above. Walking downhill, for instance, increases lumbar lordosis and tends to exacerbate the symptoms, while walking uphill reduces lordosis and relieves the pain. Cycling, with flexed lumbar spine, is well tolerated.

Neurogenic claudication can generally be distinguished from the clinical presentation of ischemic intermittent claudication by its posture-dependency. A patient with occlusive vascular disease of the lower extremities will experience intermittent claudication after walking a certain distance, and the symptoms can be relieved by standing still to rest the ischemic leg muscles. A patient with spinal stenosis will similarly experience claudication after walking for some time. In the latter case, however, merely standing still is insufficient to relieve the complaints: the posture must be changed from lordosis (erect) to kyphosis (sitting, squatting, crouching or lying down with flexed spine).

A further distinction has been proposed of spinal neurogenic claudication into a "postural"and an "ischemic" category (Wilson 1969). The pathogenesis in the first group is described above, and in the second, smaller group consisting of patients with arteriosclerosis, there is arterial insufficiency to the cauda equina as well as venous congestion due to stenosis, and symptoms are related more to exercise than to lordotic posture. In this last group, symptoms would be expected to be relieved by standing still to "rest the cauda equina".

1.4 Cauda Equina Syndrome

This is a clinical entity in which compression of the lower cauda equina including the sacral nerve roots, may result in persistent pain, loss of bladder/sphincter function and in sexual dysfunction together with dysesthesia, sometimes anaesthesia in the area of supply of the corresponding nerve roots (saddle anaesthesia). Most frequently the cause is a disc herniation large enough to occlude a spinal canal which is normal or already narrowed, and depending on the level of the occlusion motor, sensory symptoms related to involvement of lumbar nerve roots may also occur. With slowly progressive compression of the cauda equina the nerve roots have more time to adjust, and animal experiments have confirmed that in rapid onset of cauda equina compression the effects are more profound than in slow onset (Hägg and Rydevik 1999). Cauda equina syndrome is estimated to occur in up to 1% of all disc herniations, and is considered to represent a diagnostic and surgical emergency (Shapiro 2000; see also Chap. 4).

1.5 Conclusion

The pathogenesis of radicular pain has proven to be more complex than simply being the result of mechanical compression of an otherwise healthy nerve root. Various inflammatory, humoral and auto-immune factors are also involved in producing lumbosacral radicular pain, or sciatica, and much is still unclear. It does appear, however, that mechanical deformation or compression of the nerve root is an essential factor in the production of radicular pain (so-called de-afferentation pain), as opposed to "pseudoradicular" referred pain which originates in the degenerated disc, in the facet or in another spinal or even extraspinal structure such as the sacroiliac joint or hip joint.

In practical diagnostic terms, this implies the following: if a patient suffering from irradiating low back pain is shown to harbour a disc herniation which is, however, not compressing a nerve root, it appears likely that the pain is of the referred type and the response to surgical therapy is less predictable

As will be stressed in later chapters, demonstration of the presence or absence of nerve root compression forms an important aspect of diagnostic imaging in these patients, and this feature should be specified in the radiological report.

References

Beattie PF, Meyers SP, Stratford P et al (2000) Associations between patient report of symptoms and anatomic impairment visible on lumbar magnetic resonance imaging. Spine 25(7):819

Boos N, Rieder R, Schade V et al (1995) 1995 Volvo Award in clinical sciences. The diagnostic accuracy of magnetic resonance imaging, work perception, and psychosocial factors in identifying symptomatic disc herniations. Spine 20(24): 2613

Brisby H, Balague F, Schafer D et al (2002) Glycosphingolipid antibodies in serum in patients with sciatica. Spine 27(4): 380

Brisby H, Olmarker K, Rosengren L et al (1999) Markers of nerve tissue injury in the cerebrospinal fluid in patients with lumbar disc herniation and sciatica. Spine 24(8):742

Cavanaugh JM (1995) Neural mechanisms of lumbar pain. Spine 20(16):1804

Chen C, Cavanaugh JM, Ozaktay AC et al (1997) Effects of phospholipase A2 on lumbar nerve root structure and function. Spine 22(10):1057

Findlay G (2000) Neurologic compression theory. In: Gunzburg RS, Szpalski M (eds) Lumbar spinal stenosis. Lippincott Williams and Wilkins, Philadelphia

Franson RC, Saal JS, Saal JA (1992) Human disc phospholipase A2 is inflammatory. Spine 17(6 Suppl):S129

Frymoyer JW (1988) Back pain and sciatica. N Engl J Med 318 (5):291

Garfin SR, Rydevik BL, Brown RA (1991) Compressive neuropathy of spinal nerve roots. A mechanical or biological problem? Spine 16(2):162

Goh KJ, Khalifa W, Anslow P et al (2004) The clinical syndrome associated with lumbar spinal stenosis. Eur Neurol 52(4):242

Greenbarg PE, Brown MD, Pallares VS et al (1988) Epidural anesthesia for lumbar spine surgery. J Spinal Disord 1(2): 139

Haddox (1992) Lumbar and cervical epidural steroid therapy. Anesthesiol Clin N Am 10:179

Hägg O, Rydevik B (eds) (1999) Stenosis and the cauda equina syndrome. Lippincott, Williams and Wilkins, Philadelphia

Hockaday J, Whitty C (1967) Patterns of referred pain in the normal subject. Brain 90(3):481

Hou SX, Tang JG, Chen HS et al (2003) Chronic inflammation and compression of the dorsal root contribute to sciatica induced by the intervertebral disc herniation in rats. Pain 105(1–2):255

Inman V, Saunders J (1944) Referred pain from skeletal structures. J Nerv Ment Dis 99:660

Ito T, Yamada M, Ikuta F et al (1996) Histologic evidence of absorption of sequestration-type herniated disc. Spine 21(2): 230

Jinkins JR (1993) MR of enhancing nerve roots in the unoperated lumbosacral spine. AJNR Am J Neuroradiol 14(1): 193

Johnsson KE, Rosen I, Uden A (1987) Neurophysiologic investigation of patients with spinal stenosis. Spine 12(5):483

Karppinen J, Malmivaara A, Tervonen O et al (2001) Severity of symptoms and signs in relation to magnetic resonance imaging findings among sciatic patients. Spine 26(7):E149

Kawakami M, Hashizume H, Nishi H et al (2003) Comparison of neuropathic pain induced by the application of normal and mechanically compressed nucleus pulposus to lumbar nerve roots in the rat. J Orthop Res 21(3):535

Kayama S, Konno S, Olmarker K et al (1996) Incision of the anulus fibrosus induces nerve root morphologic, vascular, and functional changes. An experimental study. Spine 21 (22):2539

Kellgren J (1938) Observations on referred pain arising from muscle. ClinSci 3:175

Kuslich SD, Ulstrom CL, Michael CJ (1991) The tissue origin of low back pain and sciatica: a report of pain response to tissue stimulation during operations on the lumbar spine using local anesthesia. Orthop Clin North Am 22(2): 181

Lindahl O, Rexed B (1951) Histologic changes in spinal nerve roots of operated cases of sciatica. Acta Orthop Scand 20(3): 215

Loupasis GA, Stamos K, Katonis PG et al (1999) Seven- to 20-year outcome of lumbar discectomy. Spine 24(22): 2313

McCarron RF, Wimpee MW, Hudkins PG et al (1987) The inflammatory effect of nucleus pulposus. A possible element in the pathogenesis of low-back pain. Spine 12(8):760

Milette PC, Fontaine S, Lepanto L et al (1995) Radiating pain to the lower extremities caused by lumbar disk rupture without spinal nerve root involvement. AJNR Am J Neuroradiol 16(8):1605

Mixter W, Barr J (1934) Rupture of the intervertebral disc with involvement of the spinal canal. N Engl J Med 211:210

Modic MT, Ross JS (2007) Lumbar degenerative disk disease. Radiology 245(1):43

Modic MT, Ross JS, Obuchowski NA et al (1995) Contrast-enhanced MR imaging in acute lumbar radiculopathy: a pilot study of the natural history. Radiology 195(2):429

Mooney V, Robertson J (1976) The facet syndrome. Clin Orthop Relat Res 115:149

Mulleman D, Mammou S, Griffoul I et al (2006) Pathophysiology of disk-related sciatica. I. Evidence supporting a chemical component. Joint Bone Spine 73(2):151

Murphey F (1968) Sources and patterns of pain in disc disease. Clin Neurosurg 15:343

Murphey F (1973) Chapter 1. Experience with lumbar disc surgery. Clin Neurosurg 20:1

Myers RR, Olmarker K (1988) Pathogenesis of sciatic pain: role of herniated nucleus pulposus and deformation of spinal nerve root and dorsal root ganglion. Pain 78:99

Nygaard OP, Mellgren SI, Osterud B (1997) The inflammatory properties of contained and noncontained lumbar disc herniation. Spine 22(21):2484

Ohnmeiss DD, Vanharanta H, Ekholm J (1997) Degree of disc disruption and lower extremity pain. Spine 22(14):1600

Olmarker K, Rydevik B (1992) Single- versus double-level nerve root compression. An experimental study on the porcine cauda equina with analyses of nerve impulse conduction properties. Clin Orthop Relat Res 279:35

Olmarker K, Rydevik B, Hansson T et al (1990) Compression-induced changes of the nutritional supply to the porcine cauda equina. J Spinal Disord 3(1):25

Paine KW (1976) Clinical features of lumbar spinal stenosis. Clin Orthop Relat Res 115:77

Patel N (2002) Surgical disorders of the thoracic and lumbar spine: a guide for neurologists. J Neurol Neurosurg Psychiatry 73(Suppl 1):i42

Penning L, Wilmink JT (1981) Biomechanics of lumbosacral dural sac. A study of flexion-extension myelography. Spine 6(4):398

Penning L, Wilmink JT (1987) Posture-dependent bilateral compression of L4 or L5 nerve roots in facet hypertrophy. A dynamic CT-myelographic study. Spine 12(5):488

Piperno M, Hellio le Graverand MP, Reboul P et al (1997) Phospholipase A2 activity in herniated lumbar discs. Clinical correlations and inhibition by piroxicam. Spine 22(18): 2061

Rydevik B, Brown MD, Lundborg G (1984) Pathoanatomy and pathophysiology of nerve root compression. Spine 9(1):7

Saal JS (1995) The role of inflammation in lumbar pain. Spine 20(16):1821

Saal JS, Franson RC, Dobrow R et al (1990) High levels of inflammatory phospholipase A2 activity in lumbar disc herniations. Spine 15(7):674

Shapiro S (2000) Medical realities of cauda equina syndrome secondary to lumbar disc herniation. Spine 25(3):348

Smyth MJ, Wright V (1958) Sciatica and the intervertebral disc; an experimental study. J Bone Joint Surg Am 40-A(6):1401

Stafford MA, Peng P, Hill DA (2007). Sciatica: a review of history, epidemiology, pathogenesis, and the role of epidural steroid injection in management. Br J Anaesth 99(4):461

Takahashi H, Suguro T, Okazima Y et al (1996) Inflammatory cytokines in the herniated disc of the lumbar spine. Spine 21 (2):218

Takahashi K, Kagechika K, Takino T et al (1995) Changes in epidural pressure during walking in patients with lumbar spinal stenosis. Spine 20(24):2746

Van Akkerveeken P (1993) On painpatterns of patients with lumbar nerve root entrapment. Neuro-orthopedics 14:81

Verbiest H (1973) Chapter 23. The management of cervical spondylosis. Clin Neurosurg 20:262

Verbiest H (1975) Comment on selective nerve root infiltration for the evaluation of sciatica. Orthop Clin N Am 6:314

Wilson CB (1969) Significance of the small lumbar spinal canal: cauda equina compression syndromes due to spondylosis. 3: intermittent claudication. J Neurosurg 31(5):499

Yabuki S, Kikuchi S, Olmarker K et al (1998) Acute effects of nucleus pulposus on blood flow and endoneurial fluid pressure in rat dorsal root ganglia. Spine 23(23):2517

2.1 Introduction

All imaging techniques have one feature in common: the basis is the interaction between energy and matter. This applies even to a conventional photograph: light (electromagnetic radiation in the visible wavelength spectrum) is reflected with different frequencies (colours) and intensities (brightness) from the surface of an object, thus, producing an image visible to our eyes. This image can then be reproduced on photographic film by a camera, or captured on canvas by an artist.

In a medical diagnostic setting, ultrasound waves can be reflected from tissue interfaces within the body to produce an echographic image. Electromagnetic energy in the high-energy X-ray part of the spectrum is capable of passing through the human body but is not entirely unaffected: the X-ray photons are weakened (attenuated) to a varying degree depending on their wavelength (hardness) on the one hand, and the electron density and thickness of tissues within their path on the other. The residual radiation which has passed through the body is registered by an X-ray film or another type of photon detector, and the distribution of grey shades (contrast) in the resulting image represents local variations in the tissue density.

Besides being reflected from, or transmitted through the body, energy can also be emitted from the body itself, for instance, by injecting a substance containing a radioactive isotope into the body. This principle is the basis of nuclear medical imaging techniques.

Another emission-based technique is magnetic resonance imaging (MRI), in which the protons incorporated in water molecules of the body tissues emit radiofrequency (RF) signals under the influence of a combination of a magnetic field enclosing the body and RF energy which is beamed into the body from an external source, causing the protons to "resonate" in electromagnetic terms.

All techniques presently employed for spinal imaging have shortcomings. Conventional X-ray images have the drawback that potentially harmful radiation is employed, in addition to possessing a limited contrast resolution. In the early decades of the last century, various methods were developed to artificially enhance image contrast by injecting contrast substances with very low (air) or high radiographic density (usually iodinated fluids) into various soft tissue structures or compartments. In the spine, myelography is the best known of these techniques.

The development of new diagnostic methods, such as computed tomography and magnetic resonance imaging, has resulted in a dramatic improvement in low-contrast resolution, coupled with the advantages provided by sectional (tomographic) imaging. The downside is an increase in irrelevant detail demonstrated by these improved techniques. This applies particularly to spinal imaging. Even conventional X-ray films of the spine often demonstrate age-related and degenerative changes which are not necessarily associated with the presence of disease. An MRI study can present an even greater abundance of morphologic details whose pathologic relevance is unclear. False-positive interpretation of an incidental finding is an ever-present pitfall in all imaging studies, and this is especially the case when insufficient attention is paid to the correlation of high-resolution CT and MR imaging findings with clinical signs and symptoms.

2.2 Conventional X-ray Studies

Plain films of the spine offer a quick and inexpensive evaluation of bony structures and are frequently used as an initial screening examination in, for instance,

J. T. Wilmink, *Lumbar Spinal Imaging in Radicular Pain and Related Conditions*
DOI: 10.1007/978-3-540-93830-9_2, © Springer-Verlag Berlin Heidelberg 2010

suspected fractures, malalignment, and congenital spinal defects. Abnormal spinal curves can be assessed in scoliosis and the anatomy of individual vertebrae can be defined, although superimposition of anatomical structures is a problem. Spondylolysis and spondylolisthesis are well demonstrated. Spinal metastases can be detected on plain X-ray films, but only in a late stage, when cortical bony structures of the vertebrae are affected, or the vertebra is deformed or collapsed. Manifestations of spondylodiscitis are also detected relatively late.

At present, plain film spinal imaging is still ordered frequently in patients presenting with low back pain and neck pain, but the diagnostic value of the examination in the evaluation of such complaints is low. Contrast resolution in conventional X-ray images is limited: only four tissue densities, namely bone, water, fat, and air, can be distinguished and soft tissue pathology such as a disc herniation cannot be visualised. On the other hand, so-called degenerative features such as disc space narrowing, spondylosis, and spondylarthrosis can be demonstrated in asymptomatic as well as symptomatic individuals (Fullenlove and Williams 1957).

The diagnostic yield of plain film studies in low back pain is very limited unless so-called red flags (indicators for specific disease conditions such as neoplasm, disc herniation or infectious disease) are present (Staiger et al. 1999). As mentioned above, however, the sensitivity for early detection of specific pathology by plain films is low, and in such cases alternative techniques with higher sensitivity, such as CT or MRI, are preferable.

A plain film examination of the lumbar spine usually consists of a lateral and a postero-anterior view. Oblique views are sometimes performed of the isthmus region in case of spondylolysis, but these substantially increase the X-ray dose to the patient, and are not always necessary. Studies of the spine in flexion (kyphosis) and extension or retroflexion (lordosis) can be used in the assessment of post-traumatic or degenerative instability.

2.2.1 Contrast Studies:

The following conventional X-ray studies featuring contrast injection are presently still performed in the lumbosacral spine:

Lumbar myelography (syn. radiculography, caudography). In this examination an iodinated radiologic contrast fluid is injected into the dural sac so that the cerebrospinal fluid is opacified, outlining the dural sac, the dural root sleeves and their contents (Bates and Ruggieri 1991). Structures of interest are the conus medullaris of the spinal cord, whose tip is located approximately at the L1–2 level, and the nerve roots forming the cauda equina which originate from the conus medullaris and traverse the lumbar dural sac in craniocaudal direction. These nerve roots exit the dural sac by way of a dural root sleeve which accompanies the emerging dorsal and ventral root fibres over a variable distance (see Chap. 3). Lumbar disc herniations which are located in the central, paracentral and subarticular regions of the spinal canal (see Chap. 4) can produce impressions upon the dural sac and displacement of the intradural nerve roots, as well as cut-off of contrast filling of the root sleeve (Fig. 2.1). Sometimes also swelling of the nerve root proximal to the site of compression is seen. The myelographic image of the nerve root ends when it leaves the contrast-filled subarachnoid space. Thus, lateral disc herniations compressing the dorsal root ganglion or nerve ramus inside or outside the intervertebral foramen, and which are reported to occur in around 10% of cases, (Abdullah et al. 1988), will frequently be missed by myelography (Jackson and Glah 1987).

Contrast myelography is not a very invasive procedure, but it is not completely innocuous (Bates and Ruggieri 1991; Wilmink et al. 1984), Even in experienced hands, a lumbar puncture followed by injection of contrast fluid may be difficult and painful, especially when the dural sac is constricted or collapsed and the nerve roots are crowded together by a large herniation or by narrowing of the spinal canal at the puncture site. The iodised oils which were initially employed for myelography frequently gave rise to adhesive arachnoiditis resulting in crippling back complaints. The water-soluble contrast media which were later introduced produced better images of the root sleeves but the first generation of these agents possessed a high osmolality and neurotoxicity and could also cause adhesive arachnoiditis (Skalpe 1978). Modern low-osmolality contrast media do not share these severe side effects.

Nowadays, the most common indication to perform contrast myelography is when MRI is contraindicated or not available, and when CT does not provide an

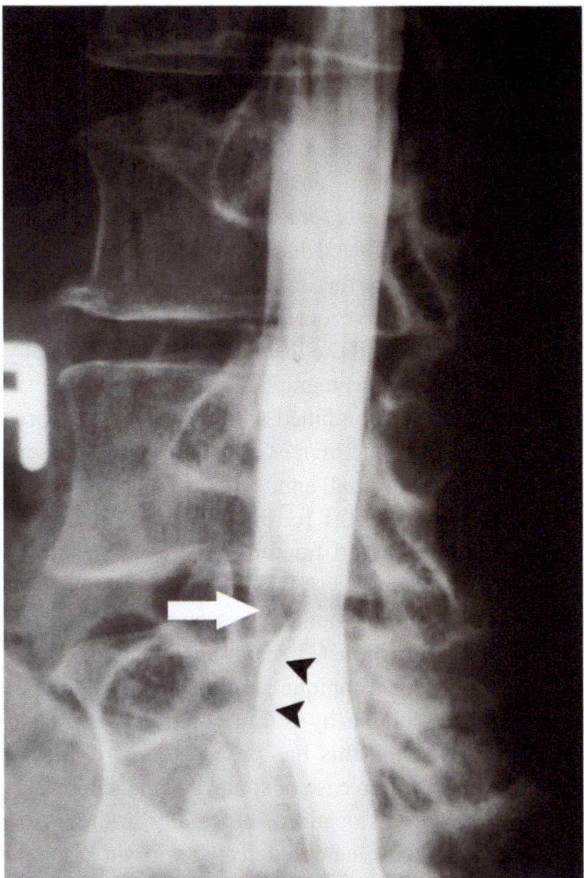

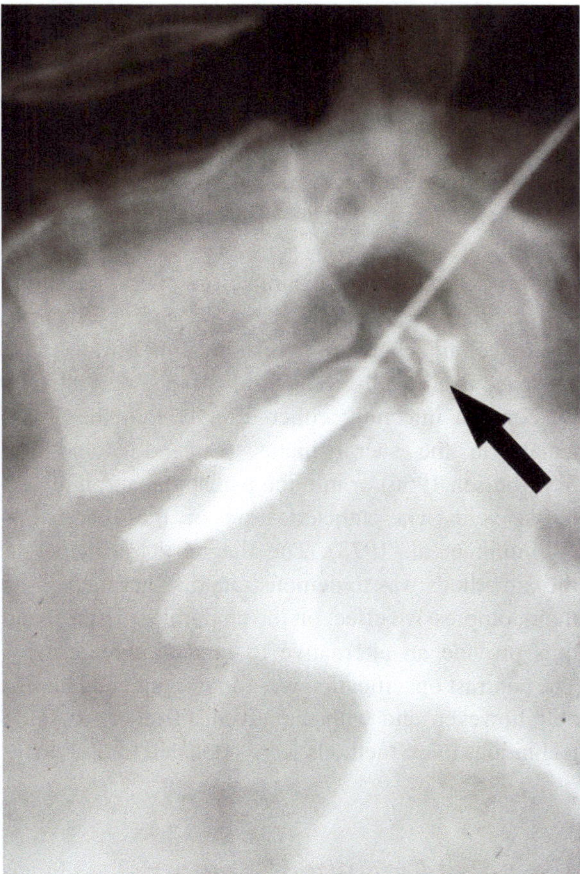

Fig. 2.1 Lumbar myelogram (radiculogram, caudogram). Right oblique projection centred on the L4 vertebra, with a water-soluble radiologic contrast medium outlining the dural sac, intradural nerve roots and root sleeves. Note ventrolateral filling defect at L4–5 disc level, mainly caused by swelling of distal intradural L5 root (*arrow*), with non-filling of L5 root sleeve. Medial displacement of intradural S1 root without compression, normal filling of S1 root sleeve (*arrowheads*)

Fig. 2.2 Lateral projection of L5-S1 discogram. Note opacification at site of nucleus pulposus, leakage of contrast medium to extruded disc (*arrow*)

adequate image of the dural sac and of possible intradural pathology. In these cases the conventional myelographic study will almost invariably be followed by CT myelography (see below).

Myelography can be employed to produce images of the dural sac and the cauda equina in the upright posture, or in lumbar flexion and extension (Penning and Wilmink 1981).

Discography. This examination technique is employed primarily to localise painful intervertebral discs responsible for lumbago or low back pain, and not to diagnose lumbosacral nerve root compression causing sciatica. A water-soluble iodinated radiologic contrast medium is injected into the nucleus pulposus of the intervertebral disc. The purpose of this is twofold. Firstly the increase in intradiscal pressure caused by the injection may reproduce or exacerbate the patient's pain complaints, thus confirming that the disc in question is the source of the pain. Secondly, X-ray images can show penetration of the contrast medium into fissures and defects in the annulus fibrosus, and sometimes also into herniated disc material (Fig. 2.2). Disc herniations and nerve root compression are diagnosed more accurately by MRI and CT however.

Discography is a controversial diagnostic procedure, with outspoken proponents as well as antagonists. The examination can be tedious and unpleasant for the patient, especially when muliple disc levels are studied. Discography is used to localise painful discs, but there are reservations because false-positive pain responses can occur, even when care is taken to apply a low injection pressure (Carragee et al. 2006), and subjective pain responses at discography should be interpreted with special caution in patients with chronic pain, social stressors and psychological disturbances (Carragee and Hannibal 2004). Annular tears or fissures can be demonstrated by discography, but MRI has shown these to occur in asymptomatic individuals as well as in low back pain sufferers with painful discs (Stadnik et al. 1998).

Two other contrast examinations, peridurography and epidural venography are no longer performed. These techniques relied on opacification of the epidural space itself, or the veins in this space respectively, by contrast injection, either directly into the spinal canal via the sacral hiatus (Luyendijk and van Voorthuisen 1966) or into the paraspinal and intervertebral veins via catheterisation of the iliac veins (Wilmink et al. 1978). The diagnostic principle of these methods was to demonstrate disc herniations by their compressive effect on the epidural structures, and thus provide an alternative to lumbar myelography. The contrast opacification was too irregular and unreliable however, and with the advent of newer imaging techniques these methods were relegated to obscurity.

2.3 X-Ray Computed Tomography

Computed tomography CT (Hounsfield 1973) revolutionised medical imaging by its introduction in the 1970s. Three innovations were combined:

- Acquisition of sectional (tomographic) images by the use of an X-ray tube rotating around the patient. This made it possible to study spinal anatomic relationships in the axial plane which could not previously be visualised. A much better insight was obtained in the morphology and classification of, for instance, spinal stenosis (see Chap. 4).
- Detection of smaller differences in X-ray attenuation (tissue density) by using more sensitive scintillation detectors instead of an X-ray film, thus, greatly improving soft tissue contrast resolution.
- Image reconstruction by a computer algorithm permitting selection of window and level settings appropriate for viewing bony or soft tissue structures as required.

The improved contrast resolution of CT made it possible to image disc herniations and other intraspinal normal and abnormal soft tissue features without the necessity of contrast injection into the dural sac (Fig. 2.4). Visualisation of intradural details by uncontrasted CT is limited; the spinal cord can sometimes be seen faintly, and intradural nerve roots not at all.

CT and myelography are complementary techniques: the first is more suitable for assessing the *cause* of radicular complaints, herniated disc, spinal stenosis etc., while the second is better for imaging the *effect*, the compressed intradural nerve root (Wilmink 1989). Techniques which combine both these features are CT myelography and MRI with MR myelography (see below).

CT can also be combined with discography to produce CT discographic images, thus improving the sensitivity with which small annular tears can be detected.

The sensitivity of CT for bony vertebral pathology such as metastasis and fracture is better than that of plain films.

A significant development has been the introduction of multi-slice spiral CT scanning with multi-planar reformatting. This technique permits rapid scanning of a large tissue volume by a thin continuous spiral or helical section, and this has proven to be of special value, for instance, in case of spinal trauma where subtle fractures and dislocations, especially in the posterior spinal elements, can be detected with an ease and accuracy unrivalled by any other imaging method.

CT can provide an acceptable diagnostic alternative to MRI in many cases with disc herniation or spinal stenosis (Figs. 2.3, 2.4). Soft tissue resolution by CT, however, is less than when MRI is employed, and some disc herniations can be overlooked (see Sect. 2.4). Anatomical detail is also less in reformatted sagittal CT images when compared to direct sagittal MRI cuts; in addition bone marrow pathology annular fissures and other subtle changes cannot be detected by CT. Intraspinal details usually are less well-depicted by CT at the level of the vertebral pedicles and lamina, where the dural sac is entirely surrounded by a ring of bony structures (see Chap. 3), where there is little epidural fat to outline the dural sac and migrated disc fragments may be missed. At the disc level the structures bordering the spinal canal are ligamentous and less dense, and there is usually more intraspinal fat present to act as a natural contrast agent.

CT has for many years formed the mainstay of diagnostic imaging in patients with radicular pain and related conditions, despite the drawback that compression of the intradural nerve root could not be visualised directly.

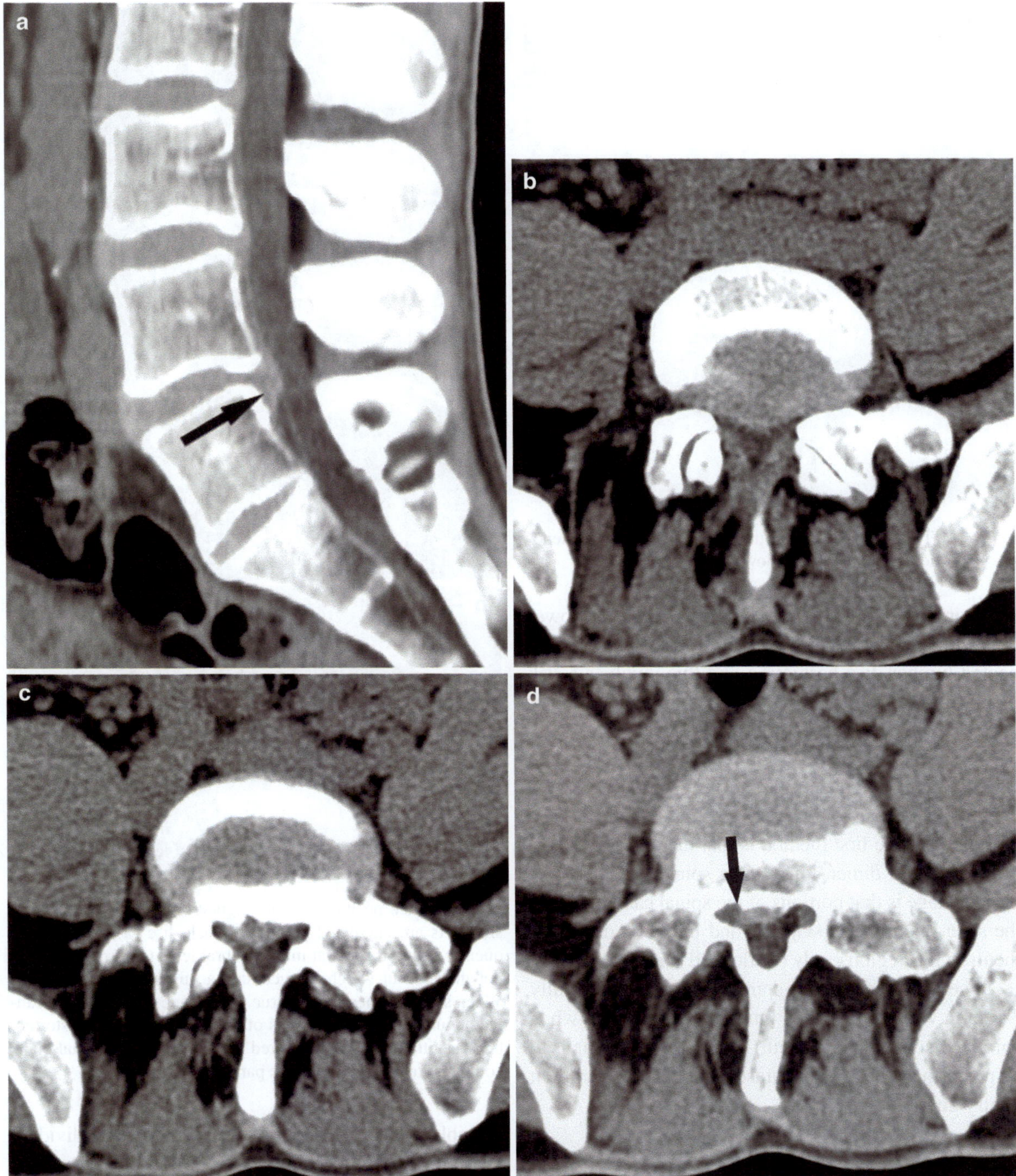

Fig. 2.3 Spiral CT study with multiplanar reformat. Patient with L4–5 disc herniation (**a**) mid-sagittal reformat showing extrusion migrating below disc level (*arrow*), axial 2 mm cuts at level of posterior disc (**b**), L5 endplate (**c**), and L5 lateral recess (**d**) show extrusion migrating laterally towards right L5 root in lateral recess (*arrow*). Left L5 root normally outlined by fat

Indirect evidence of compression of the intradural root in non-myelographic CT images can be derived from features such as flattening of the ventrolateral angle of the dural sac at disc level, as well as displacement by the herniation and disappearance of the epidural fat adjacent to the dural sac (Wilmink 1989).

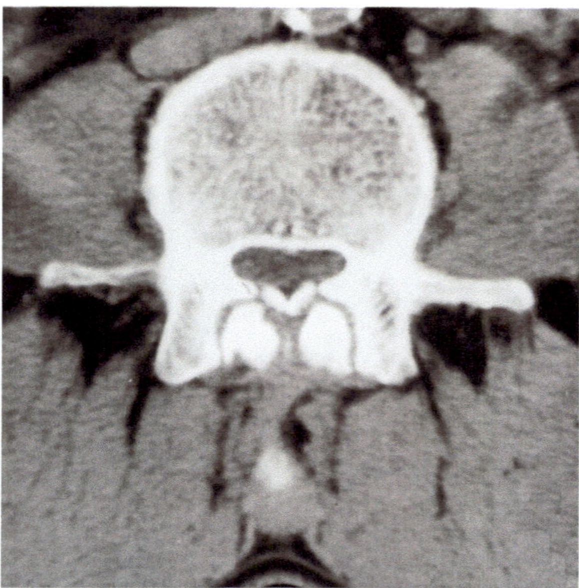

Fig. 2.4 CT of lumbar vertebra in developmental spinal stenosis. Note short pedicles and shallow spinal canal

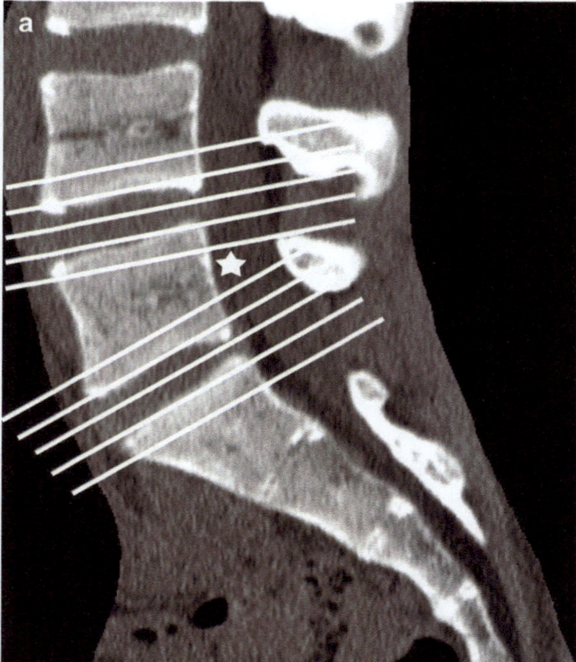

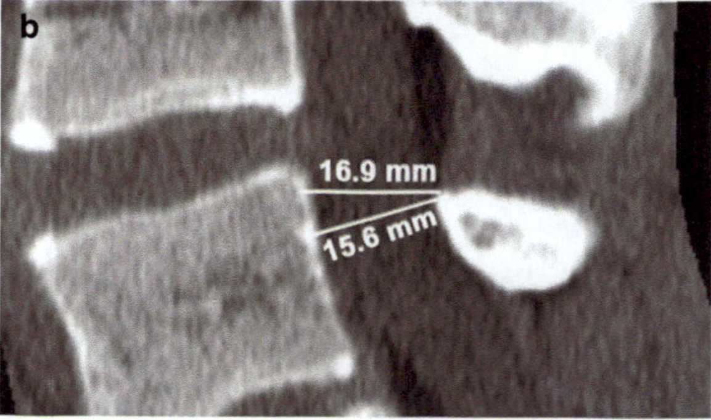

In order to limit the radiation dose, only the lower three lumbar disc levels are routinely scanned in suspected lumbar disc herniation and this involves a risk of missing a herniation which is situated at a higher lumbar level (see also Chap. 3).

CT slices can either be acquired in separate sets with the CT gantry angulated parallel to each disc, or as a continuous or overlapping series of parallel slices. The advantage of the first method is that there is less distortion of sagittal dimensions of the spinal canal, but the disadvantage is that portions of the spinal canal between the slice sets may be skipped, and migrated disc fragments in this region easily overlooked (Fig. 2.5).

Slice thickness in non-spiral lumbar CT is usually 3–5 mm, with thinner 2 or 1 mm slices preferred when spiral CT scanning with multi-planar reformatting is to be performed. The spiral datasets are acquired without gantry angulation.

Fig. 2.5 Slice positioning and angulation in spinal CT. When slice sets are angulated parallel to each disc (**a**), there is frequently a "blind spot" at mid-vertebral level (*asterisk*) which is not imaged but which may contain a migrated disc fragment. When slices are acquired in true axial plane without craniocaudal angulation (**b**) dimensions of the spinal canal are distorted: bony sagittal diameter measured as 16.9 mm in true axial plane compared to 15.6 mm in plane parallel to L4–5 disc

2.3.1　CT Myelography

This technique which was first reported by Di Chiro and Schellinger (1976) is a useful adjunct to conventional myelography as well as to non-contrast CT. The presence of an intrathecal contrast medium makes it possible to clearly discern the spinal cord and individual nerve roots within the dural sac, which is not possible on non-contrasted CT images. These structures are presented in the axial plane, which is not possible on conventional myelograms. The conventional myelographic image of the nerve root ends after its departure from the dural root sleeve, whereas with CT myelography the root can first be followed through the CSF compartment where it is outlined by the contrast medium in the

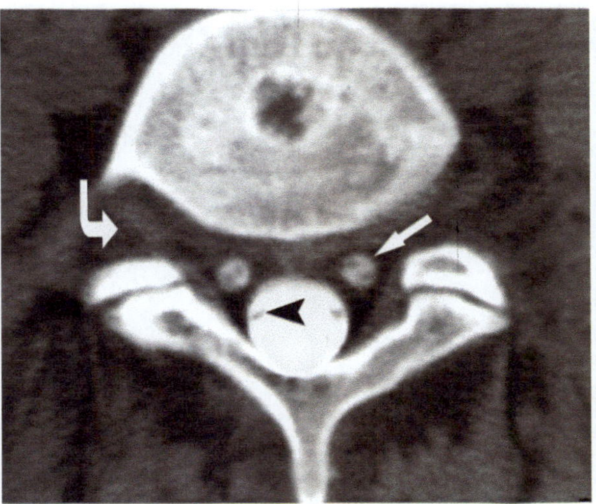

Fig. 2.6 CT myelography. 4.5 mm CT section through L5 end-plate after intradural contrast injection. Note dural sac and root sleeves opacified by contrast medium, with intradural details shown which are not depicted in plain CT: ventral and dorsal root components seen as *dark dots* within contrast-filled S1 root sleeve (*arrow*) and S2 root in dural sac (*arrowhead*). Curved arrow indicates right extradural L5 spinal nerve ramus exiting foramen and outlined by fat and seen only faintly at wide window setting

arachnoid space, then more distally through the foramen and beyond, where it is outlined by fat (Fig. 2.6).

When MRI is not available or contraindicated, CT myelography can be used for the detection of intraspinal space occupying lesions: intradural (intramedullary neoplasm or cyst, extramedullary meningioma or nerve root tumour) extradural (disc herniation, vertebral neoplasm or extradural hematoma) or both (dumbbell schwannoma). Cord atrophy or transection can also be demonstrated, but spinal cord lesions without mass effect, such as cord infarct or multiple sclerosis plaques can only be visualised by MRI. Other drawbacks of CT myelography compared to MRI are the necessity for intrathecal contrast injection and the employment of ionising X-rays.

On the other hand, spatial resolution in CT myelographic images is usually better than in axial MR images, and this is especially important in diagnosis of nerve root compression, for instance in the lateral recess of the spinal canal, where MRI often does not provide sufficient detail. CT is more accurate than MRI for the assessment of calcified herniations as well as bony spurs emanating from the vertebral bodies or encroaching upon the foramen as well as for demonstrating the presence of gas in a degenerated disc or joint (see Fig. 4.18).

2.4 Magnetic Resonance Imaging (MRI)

Imaging by nuclear magnetic resonance (NMR) (Mansfield and Maudsley 1977), presently better known as magnetic resonance imaging or MRI, produces computed tomographic sections similar to X-ray CT, but makes use of a different imaging principle. In X-ray CT, image contrast is derived from differences in X-ray attenuation due to variations in electron density in various structures within the body. In MRI the protons of the body are induced to act as radiofrequency (RF) transmitters by being positioned in a magnetic field and subjected to RF energy directed from an antenna, or coil. The electromagnetic resonance of the protons is analogous to the resonance of a tuning fork when exposed to sound of the appropriate frequency. The RF signals from the protons can be manipulated or "weighted" to selectively amplify signal intensity of various substances and structures within the body, and are spatially encoded to produce an image.

An MR image in which contrast is dependent on differences in longitudinal magnetic relaxation times as defined by so-called T1 values between various tissues is called "T1-weighted". When image contrast is predominantly determined by differences in transverse magnetic relaxation values (T2), the image is called "T2-weighted".

For spinal imaging, MRI has significant advantages over CT: soft tissue contrast resolution is better (Fig. 2.7) and there are no artefacts due to high-density skeletal structures. The signal intensity of bony spinal structures is less bright in MR than in CT images, and the latter method is better for diagnosing bony cortical lesions such as in vertebral fractures. Although some consider that spinal stenosis is better demonstrated by CT than by MRI, in fact cortical bone can be well-distinguished as a dark line bordering the brighter bone marrow in T1-weighted MR images. Also, spinal stenosis has an important ligamentous as well as a bony component. Even in cases with severe developmental stenosis, compression of the dural sac and the cauda equina takes place mainly at the level of the intervertebral disc, and is not due only to bony narrowing of the spinal canal but rather to superimposed ligamentous encroachment by bulging of the annulus fibrosus and hypertrophy of the flaval ligaments (Fig. 2.8, see also Chap. 4, Fig. 4.1.b and d), and

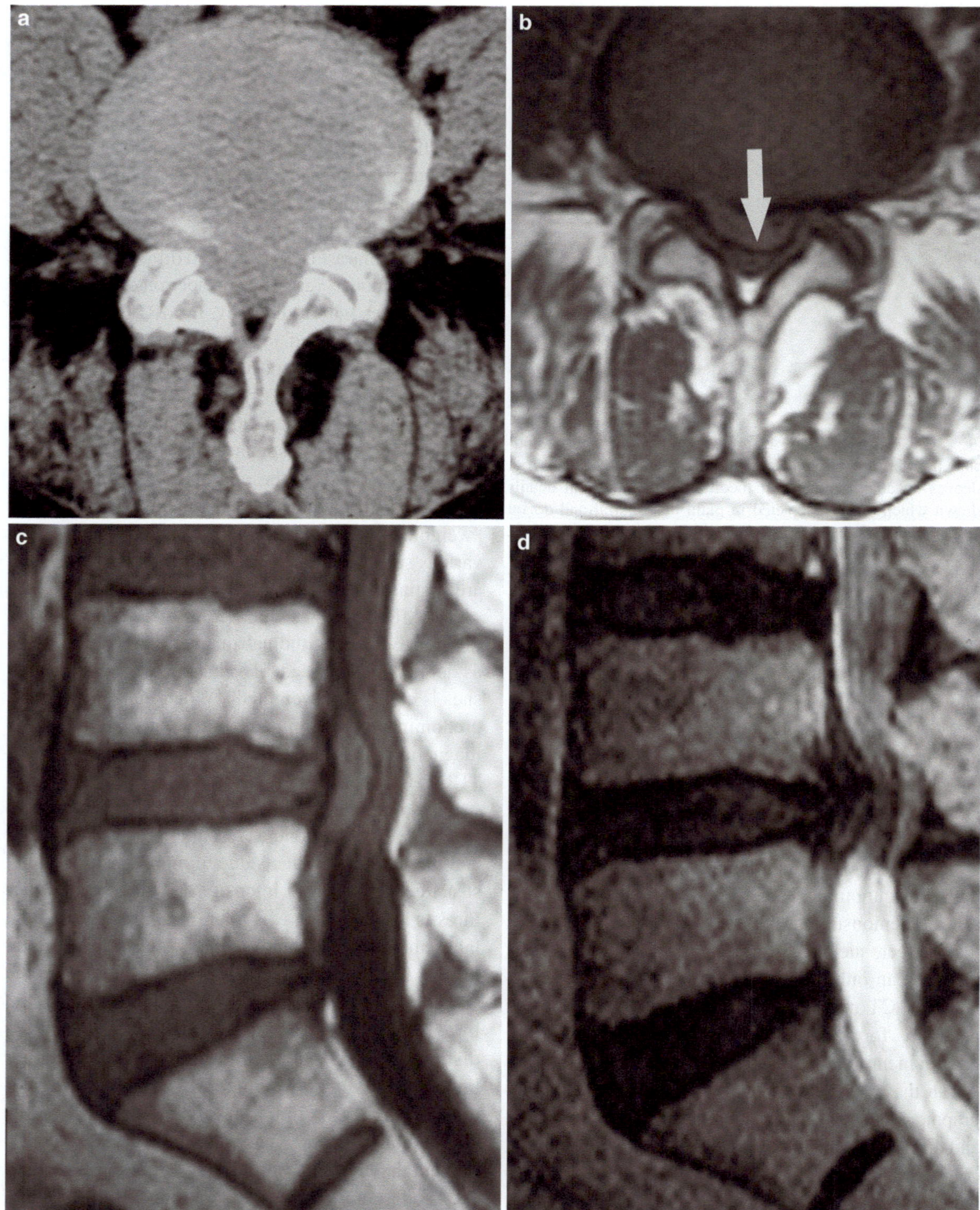

Fig. 2.7 CT compared to MRI. CT and MRI of same large L4–5 disc extrusion. Axial 5 mm CT section (**a**) shows apparently normal L4–5 disc. Axial T1-weighted 4.5 mm MRI section (**b**) shows large extrusion almost completely collapsing dural sac (*arrow*), also well-depicted in sagittal T_1-(**c**) and T_2-weighted images (**d**). Note that in retrospect remnant of collapsed dural sac is very faintly visible on CT section

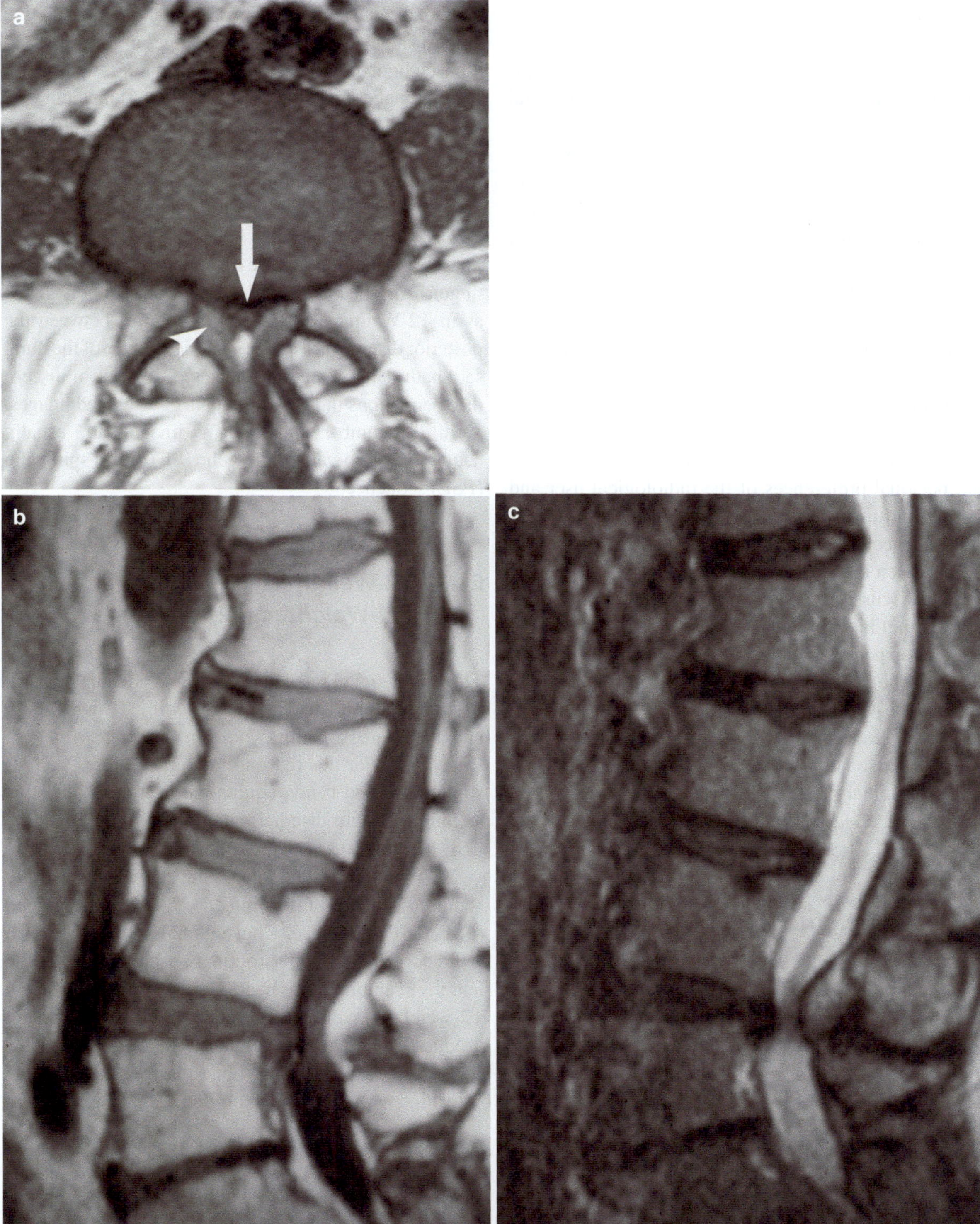

Fig. 2.8 T1-weighted axial MR image (**a**) in patient with localised narrowing of spinal canal at L4–5 showing almost complete CSF block on sagittal images (**b, c**) best seen on T2-weighted image (**c**). Note that axial cut clearly shows bony details such as facets on the one hand, as well as soft tissue structures such as annulus fibrosus (*arrow*) and flaval ligament (*arrowhead*) on the other

sometimes deformation of the spinal canal by degenerative anterolisthesis.

Subtle changes in shape and composition of the spinal cord can be demonstrated by MRI, and intradural nerve roots can be seen without the necessity for contrast injection into the dural sac (MR myelography, see below). MR images can be acquired in any plane desired, and are superior to reformatted sagittal or coronal CT images of the spine, especially for showing soft tissues.

The largest single indication for spinal MR imaging is presently in degenerative spinal disease, usually performed to diagnose a possible disc herniation.

A number of options for lumbar spinal MR imaging will now be discussed. It will be clear that there are many methods to produce good-quality diagnostic spinal images (Ruggieri 1999), and the selection depends upon the characteristics of the MRI system employed and personal preferences of the radiological user and clinical end-user. An example of a typical set of imaging sequences for use in lumbar degenerative disc disease is given in Fig. 2.9.

The discussion of the various techniques set out below is not intended to be exhaustive, and reflects the personal experience of this author. For more detailed information regarding technical aspects of MR imaging and the various acquisition sequences mentioned below, the reader is referred to specialised texts dealing with these subjects. A review of recent developments in spinal MR imaging sequences is given by Vertinsky et al. (2007).

2.4.1 T1-Weighted (T1-W) Images

In these images the CSF-filled dural sac is darker than the disc and vertebrae (Fig. 2.9a). Normal adult bone marrow has a light grey shade, with somewhat brighter signal intensity than that of the intervertebral disc. The fat seen in the epidural pockets dorsal to the dural sac, in

the sacral canal and in the intervertebral foramina has the highest signal intensity in T1-W images of the spine, and T1-weighting is popularly said to produce a "fat image". In such images fat acts as a natural contrast medium, and structures bordered by fat are clearly outlined: dorsal and caudal borders of the lumbar dural end-sac, foraminal borders and intraforaminal contents such as dorsal root ganglia, as well as laterally migrated disc extrusions.

Due to the low signal intensity of CSF on T1-W images, the intradural nerve roots can only be faintly distinguished. The spinal cord can be seen, but not as well as in T2-W images. The lack of contrast between the posterior disc surface and the anterior border of the dural sac, both dark, sometimes makes it difficult to discern disc herniations in this location on T1-weighted images.

In the lumbar spine T1-W images are usually acquired by a so-called spin-echo (SE) or fast spin-echo (FSE) sequence.

2.4.2 T2-Weighted (T2-W) and T2*-Weighted (T2*-W) Images

The bright signal intensity of water (CSF, nucleus pulposus) predominates in images with T2-weighting, and these are sometimes known as "water images" (Fig. 2.9b). For this reason intradural features such as spinal cord and cauda equina are best seen with this technique, as are disc herniations impinging upon the CSF-filled dural sac or the root sleeve.

T2-W lumbar spinal images are at present generally acquired with a 2D fast spin-echo, syn. turbo spin-echo (FSE, TSE) sequence. Conventional spin-echo (CSE) sequences are no longer routinely used because of the lengthy scanning times necessary to produce sufficient T2-weighting with this technique. CSE and FSE do not produce identical T2-weighted images; in a CSE sequence epidural fat and bone marrow fat have low signal intensity, while FSE produces a much higher fat

Fig. 2.9 Images from normal lumbar spinal MRI examination at 1.5 T. (**a**) Mid-sagittal 4 mm T1-weighted spin-echo image showing bright signal from epidural and subcutaneous fat, dark CSF signal. (**b**) Mid-sagittal 4 mm T2-weighted fast spin-echo image showing bright fluid signal from CSF and nucleus pulposus, also from epidural and subcutaneous fat. Note better depiction of posterior disc contour compared to (**a**). (**c**) Axial 4 mm T2-weighted fast spin-echo image at L4–5 produced with 3D DRIVE technique. Note good depiction of intradural cauda equina fibres by surrounding CSF (*white arrow*), also of dorsal root ganglion in foramen by surrounding fat (*white arrowhead*). Borders of dural sac (*small black arrows*) are less well-defined, however (**d**). Right and left oblique MR myelographic images presenting 3D projections of dural sac acquired with single-shot, single-slice technique (see below). Note good depiction of intradural nerve roots and root sleeves. Vertebral structures not imaged due to heavy T2 weighting

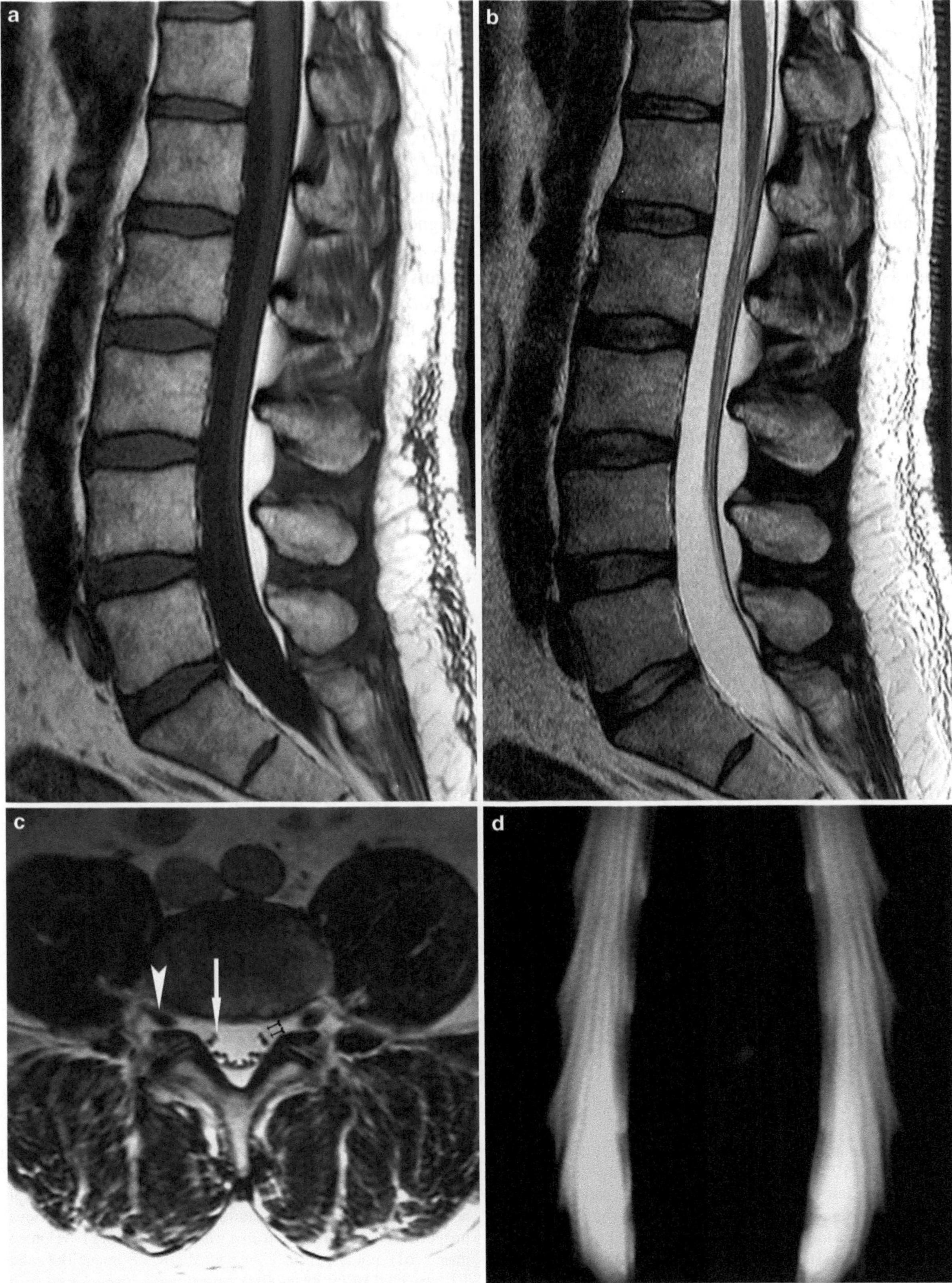
a
b
c
d

signal. In FSE T2-weighted images epidural and foraminal fat may be almost iso-intense to CSF (Fig 2.9b, c). This has the advantage that extradural disc fragments in the intervertebral foramen are well-outlined by bright fat; almost as well as in T1-W images. One could say that FSE T2-W images provide "water contrast" as well as "fat contrast". The disadvantage of this is that the CSF-filled dural sac can be difficult to distinguish from the surrounding epidural fat, as both are now bright (Fig. 2.9c).This can create a problem when assessing, for instance, abnormal increase in epidural fat (lipomatosis) on T2-W FSE images (see Chap. 4). In addition, bone marrow lesions with high water content, such as in certain degenerative changes, metastases or osteomyelitis, which classically appear hyperintense to normal bone marrow in a T2-weighted

CSE image, may be almost invisible on T2-weighted FSE images because the normal fatty bone marrow is now iso-intense to the lesions. Application of fat-suppression can be useful here (see below).

An FSE T2-W 3D driven equilibrium technique (DRIVE) presently used in our department for axial spinal imaging employs a desaturating pulse after acquisition of the spin-echo, in order to null residual magnetisation and so reduce the repetition time. In this way heavy T2 weighting can be produced in a rapid acquisition (Fig. 2.9c).

An alternative option for producing "water images" is by the use of a $T2^*$-weighted gradient-echo (GRE) sequence which also produces a high water signal. This technique is sometimes used for axial spinal imaging, most frequently in the cervical region.

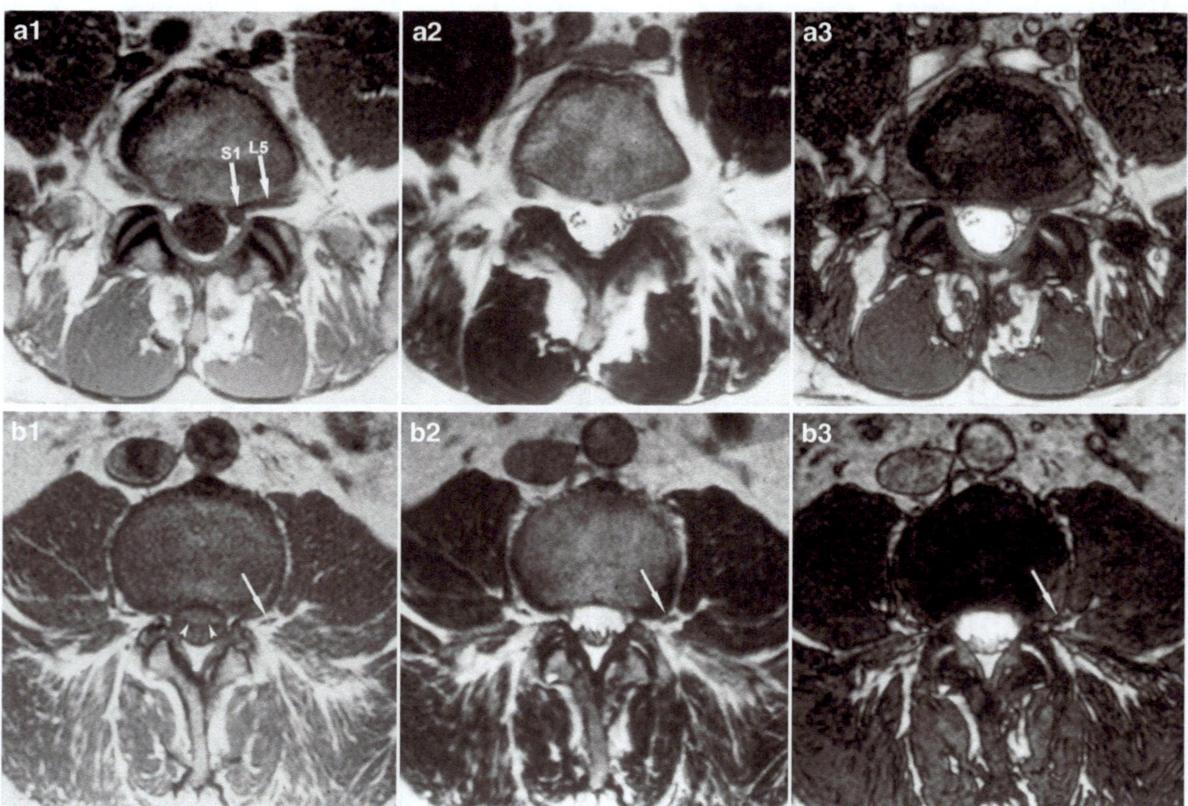

Fig. 2.10 Comparative axial images acquired by T1 SE, T2 DRIVE, and $T2^*$BFFE techniques respectively. (**a1–3**) Case with conjoint left L5 and S1 root sleeves. T1-weighted image (**a1**) shows no intradural detail due to low CSF signal. Dural sac, root sleeves and foraminal details well-depicted due to high fat signal. T2-weighted DRIVE image (**a2**) produced by FSE sequence giving high CSF signal as well as high fat signal shows good depiction of intradural nerve roots as well as dorsal root ganglia in foramina. Outline of dural sac less well shown, however. $T2^*$-weighted BFFE image (**a3**) produced with gradient-echo sequence shows good depiction of dural sac, root sleeve and intradural nerve roots, but foraminal structures are less well shown. Spurious image of L3–4 disc protrusion (*arrowheads*) shown in T1-weighted image (**b1**), not shown in T2-weighted DRIVE image (**b2**) and $T2^*$-weighted BFFE image (**b3**). Spinal nerve (*arrow*) well seen outlined by fat in (**b1**) and (**b2**), not in (**b3**)

Figure 2.10 shows a comparison of imaging features of three techniques for axial lumbar spinal imaging: T1-W fast spin-echo, T2-W DRIVE and T2*-W balanced fast-field echo (BFFE). We have found the second option the most useful.

2.4.3 Proton Density-Weighted (PD-W) Images

MRI is a highly versatile method for assessing various tissue characteristics and transforming these characteristics into image contrast. Beside producing images weighted for differences in T1 or T2 relaxation times, the MR acquisition sequence can be so arranged that neither of these two tissue parameters plays a significant role in image contrast; variations in signal intensity (brightness) producing image contrast now depend mainly on variations in proton density within the tissues. Ligamentous structures containing bound protons (ligaments, cortical bone) are then clearly discernible by their low signal intensity. Ruptures in ligamentous structures such as the outer annulus fibrosus are very clearly seen (Fig. 2.11) but this is the only especially useful diagnostic feature of proton density weighting and the technique is at present not routinely used in spinal imaging.

2.4.4 Fat-Suppressed Images

Suppression of bright fat signal in the MR image can be achieved in several ways. Short TI inversion recovery (STIR) is very effective in nulling the fat signal from epidural fat and bone marrow, and is helpful in the analysis of bone marrow signal changes (Fig. 2.12). Spectral fat suppression by pre-saturation (SPIR, fatsat) can also be used in T2-W fast spin-echo sequences to produce the same effects.

Post-gadolinium T1-weighted images can be acquired with a spectral fat-saturation pre-pulse (SPIR or fatsat). This is useful when bright fat signal (bone marrow, epidural fat) is a hindrance to assessing contrast enhancement of vascular structures (Fig. 2.13), but also infectious or metastatic bone marrow enhancement, or enhancement of post-operative epidural scar tissue can be better identified in this way (see also Chaps. 4 and 5). STIR

cannot be used in T1-W post-gadolinium MR imaging because the bright gadolinium signal is suppressed by this technique together with the fat signal.

2.4.5 MR Myelography:

The purpose of producing MR myelographic images is not to satisfy nostalgic feelings in elder colleagues but to provide a better diagnostic image of the intradural nerve root. The course of a traversing nerve root as it passes from the dural sac into the root sleeve in the lateral recess region of the spinal canal is often hard to follow in sagittal or axial MRI sectional images. Sagittal sections suffer from partial volume effects in the lateral recess region, and even thin axial cuts can fail to identify the root, especially when the lateral recess is not roomy. Individual cauda equina fibres can be discerned on thin (2 mm)-section T1-weighted volume scans and traced over some distance in oblique reformats (Hofman and Wilmink 1995) but comparison of the aspect of a single nerve root and root sleeve with the contralateral root or the adjacent root above or below is not possible with flat sections through a curved tubular banana-shaped object such as the lumbosacral dural sac. Curved reformatted sections can be constructed but the production is time-consuming.

A presentation of a virtual 3D image of the dural sac and root sleeve allows a better assessment of the course of the root, and an easier comparison with adjacent and contralateral roots. MR myelographic images are generally acquired with heavy T2-weighting, which produces a very bright water signal from the CSF in the dural sac and (virtually) no signal from other spinal structures. The dural sac is then easily segmented by a maximum intensity projection (MIP) technique similar to that used in MR angiography, and presented as a virtual 3D object with the root sleeves well shown and the intradural roots visible as dark linear structures (Krudy 1992; el Gammal et al. 1995; Ferrer et al. 2004). This technique compares well with conventional contrast myelography; (Ramsbacher et al. 1997; Kuroki et al. 1998), and patient acceptance of an MRI study is better than is the case with conventional myelography (Albeck and Danneskiold-Samsoe 1995).

Figure 2.14 shows an example of adjacent oblique T2-weighted MRI sections fused to produce a virtual 3D representation of the dural sac and emerging root

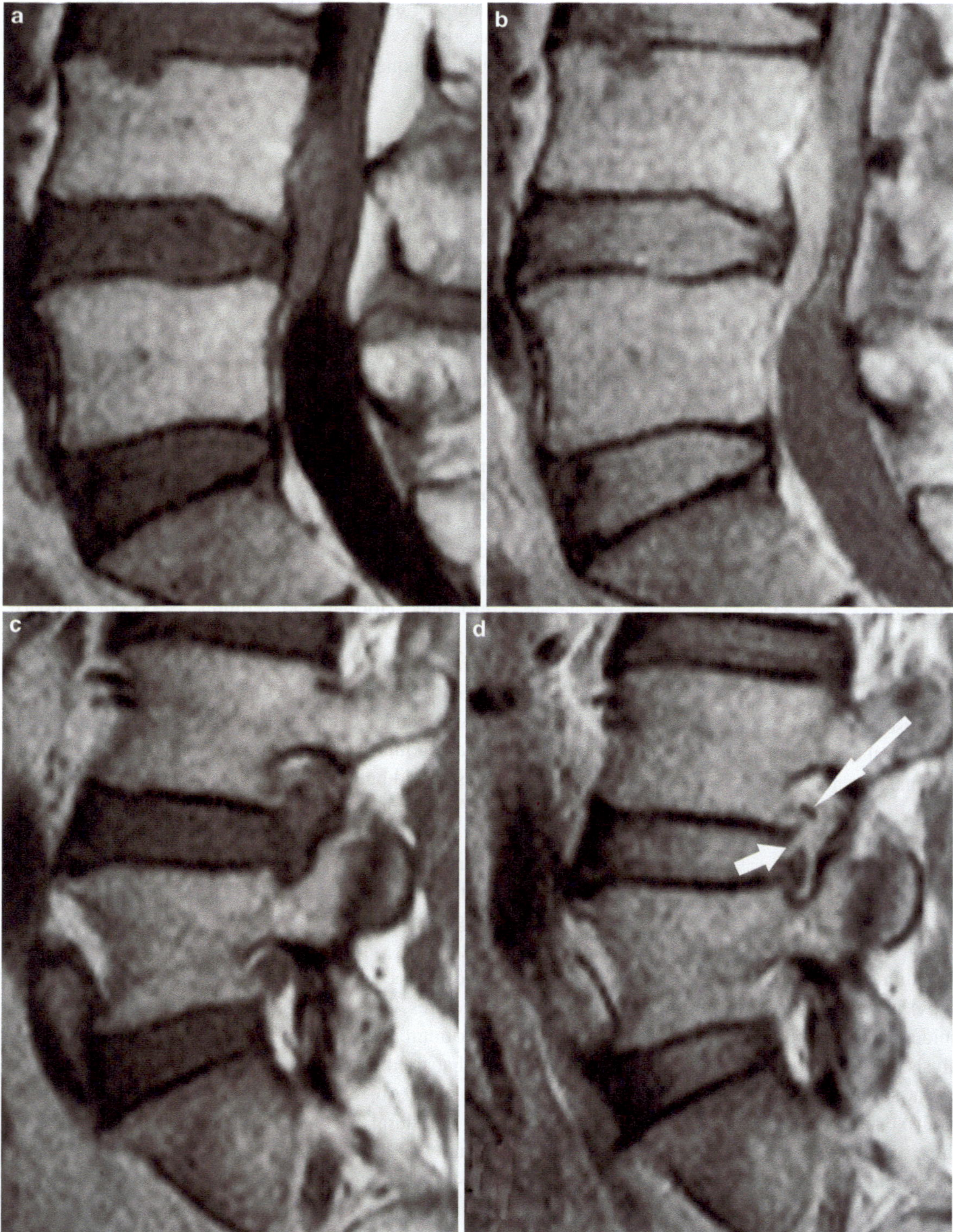

Fig. 2.11 Imaging of annular rupture by proton density compared to T1-weighting. Midsagittal T1-(**a**) and proton density-weighted images (**b**) show extruded disc material behind intact L4–5 posterior longitudinal ligament. Lateral sagittal cuts through foramen with similar weighting (**c, d**) show ruptured annulus, more clearly in proton density weighted image (**d**) (*arrow*). Note small fragment of annulus displaced upwards into foramen (*long arrow*)

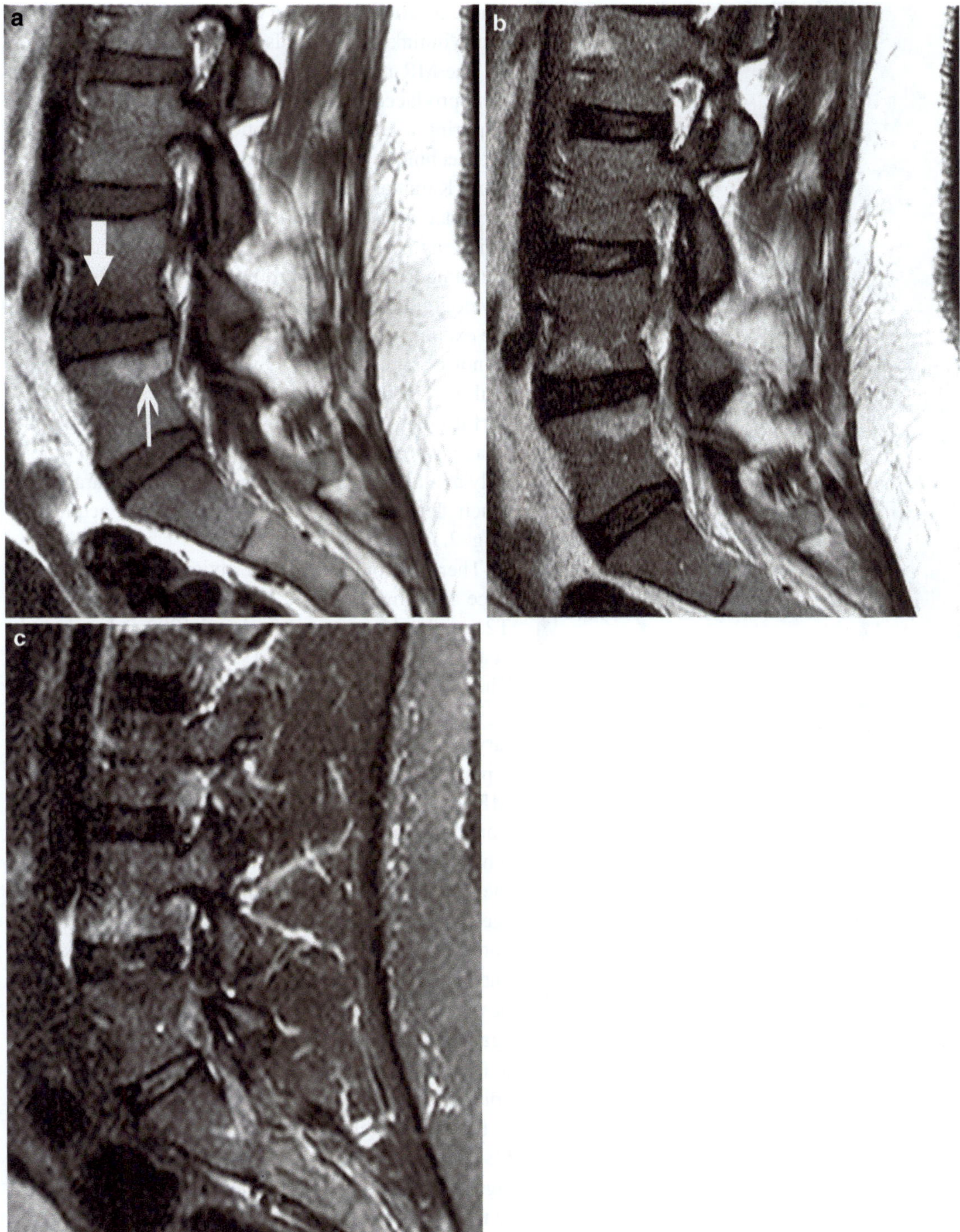

Fig. 2.12 Fat suppression in degenerative bone marrow changes. T1-weighted image (**a**) shows area of signal loss due to increase in bone marrow water content above L4 endplate (*arrow*); area of increased bone marrow fat signal below L5 endplate (*thin arrow*). T2-weighted fast spin-echo image (**b**) shows areas with increased fat as well as water content now hyperintense. STIR fat-suppressed image (**c**) confirms high water signal in bone marrow above L4 endplate indicating Modic type 1 degenerative changes; also suppression of fat signal from area below L5 endplate indicating Modic type 2 fatty degenerative changes here. Decrease in bone marrow fat signal combined with increase in water signal is seen in Modic type I changes but also in for instance metastasis or spondylitis. Follow-up in this case revealed no progression over time

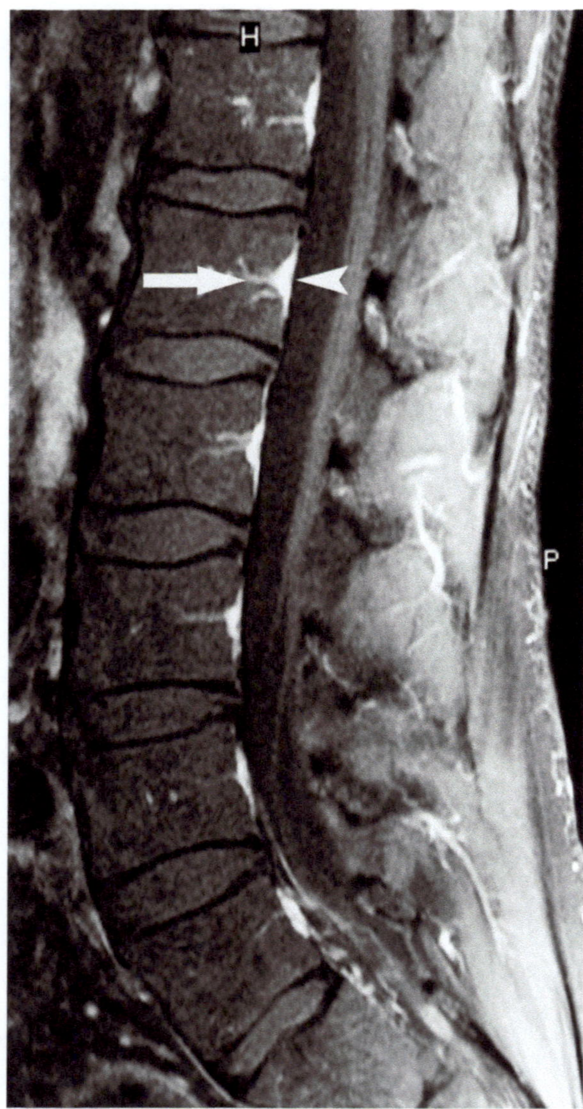

Fig. 2.13 Fat-suppressed post-gadolinium imaging. Mid-sagittal T1-weighted spin-echo image with SPIR fat suppression by spectral pre-saturation, post-gadolinium injection. Note signal loss from fat in subcutaneous and epidural regions, bright enhancement of basivertebral veins (*arrow*) and epidural veins (*arrow head*)

sleeves. Such a presentation makes MR myelography a valuable adjunct in cases where disc or canal pathology is seen to be present on the standard MR images, but

where its effect on the nerve root is not clear (Hofman and Wilmink 1996; see also Chaps. 4 and 5).

The MR myelographic dataset shown in Fig. 2.14 were produced with a multi-slice, multi-shot technique requiring a lengthy acquisition 6 min. 30s. A single-shot technique can be employed to reduce acquisition time (Karantanas et al. 2000), and a refinement of this sequence is used in our department. When the echo-train length of an FSE sequence is increased to equal the number of acquired profiles, a strongly T2-weighted myelographic image can be produced with only a single excitation. Such an image possesses a poor signal-to-noise ratio (SNR), however (Fig. 2.15). When multiple, successive, single-shot excitations are now performed to improve the SNR, an MR myelographic image is produced requiring a total acquisition time of only about 30 s, with an image quality comparable to a much lengthier multi-slice, multi-shot acquisition (Fig. 2.16).

There are other technical options available to produce MR myelographic images, using gradient-echo T2*weighted sequences (Zisch et al. 1992; Schnarkowski et al. 1993; Eberhardt et al. 1997; Baskaran et al. 2003). These will not be discussed in detail here.

It must be stressed that MR myelography is ancillary to the standard MRI investigation, and can never replace it (Thornton et al. 1999; O'Connell et al. 2003). MR myelography has the same drawbacks as conventional contrast myelography: false negatives occur when the root is compressed distal to the root sleeve, in the foramen or the sacral canal, and false positives are seen when non-filling of a root sleeve is not due to compression (see Chap. 3, Fig. 3.5). The standard MRI cuts and the MR myelographic images should always be carefully matched against each other, and also against the clinical presentation. If a small L5-S1 herniation for instance is seen to be extending into the epidural fat ventral to the dural sac but the root sleeve at the same level is normally depicted and filled with CSF on the MR myelogram (see Fig. 4.3), the clinical signs and symptoms of the patient should be reviewed with extra caution because a chance finding of an asymptomatic herniation is then quite likely.

Fig. 2.14 MR myelography. Two sections (**a, b**) selected from a 4-mm overcontiguous multi-shot, multi-slice oblique T2-weighted FSE MR myelographic acquisition, fused by MIP to produce a 3D image of virtual dural sac (**c**); acquisition time 6 min. 30s. Better detail of intradural roots in individual sections (**a**) and (**b**), but better appreciation of entire dural sac and all root sleeves in (**c**) (*arrows*)

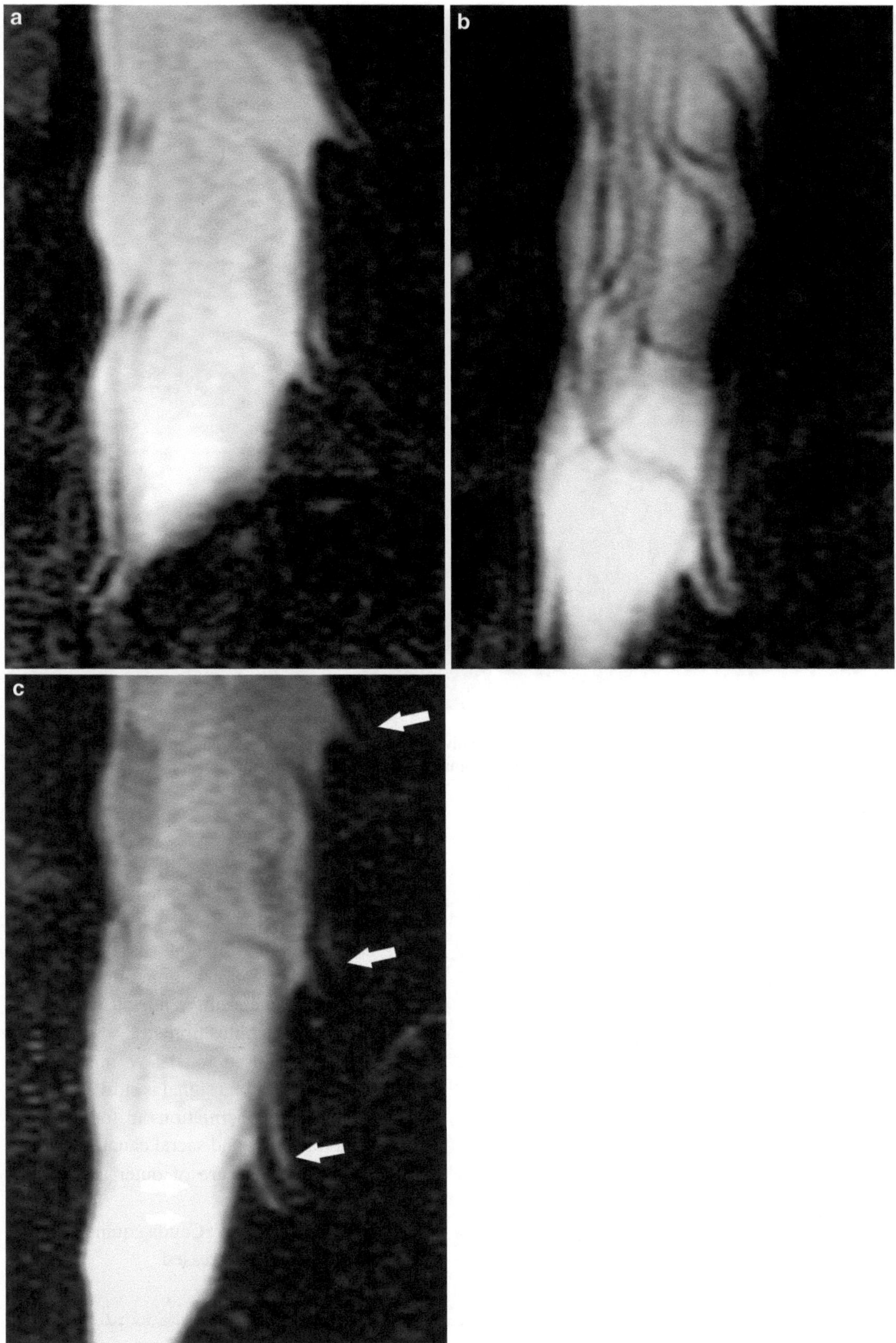

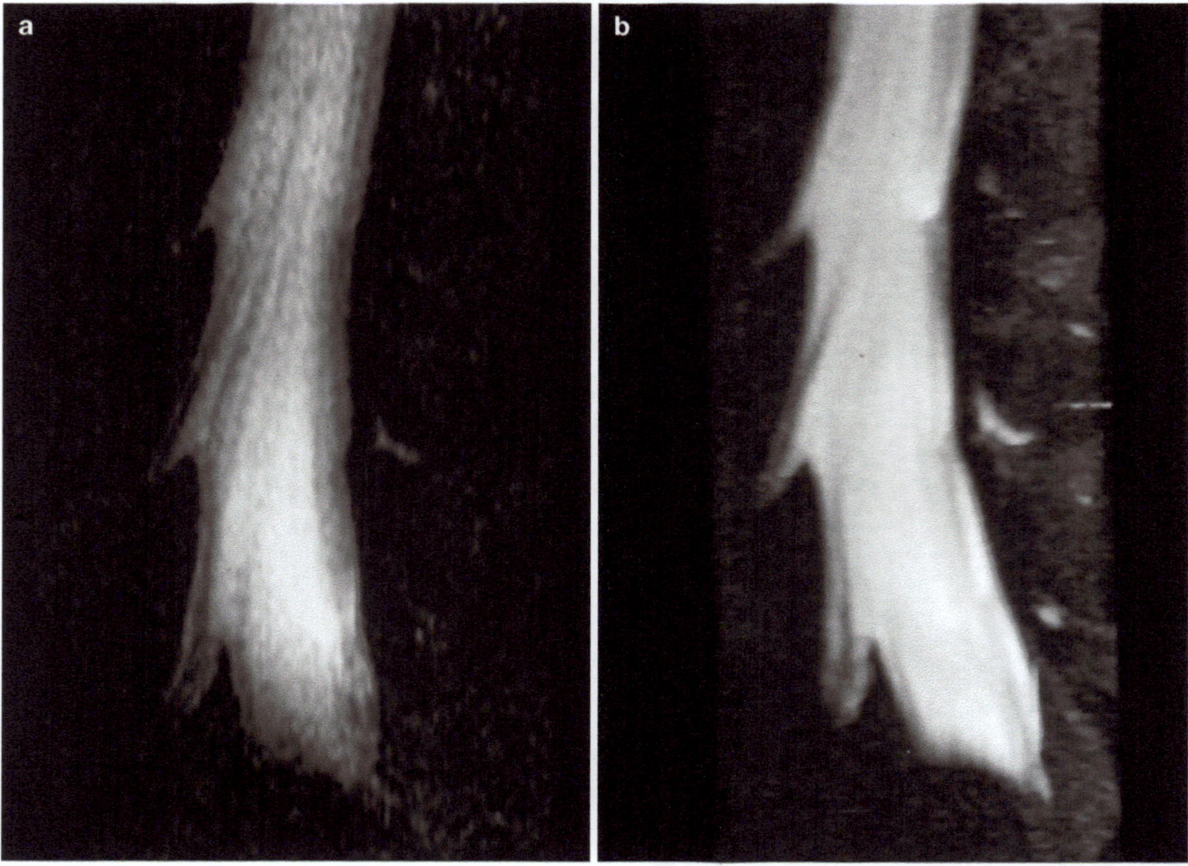

Fig. 2.15 MR myelography. Single-shot, single-slice MR myelographic images in normal spinal canal (**a**), acquisition time 1.5 s, compared to multi-shot, multi-slice MIP image in same individual (**b**), acquisition time 6 min. 30 s. Note much poorer signal-to-noise ratio in single-shot image

Summary

Imaging sequences and features best shown by these in degenerative conditions.

> *T1-W*: Epidural and foraminal fat; lateral and foraminal disc herniations in regions containing fat (foramen, lumbosacral transition and sacral canal). Disc herniations adjacent to dural sac are not well seen; intradural nerve roots are not well seen.

> *T1-W + Gd*: Epidural veins; enhancing annular fissures; inflammatory epidural reaction around an extruded disc fragment, inflamed nerve root, post-operative epidural scarring or spondylodiscitis. Epidural scar or bone marrow enhancement is usually better seen with spectral fat suppression.

> *T2-W*: Dural sac and contents; central and paracentral disc herniations impinging on the dural sac; water content of the nucleus pulposus; fissures in the annulus fibrosus.

> NB: When FSE is used for T2-W imaging, epidural and foraminal fat signal is sufficiently bright to outline disc herniations in foramen, lumbosacral transition and sacral canal.

> Proton density-W: Rupture of outer annulus fibrosus.

> T2++W MR myelography: Cauda equina, root sleeves, normal and compressed.

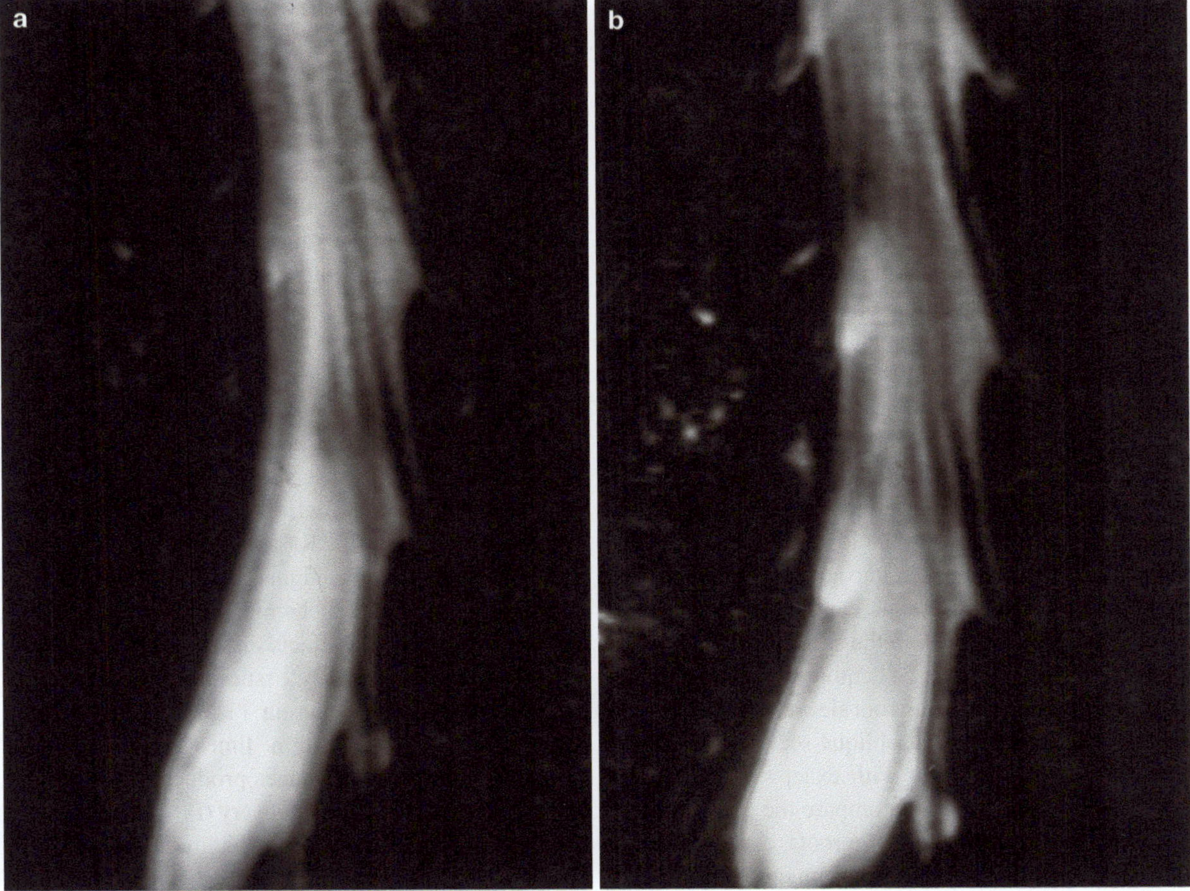

Fig. 2.16 MR myelography. Single-shot, single-slice multi-excitation MR myelographic image (**a**), acquisition time 32 s compared to multi-shot, multi-slice image in same individual (**b**), acquisition time 6 min. 30 s. Note comparable image quality despite much more rapid acquisition in (**a**)

2.4.6 Imaging Planes

As a general rule, in sectional imaging, anatomic surfaces or structures are best imaged in a plane which lies perpendicular to the surface of interest, and least well in a plane parallel to this surface. Thus, vertebral endplates are best seen in sagittal and coronal sections, and not well in the axial plane because of partial volume effects. The inner pedicular borders are best seen in axial and coronal sections, and not well in sagittal cuts.

Sagittal: Images in this plane are best for demonstrating disc herniations and distinguishing between "contained" protrusions (whose maximum height does not exceed the height of the parent disc) and extrusions, in which the displaced disc material passes through a rupture in the outer annulus fibrosus and extends cranial and/or caudal to the vertebral endplates bordering the disc space (see Chap. 4 and Fig. 4.3). The distinction between diffuse disc bulging and broad-based herniation is often difficult to make in the sagittal plane, and the lateral recesses and the root sleeves are not well imaged. The foraminal borders on the other hand are best defined in sagittal images, as is cranial migration of extruded material in the foramen with compression of the dorsal root ganglion against the pedicle (see Fig. 4.5). The mid-sagittal diameter of the spinal canal is better assessed in the sagittal plane than on axial images, as are spinal deformities such as anterolisthesis and retrolisthesis. Isthmic fractures in spondylolysis may be detected, as well as increase or decrease in sagittal diameter of the spinal canal which is associated with spondylolytic and degenerative anterolisthesis, respectively (see Chap. 4 and Fig. 4.20).

Axial: Images in this plane permit the best classification of the axial location and extent of a disc abnormality, diffuse, broad-based or focal (see Chap. 4 and Fig. 4.2). Migration of extruded disc material cranial or caudal to the level of the endplates can be hard to assess due to partial volume effects. The lateral recesses of the spinal canal are best studied in the axial plane, as well as lateral encroachment upon the spinal canal due to hypertrophy of the facets and flaval ligaments, and the passage of the traversing nerve roots through these regions may be traced. Isthmic fractures in spondylolysis can often be seen in axial images. When measurements of the sagittal diameter of the spinal canal are performed in the axial plane, error due to tilting of the plane of section relative to the longitudinal axis of the spinal canal should be taken into account (see Fig. 2.5). The foramen and its contents can be studied in axial images, but less well than in the sagittal plane.

Oblique: Sections can be acquired or reconstructed in the plane of the emerging root sleeve, usually 20–30° off-coronal. Left and right oblique sections are sometimes difficult to position with exact symmetry, and this can make it difficult to compare the course of left and right root sleeves and nerve roots, especially with thin sections. Oblique 3D virtual images of the dural sac acquired in T2-weighted MR myelographic projections do not suffer from this drawback.

Coronal: This imaging plane is used only rarely in diagnosis of degenerative disease. Some spinal deformities such as scoliosis or hemivertebra are imaged best in the coronal plane.

2.4.7 Upright Imaging

The introduction of open MRI systems has made upright weight-bearing MRI studies possible, with the additional option of dynamic flexion-extension imaging of the spine (Weishaupt and Boxheimer 2003; Jinkins et al. 2005). As discussed in detail in Chapters 3 and 4, the effect of such postural changes on normal and pathologic spinal anatomy makes this a valuable addition to our diagnostic arsenal, most likely to be useful in cases with spinal developmental stenosis or another form of narrowing of the spinal canal.

2.4.8 Considerations of Field Strength

Increasing the field strength of the magnet used for MRI produces an equivalent increase in signal-to-noise ratio and hence in low-contrast resolution in the MR image. A study comparing image quality at 0.5, 1 and 1.5T showed image quality at the two higher field strengths to be superior to that obtained at 0.5T (Maubon et al. 1999). If desired, the increase in signal can also be traded off against other image properties: thinner slices or an increase in matrix size to improve spatial resolution, or a larger field of view to expand anatomic coverage without sacrificing image quality. Alternatively, the acquisition time can be reduced.

There are other factors beside field strength affecting image quality in MRI, the most important being the characteristics of the RF antenna or coil employed. In addition, imaging at higher field strengths such as 3T produces increased chemical shift artefacts, susceptibility and flow artefacts and also problems with energy deposition in body tissues. A drawback is the loss of fluid-tissue contrast in T1-W FSE images due to increased T1 relaxation times at higher field strengths. T1-weighted images produced by GRE and fluid-attenuated inversion recovery (FLAIR) sequences suffer less from this problem (Shapiro 2006).

2.4.9 Abbreviated Scanning Protocols

The suggestion has been made to reduce the number of acquisition sequences per spinal MRI study, in the interest of increasing patient throughput. In a study comparing a rapid two-sequence screening protocol lasting 2 min. 30s and a detailed four-sequence protocol requiring 28 min, all moderate and severe bulges and herniations were detected by the rapid protocol but more subtle changes were better seen in the detailed examination (Robertson et al. 1996). Another study (Chawalparit et al. 2006) showed disc herniations to be demonstrated equally well by the two imaging protocols, but sensitivity for nerve root compression was significantly poorer in the screening protocol. In a study comparing a rapid MRI examination with spinal radiographs in a group of 380 patients with low back pain (Jarvik et al. 2003), clinical outcomes were the same for both groups but costs were greater in the MRI group while more patients were operated (10 in the MRI group versus four in the radiography group). Costs of rapid MRI were about half those of a conventional MRI study (Gray et al. 2003).

References

Abdullah AF, Wolber PG, Warfield JR et al (1988) Surgical management of extreme lateral lumbar disc herniations: review of 138 cases. Neurosurgery 22:648–653

Albeck MJ, Danneskiold-Samsoe B (1995) Patient attitudes to myelography, computed tomography and magnetic resonance imaging when examined for suspected lumbar disc herniation. Acta Neurochir (Wien) 133:3–6

Baskaran V, Pereles FS, Russell EJ et al (2003) Myelographic MR imaging of the cervical spine with a 3D true fast imaging with steady-state precession technique: initial experience. Radiology 227:585–592

Bates D, Ruggieri P (1991) Imaging modalities for evaluation of the spine. Radiol Clin North Am 29:675–690

Carragee EJ, Alamin TF, Carragee JM (2006) Low-pressure positive Discography in subjects asymptomatic of significant low back pain illness. Spine 31:505–509

Carragee EJ, Hannibal M (2004) Diagnostic evaluation of low back pain. Orthop Clin North Am 35:7–16

Chawalparit O, Churojana A, Chiewvit P et al (2006) The limited protocol MRI in diagnosis of lumbar disc herniation. J Med Assoc Thai 89:182–189

Di Chiro G, Schellinger D (1976) Computed tomography of spinal cord after lumbar intrathecal introduction of metrizamide (computer-assisted myelography). Radiology 120:101–104

Eberhardt KE, Hollenbach HP, Tomandl B et al (1997) Three-dimensional MR myelography of the lumbar spine: comparative case study to X-ray myelography. Eur Radiol 7:737–742

el Gammal T, Brooks BS, Freedy RM et al (1995) MR myelography: imaging findings. AJR Am J Roentgenol 164:173–177

Ferrer P, Marti-Bonmati L, Molla E et al (2004) MR-myelography as an adjunct to the MR examination of the degenerative spine. Magma 16:203–210

Fullenlove TM, Williams AJ (1957) Comparative roentgen findings in symptomatic and asymptomatic backs. Radiology 68:572–574

Gray DT, Hollingworth W, Blackmore CC et al (2003) Conventional radiography, rapid MR imaging, and conventional MR imaging for low back pain: activity-based costs and reimbursement. Radiology 227:669–680

Hofman PA, Wilmink JT (1995) 3-D volume scanning. A new technique for lumbar MR imaging. Acta Neurochir (Wien) 134:108–112

Hofman PA, Wilmink JT (1996) Optimising the image of the intradural nerve root: the value of MR radiculography. Neuroradiology 38:654–657

Hounsfield GN (1973) Computerized transverse axial scanning (tomography). 1. Description of system. Br J Radiol 46:1016–1022

Jackson RP, Glah JJ (1987) Foraminal and extraforaminal lumbar disc herniation: diagnosis and treatment. Spine 12: 577–585

Jarvik JG, Hollingworth W, Martin B et al (2003) Rapid magnetic resonance imaging vs radiographs for patients with low back pain: a randomized controlled trial. JAMA 289: 2810–2818

Jinkins JR, Dworkin JS, Damadian RV (2005) Upright, weight-bearing, dynamic-kinetic MRI of the spine: initial results. Eur Radiol 15:1815–1825

Karantanas AH, Zibis AH, Papanikolaou N (2000) Single-shot turbo spin-echo MR myelography: comparison with 3D-turbo spin-echo MR myelography and T2-turbo spin-echo at 1 T. Comput Med Imaging Graph 24:37–42

Krudy AG (1992) MR myelography using heavily T2-weighted fast spin-echo pulse sequences with fat presaturation. AJR Am J Roentgenol 159:1315–1320

Kuroki H, Tajima N, Hirakawa S et al (1998) Comparative study of MR myelography and conventional myelography in the diagnosis of lumbar spinal diseases. J Spinal Disord 11:487–492

Luyendijk W, van Voorthuisen AE (1966) Contrast examination of the spinal epidural space. Acta Radiol Diagn (Stockh) 5:1051–1066

Mansfield P, Maudsley AA (1977) Medical imaging by NMR. Br J Radiol 50:188–194

Maubon AJ, Ferru JM, Berger V et al (1999) Effect of field strength on MR images: comparison of the same subject at 0.5, 1.0, and 1.5 T. Radiographics 19:1057–1067

O'Connell MJ, Ryan M, Powell T et al (2003) The value of routine MR myelography at MRI of the lumbar spine. Acta Radiol 44:665–672

Penning L, Wilmink JT (1981) Biomechanics of lumbosacral dural sac. A study of flexion-extension myelography. Spine 6:398–408

Ramsbacher J, Schilling AM, Wolf KJ et al (1997) Magnetic resonance myelography (MRM) as a spinal examination technique. Acta Neurochir (Wien) 139:1080–1084

Robertson WD, Jarvik JG, Tsuruda JS et al (1996) The comparison of a rapid screening MR protocol with a conventional MR protocol for lumbar spondylosis. AJR Am J Roentgenol 166:909–916

Ruggieri PM (1999) Pulse sequences in lumbar spine imaging. Magn Reson Imaging Clin N Am 7:425–37, vii

Schnarkowski P, Wallner B, Goldmann A et al (1993) [MR-myelography of the lumbar spine using a PSIF sequence: first experiences]. Aktuelle Radiol 3:53–56

Shapiro MD (2006) MR imaging of the spine at 3T. Magn Reson Imaging Clin N Am 14:97–108

Skalpe IO (1978) Adhesive arachnoiditis following lumbar myelography. Spine 3:61–64

Stadnik TW, Lee RR, Coen HL et al (1998) Annular tears and disk herniation: prevalence and contrast enhancement on MR images in the absence of low back pain or sciatica. Radiology 206:49–55

Staiger TO, Paauw DS, Deyo RA et al (1999) Imaging studies for acute low back pain. When and when not to order them. Postgrad Med 105:161–162, 165–166, 171–172

Thornton MJ, Lee MJ, Pender S et al (1999) Evaluation of the role of magnetic resonance myelography in lumbar spine imaging. Eur Radiol 9:924–929

Vertinsky AT, Krasnokutsky MV, Augustin M et al (2007) Cutting-edge imaging of the spine. Neuroimaging Clin N Am 17:117–136

Weishaupt D, Boxheimer L (2003) Magnetic resonance imaging of the weight-bearing spine. Semin Musculoskelet Radiol 7:277–286

Wilmink JT, Penning L, Beks JW (1978) Techniques in transfemoral lumbar epidural phlebography. Neuroradiology 15:273–286

Wilmink JT, Lindeboom SF, Vencken LM et al (1984) Relationship between contrast medium dose and adverse effects in lumbar myelography. Diagn Imaging Clin Med 53:208–214

Wilmink JT (1989) CT morphology of intrathecal lumbosacral nerve-root compression. AJNR Am J Neuroradiol 10:233–248

Zisch RJ, Hollenbach HP, Artmann W (1992) Lumbar myelography with three-dimensional MR imaging. J Magn Reson Imaging 2:731–734

In this chapter, the presentation centres around the lumbosacral nerve roots and spinal nerves, and the anatomical structures and relationships which these encounter from the origin at the conus medullaris, along their intrathecal course as dorsal or ventral roots of the cauda equina, and after their departure from the dural sac and spinal foramina as ventral rami of the spinal nerves, which eventually combine to form the lumbosacral plexus.

The paragraph on *topographic anatomy* provides an overview of anatomic features in the trajectory of the coursing nerve roots and nerves which are of significance for planning and interpreting imaging procedures and for an understanding of the factors involved in nerve root compression.

Sectional anatomy illuminates the same aspects from a different viewpoint, more directly linked to modern diagnostic imaging.

Functional anatomy provides insight into the effects of postural changes upon intraspinal structures, and the way in which posture-dependent nerve root compression may come about.

3.1 Topographic Anatomy

The nerve roots servicing the lumbosacral region originate from or terminate in the conus medullaris (Figs. 3.1 and 3.2), the cone-shaped lower ending of the spinal cord whose tip is usually located at approximately the L1–2 intervertebral level. This long bundle of lumbosacral nerve roots is called the cauda equina or horse's tail, which resembles in the anatomical preparation (Fig. 3.2). Proceeding caudally, a sensory dorsal and motor ventral nerve root come together in the lateral region of the dural sac, finally departing from the dural sac via the dural root sleeve which contains an extension of the subarachnoid space. At the termination of the root sleeve, the roots divide into a number of fascicles. The sensory root fascicles merge into the dorsal root ganglion, and the motor fascicles blend in distal to the dorsal root ganglion as the mixed spinal nerve is formed, the ventral ramus of which goes on to become part of the lumbosacral plexus (Kostelic et al. 1991, 1992; Wiltse 2000). The dorsal ramus provides innervation of local spinal structures.

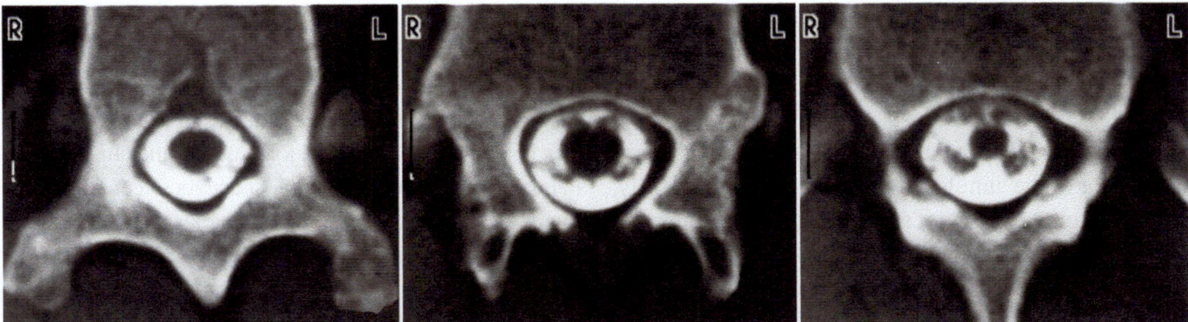

Fig. 3.1 CT myelographic images of conus medullaris and adjacent structures. Axial sections showing spinal cord just above conus, surrounded by small veins (*left*); through intumescence of conus with adjacent dorsal sensory and ventral motor roots (*centre*) and just above termination of conus (*right*)

J. T. Wilmink, *Lumbar Spinal Imaging in Radicular Pain and Related Conditions*
DOI: 10.1007/978-3-540-93830-9_3, © Springer-Verlag Berlin Heidelberg 2010

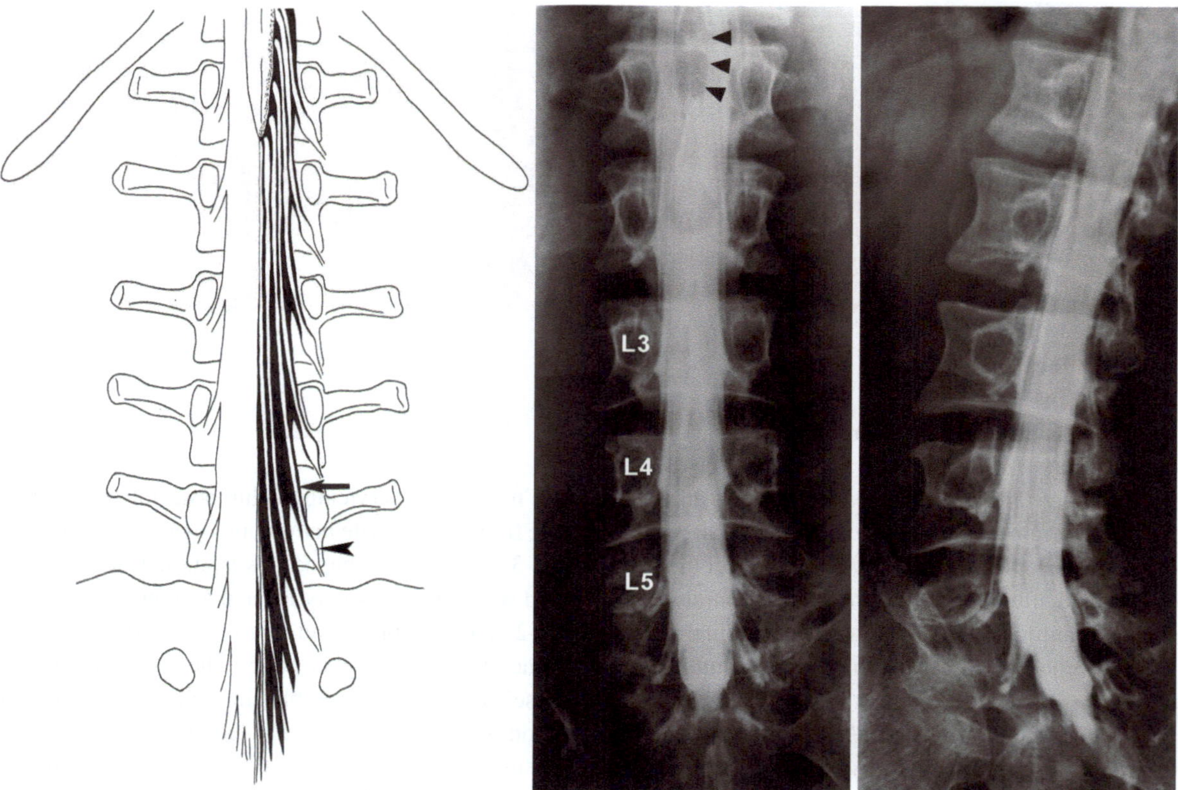

Fig. 3.2 Images of cauda equina. Diagram (*left*) showing outline of dural sac with root sleeves in left half of drawing, CSF in black at right outlining nerve roots. Note root and root sleeve outlined by CSF (*arrow*); myelographic image ends at intumescence of dorsal root ganglion (*arrowhead*). Conventional myelographic image in P-A projection (*centre*), showing conus medullaris (*arrowheads*), cauda equina and root sleeves. Because of their oblique anterior course, root sleeves are best seen in oblique projection (*right*)

Each exiting lumbar nerve root is numbered according to the vertebra under whose pedicle it enters the lumbar intervertebral foramen. For instance, the L5 root passes under L5 pedicle to emerge from the L5-S1 foramen as fifth lumbar nerve. More caudally, the S1 nerve exits the sacral canal via the first sacral foramen. Figure 3.3 demonstrates this and also shows that each intervertebral disc is anatomically related to two nerve roots: thus, the L5 root within the spinal canal passes adjacent to the subarticular region of the L4–5 dorsal annulus fibrosus, and the L4 spinal nerve outside the L4–5 foramen lies against the extraforaminal sector of the annulus of the same disc. Conversely, each emerging nerve root and nerve pass two intervertebral discs: one disc being traversed within the spinal canal when the root is emerging from the dural sac, and the next disc being passed further caudally and laterally when the nerve has exited the intervertebral foramen.

The *dural sac* is a tube which is connected with the intracranial dura mater via the foramen magnum, and which extends over the entire length of the cervical, thoracic, and lumbar sections of the spinal canal, tapering gradually to terminate in an end-sac or cul-de-sac, usually at about the upper one-third of the S2 body (Binokay et al. 2006) but sometimes considerably higher or lower (Fig. 3.4).

The spinal dura mater is reported to consist of three concentric layers (Vandenabeele et al. 1996), with the inner border cell layer closely adherent to the outer barrier cell layer of the arachnoid membrane. In man, no naturally occurring subdural space between the dura mater and the arachnoid membrane exists (Haines 1991; Reina et al. 2002; Vandenabeele et al. 1996), but such a space can be artificially created, for instance, by the subdural injection of a contrast agent or anesthetic fluid. The *spinal pia mater* invests the spinal cord and proximal portions of the nerve roots and is thicker and denser

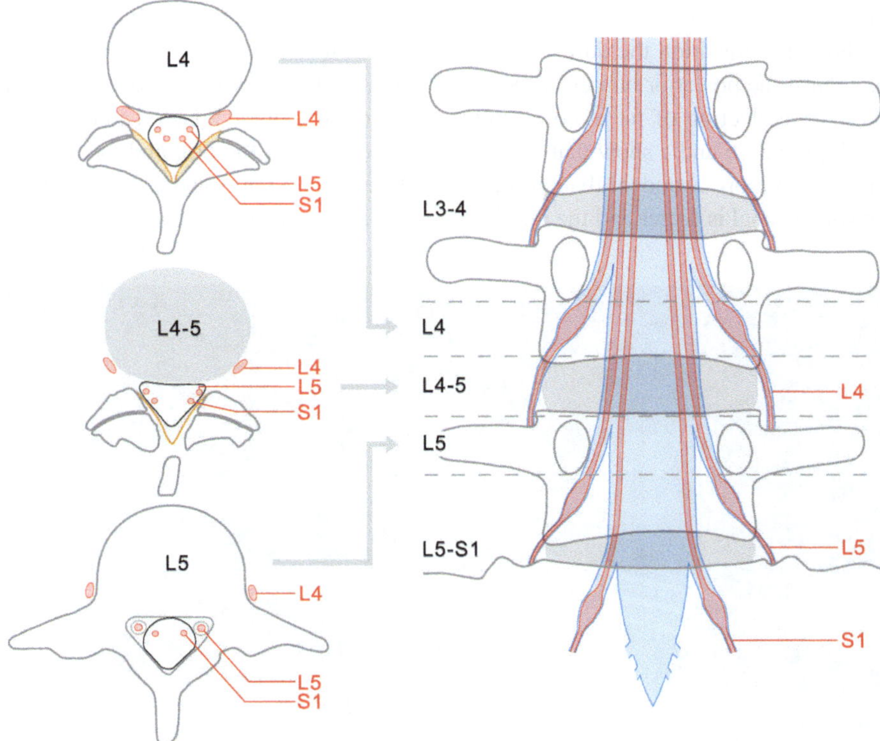

Fig. 3.3 Intradural roots, root sleeves and dorsal root ganglia in axial sections. *Left*: sections centred around L4–5 disc as indicated by *dotted lines* in coronal image at *right*. Note that intradural L5 root traverses sub-articular region of L4–5 disc, while L4 nerve passes same disc in extraforaminal region. In the same way L5 nerve lies adjacent to extraforaminal segment of L5-S1 disc

here than in the cranium, due to the addition of an outside layer. The *subarachnoid space* between the arachnoid membrane and the pia mater is filled with cerebrospinal fluid or CSF, which bathes the spinal cord and nerve roots, and is in communication with the intracranial CSF spaces. In the recumbent position of the body, the conus medullaris may be seen to sink to the dependent portion of the spinal canal, but if the specific gravity of the fluid in the arachnoid space is sufficiently increased by the injection of a dense myelographic contrast medium, the conus and cauda equina will float.

The *root sleeves* contain an extension of the subarachnoid space containing CSF, as well as a dorsal and ventral nerve root, and these depart from the dural sac at every vertebral segment (Fig. 3.5). The level of departure is variable, however (Bogduk and Twomey 1991; Rauschning 1991; Hasegawa et al. 1996). In the upper lumbar region, the root sleeves are usually formed well below the level of the disc and depart with a more transverse inclination (Bose and Balasubramaniam 1984).

At L4–5 the axilla or point of emergence of the root sleeve is located higher, usually at about the level of the upper L5 end-plate, and at L5-S1 above the disc level in the majority of cases (Suh et al. 2005) (Fig. 3.6, see

also Fig. 3.3) and with a more longitudinal inclination. An unusually high or low position of the dural end-sac will lead to a similarly high or low departure of the root sleeves relative to the disc (see Fig. 3.4). This relationship affects the mobility of the intradural nerve root at the level of the intervertebral disc, and thus the liability of the nerve root to compression at various spinal disc levels, as will be discussed in more detail in Chap. 4.

The length of the root sleeve visible at (MR) myelography is variable, from almost non-existent to 5 mm or more in length (Fig. 3.7, see also Fig. 3.5).

The epidural space surrounding the dural sac contains fat, various ligaments and a venous plexus.

The *epidural fat* is present in quantities which vary according to individual and localisation. In almost the entire lumbar region collections of fat occur dorsal to the dural sac at the interlaminar (disc) level. The function of the fat here appears to be to smooth or fair the posterior border of the spinal canal, which forms an irregular bony and ligamentous contour (Fig. 3.8a). The fat may also act as a lubricant, allowing some craniocaudal movement of the dural sac relative to the walls of the spinal canal (see Sect. 3.3). The retrodural fat pads can be seen to decrease in depth as we pass from the higher to the lower lumbar region. At about the lumbosacral transition the dural sac moves dorsally to lie against the posterior border of the spinal canal, and the main collection of fat is now ventral to the dural sac. Figure 3.8b and c show that at L5-S1 the epidural fat is much more abundant than at the higher levels as the spinal canal is larger and the dural end-sac smaller.

A body of literature is available about the *intraspinal ligaments*. The posterior longitudinal ligament (PLL) presents a cruciate aspect seen from behind, with a broad bilateral attachment to the dorsal annulus fibrosus of the disc and the adjacent end-plates, narrowing to a craniocaudal strip behind the vertebral body, to which it is not attached. The PLL consists of two, possibly three

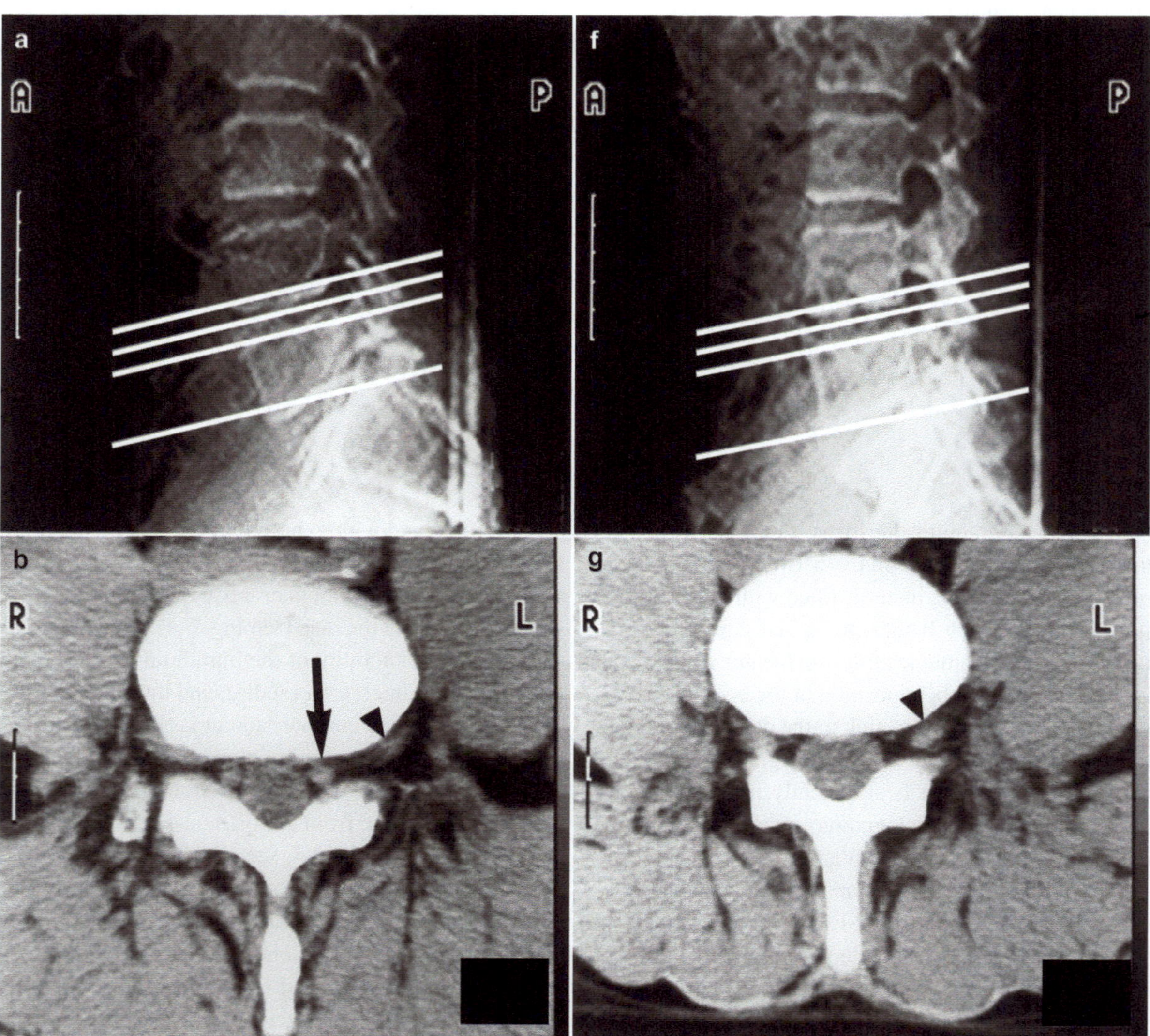

Fig. 3.4 Individual variability in level of root sleeves and dural end-sac in two individuals; with high end-sac in left column (**a–e**), low end-sac at in right column (**f–j**). *Top row*: Digital scoutviews with lines showing slice positioning. *Second row*: L4 end-plate level. *Arrowheads* indicate L4 spinal nerve leaving foramen. *Arrow* in *left image* shows high departure of L5 root sleeve from dural sac. No L5 root sleeve yet visible at *right*. *Third row*: L4–5 disc level. L4 extraforaminal nerve shown by *arrowheads*. *Arrow* in *left* image indicates L5 root sleeve coursing caudally and laterally. No root sleeve yet visible in image at *right*. *Fourth row*: L5 lateral recess level. *Arrow* in image at *left* shows L5 root sleeve in lateral recess outlined by fat. Open arrowhead shows high departure of S1 root sleeve from terminal dural sac. In image at *right* L5 root is still invisible within dural sac (*arrow*). *Bottom row*: Lower cuts at S1 lateral recess level. In image at left, section passes below dural end-sac; only sacral nerve roots seen. In image at right, section passes through end-sac well above its tip. *Arrows* indicate extraforaminal L5 nerve, *open arrowhead* in image at *left* points to high S1 dorsal root ganglion; in image at *right open arrow* indicates S1 root sleeve just emerging from dural sac

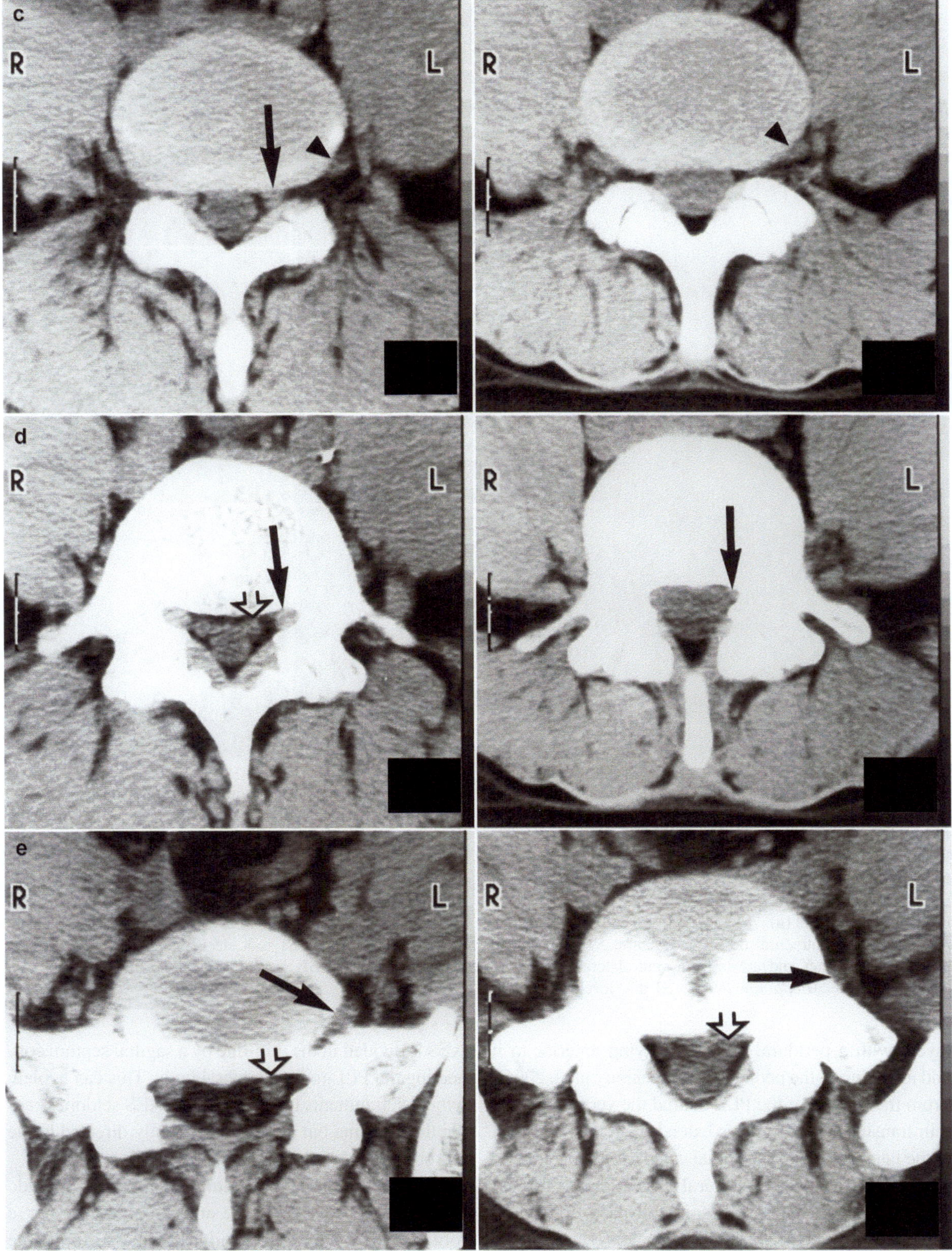

Fig. 3.4 (continued)

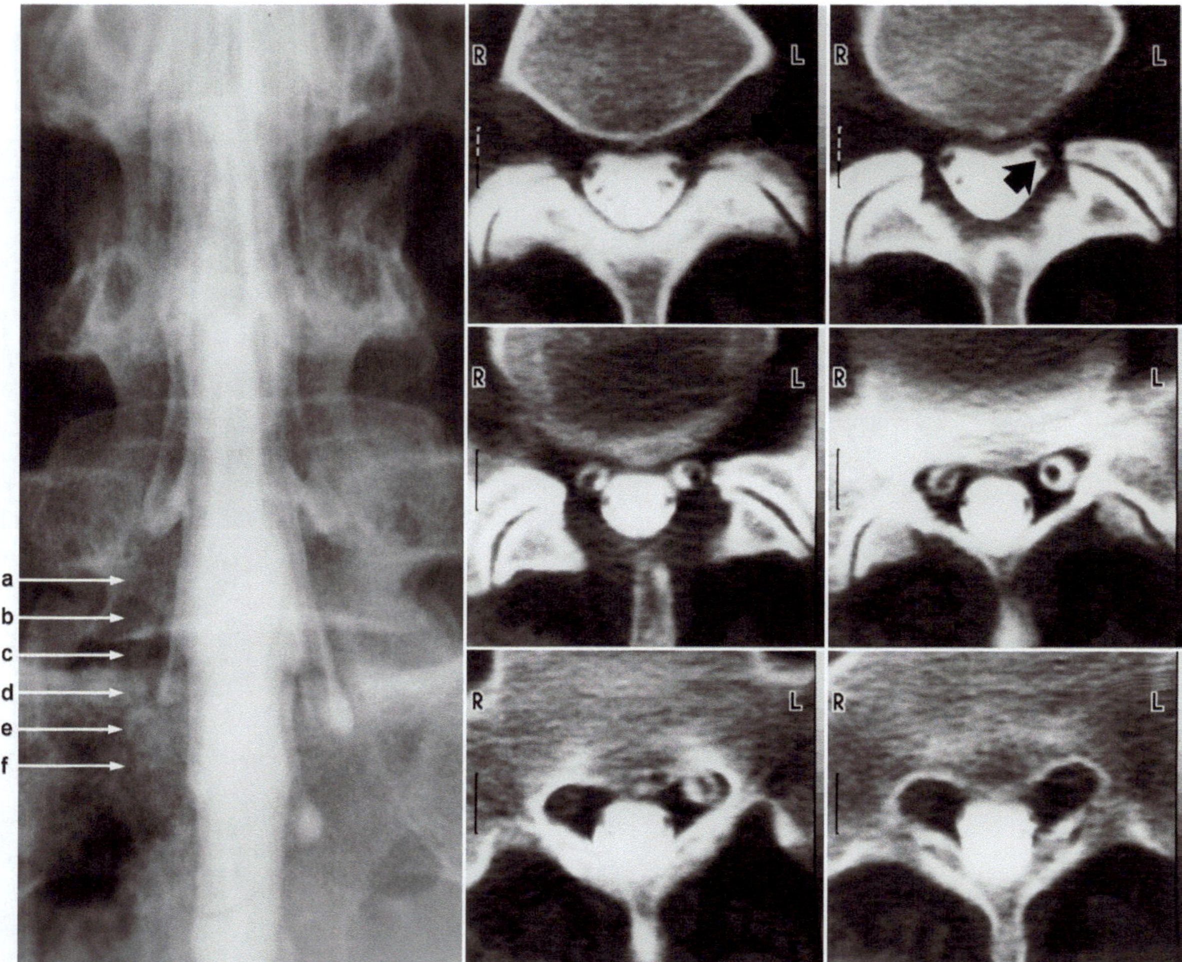

Fig. 3.5 Root sleeve anatomy and asymmetry without compression. *Left*: P-A lumbar myelogram with arrows (**a-f**) indicating levels of CT myelographic sections, centred around L5-S1 disc level. Note earlier termination of right S1 root sleeve contrast filling between levels of *arrows* (**d**) and (**e**). *Right*: Six adjacent CT myelographic sections in same individual. *Top row left*: L5 upper foraminal level (**a**). *Top row right*: L5 end-plate level (**b**). *Arrow* indicates intradural dorsal and ventral S1 roots which have come together and are moving ventrolaterally, about to enter root sleeve. *Middle row left*: L5-S1 disc level (**c**). S1 root sleeves are separating from dural sac, with S1 roots still visible within. *Middle row right*: S1 lateral recess level (**d**). Asymmetric aspect of S1 root sleeves, with diminution of CSF space around right S1 roots which are still just visible. *Bottom row left*: Sacral canal level (**e**). *Right* S1 root sleeve now only very faintly visible due to lack of contrast, but without signs of compression. Normal roots in root sleeve at *left*. *Bottom row right*: Level of S1 dorsal root ganglia (**f**). Both S1 root sleeves now no longer contain contrast-enhanced CSF

layers with a peridural membrane lying anterior to it and attaching to the pedicles (Loughenbury et al. 2006). From the section of the PLL behind the vertebral body, thin translucent membranes extend bilaterally to insert at the lateral walls of the spinal canal (Schellinger et al. 1990). Thus, an anterior epidural space (AES) is formed separate from the rest of the epidural space, containing the mid-line part of the epidural venous plexus (see below) and bordered posteriorly by the PLL and the lateral membranes, anteriorly by the vertebral body. The AES is divided in the mid-line by a sagittal septum connecting the PLL to the vertebral body. This can explain why disc fragments migrating to the AES seldom straddle the mid-line but are most frequently directed to the left or the right (Schellinger et al. 1990).

Other extradural ligamentous connections include those between the dural sac and the emerging nerve root sleeves on the one hand, with the walls of the spinal canal, the PLLs and the facet capsule, on the other. Reports are frequently contradictory, especially

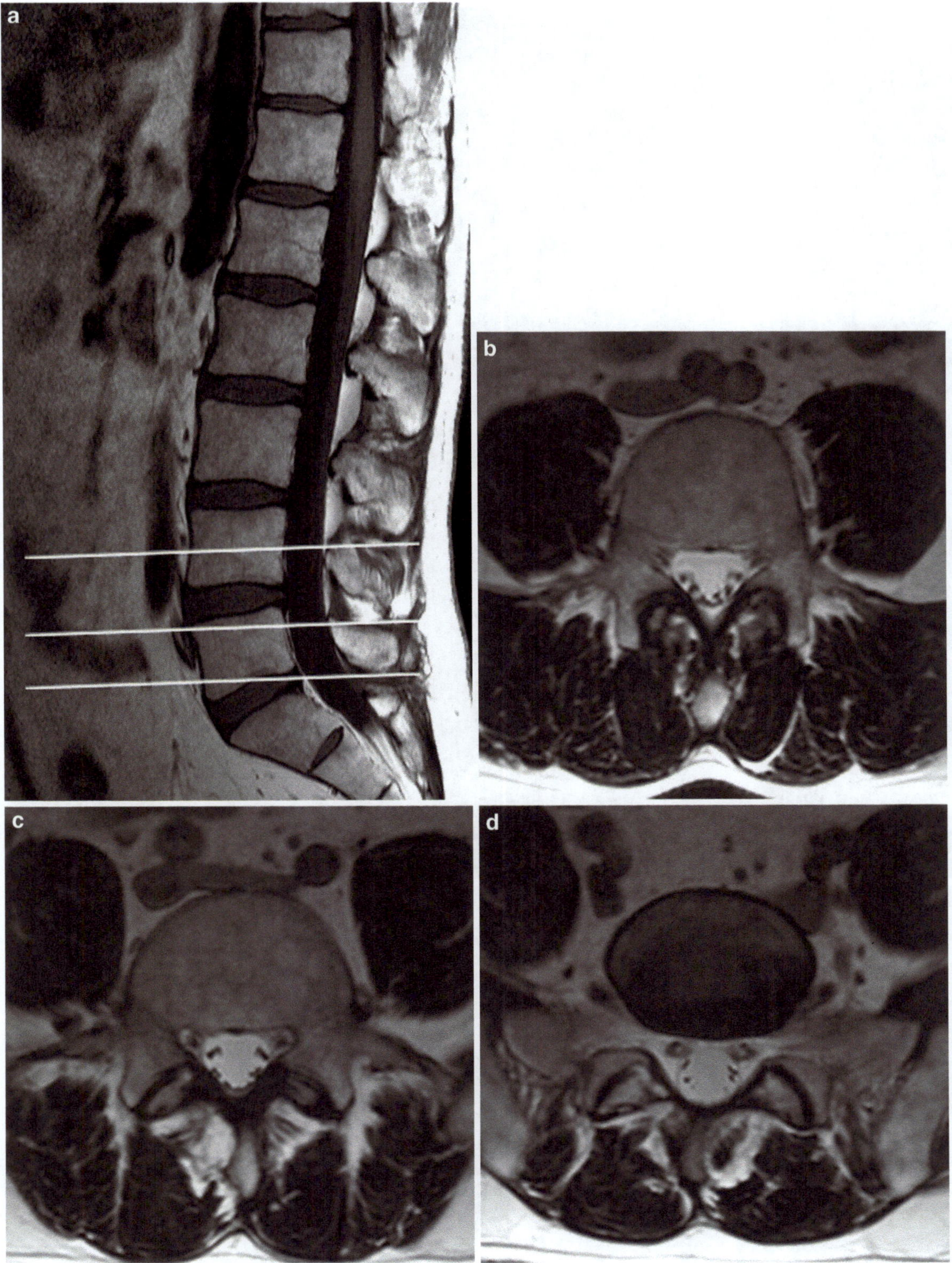

Fig. 3.6 Levels of root sleeve departure relative to disc at lower lumbar levels. (**a**) Sagittal T1-weighted image indicating axial slice levels. (**b-d**) Axial T2-weighted slices through levels of emergence (axilla) of root sleeves. (**b**) Axilla of L4 root sleeve 22 mm caudal to L3–4 disc. (**c**) Axilla of L5 root sleeve 5 mm caudal to L4–5 disc. (**d**) Axilla of S1 root sleeve at L5-S1 disc level

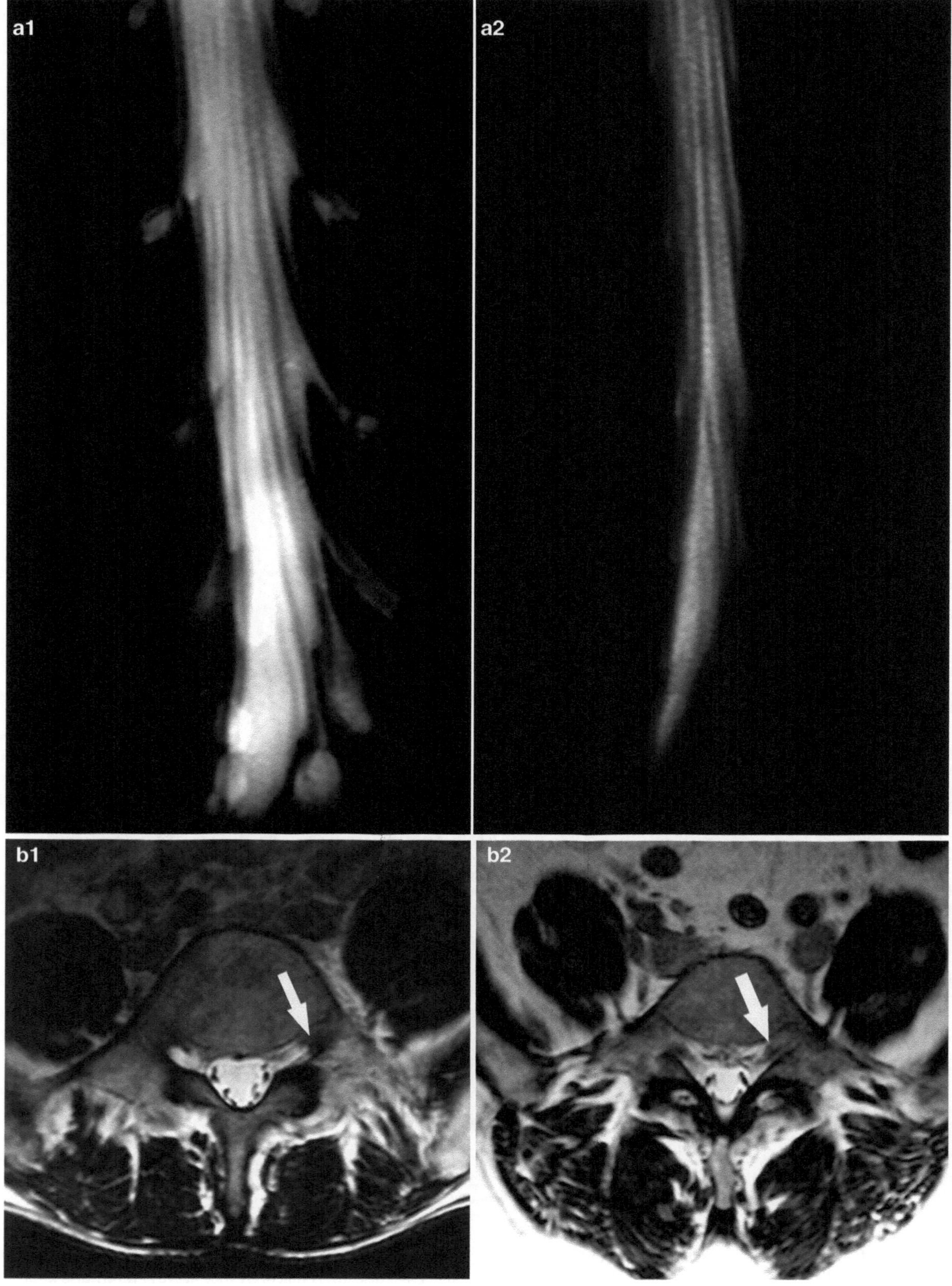

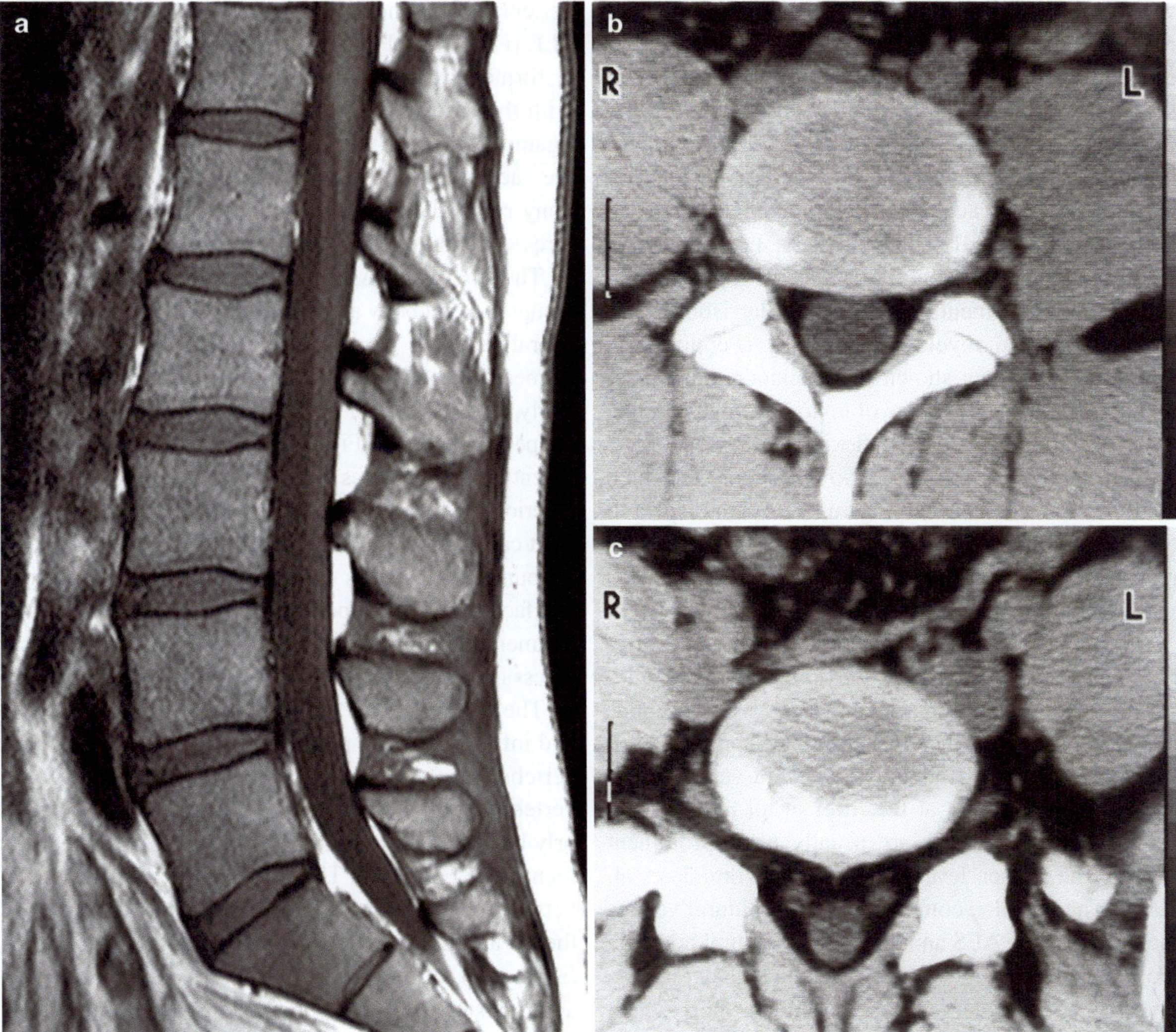

Fig. 3.8 Dural and epidural relationships at L4–5 and L5-S1. (**a**) Sagittal T1-weighted MR image illustrating distribution of epidural fat, craniocaudal tapering of dural sac in lumbosacral transition with relative increase in surrounding fat. In middle and upper lumbar regions fat is only present in dorsal interlaminar spaces. In lower lumbar to upper sacral region dural sac tapers to cul-de-sac and moves dorsally within spinal canal, with fat filling in ventral epidural space. (**b**) Axial CT section at L4–5. Area of spinal canal was measured as approximately 450 mm^2 and area of dural sac as 300 mm^2. (**c**) Section at L5-S1 with area of canal measured as approximately 700 mm^2 and area of dural sac and S1 roots as 175 mm^2. Anterior epidural veins and midline ligament faintly seen. Depth of anterior epidural space (AES) at L5-S1 appears to protect S1 roots against early compression by small disc herniations (see also Chap. 4)

Fig. 3.7 Variable length of root sleeves at lumbar MR myelography. (**a1**) Image at *left* shows dural sac with exceptionally long root sleeves, multiple root sleeve cysts. Axial cut (**b1**) of same case shows long distance between dural sac and dorsal root ganglion (*arrow*). Slight obliquity of cut tilted towards plane of left root sleeve accentuates this.Image at *right* in (**a2**) shows short, almost nonexistent root sleeves and axial cut (**b2**) shows dorsal root ganglion (*arrow*) close dural sac

with regard to terminology. Several groups have reported the presence of meningovertebral ligaments especially in the lumbar region, fixing the dural sac to the spinal canal and the PLL (Spencer et al. 1983; Barbaix et al. 1996; Bashline et al. 1996), also immobilising the emerging nerve root sleeves in the anterior part of the spinal canal and the foramen (Grimes et al. 2000; Spencer et al. 1983). Others, however, have mentioned the possibility of displacement of the dural sac during movements (Parkin and Harrison 1985), and a functional myelographic study (Penning and Wilmink 1981) has shown that caudocranial movement of the dural cul-de-sac of up to 25 mm is possible in some individuals during flexion–extension of the lumbar spine (see Sect. 3.3). So the degree to which the dural sac and root sleeves are fixed with respect to the surrounding bony and ligamentous structures is not clear, and there appears to be considerable individual variability.

The *anterior epidural veins* (anterior internal vertebral veins AIVV, or Batson's plexus), are located anterior to the dural sac (Fig. 3.9a). This valveless venous plexus presents a typically ladder-like appearance in the frontal view, with the rungs at the mid-vertebral levels and a fenestration at the level of all discs except L5-S1, where the veins are usually more prominent than at the higher levels (Fig. 3.9b; Wilmink et al. 1978). The mid-line component of the epidural venous plexus lies in the AES and drains the vertebral body via the basivertebral vein (Fig. 3.9a) while the lateral parts give rise to the intervertebral foraminal veins which connect with the ascending lumbar veins outside the vertebral column (Fig. 3.9b). Each intervertebral foramen therefore contains one or two veins as well as the dorsal root ganglion, surrounded by foraminal fat which is continuous with the epidural fat within the spinal canal as well as the paravertebral fat outside.

The *walls of the spinal canal* are partly bony and partly ligamentous. The anterior wall consists of the vertebral body and intervertebral disc, covered by the PLL (Fig. 3.10). Posteriorly the boundary of the canal is formed by the lamina and interspinous ligament, with the latter blending ventrolaterally into the flaval ligament which in its turn continues ventrolaterally as the facet joint capsule. Figure 3.10 also shows that bony rings alternate with rings of ligamentous structures which line the walls of the spinal canal.

The *lateral recess of the spinal canal* is similarly composed of a bony and ligamentous portion. The bony lateral recess is located at the pedicular level and is formed by the dorsal surface of the vertebral body anteriorly, by the superior articular process posteriorly and the pedicle laterally (Fig. 3.11, upper diagram). The 'ligamentous lateral recess' located more cranially is formed anteriorly by the disc surface and posteriorly by the facet joint capsule. Laterally, the lower half of the foramen is encountered, which is often narrowed by disc bulging and facet and flaval hypertrophy, with the exit filled in by ligamentous strands so that a true ligamentous lateral recess is formed (Fig. 3.11 lower diagram).

The *intervertebral foramen* is bordered superiorly and inferiorly by the pedicular borders of the adjacent vertebrae, anteriorly by the posterior surface of the vertebral body and the intervertebral disc and posteriorly by the articular processes and their covering ligaments (see Fig. 3.10). There are significant differences between the upper and the lower lumbar foramina. At the L1 and L2 levels the pedicle attaches to the posterior aspect of the vertebral bodies and is oriented anteroposterioly, corresponding to a sagittally oriented foramen. At the lower lumbar levels the intervertebral compartment more resembles a canal than a foramen, as the attachment of the pedicle moves laterally and ventrally on the vertebral body, and the pedicle is more obliquely oriented in the coronal as well as the axial plane (Pfaundler et al. 1989).

The shape and dimensions of the foramina vary per lumbar spinal level and are also influenced by the

---

Fig. 3.9 Venous spinal structures. (**a**) Diagram showing anterior epidural veins covering anterior border of bony spinal canal (*arrows*). This valveless venous plexus drains vertebral body via basivertebral vein (*dotted tubular structures*), connects with paravertebral ascending lumbar veins (*short arrow*) by way of foraminal veins (*arrowhead*). Lumbar veins (*curved arrow*) connect vertebral venous system with inferior vena cava. (**b**) Subtracted catheter epidural venogram shows epidural venous plexus resembling stack of ovals, or ladder with rungs at mid-vertebral level where basivertebral veins connect. Note that venous plexus approaches mid-line at mid-vertebral levels, veins move laterally at disc levels to join intervertebral veins. Paravertebral ascending lumbar veins incompletely opacified. At L5-S1 level (*arrow*) anteriror epidural space is deeper and veins cover disc in mid-line (see also Fig. 3.8; Fig. 3.18). (**c**) Axial post-contrast CT sections around L4–5 show position of enhancing anterior epidural veins. At mid-vertebral level (**c1**), veins are grouped around mid-line (*arrows*). Structure in lateral recess indicated by curved arrow is nerve root, not vein. At intervertebral level (**c2**), veins are located more laterally in spinal canal (*arrows*)

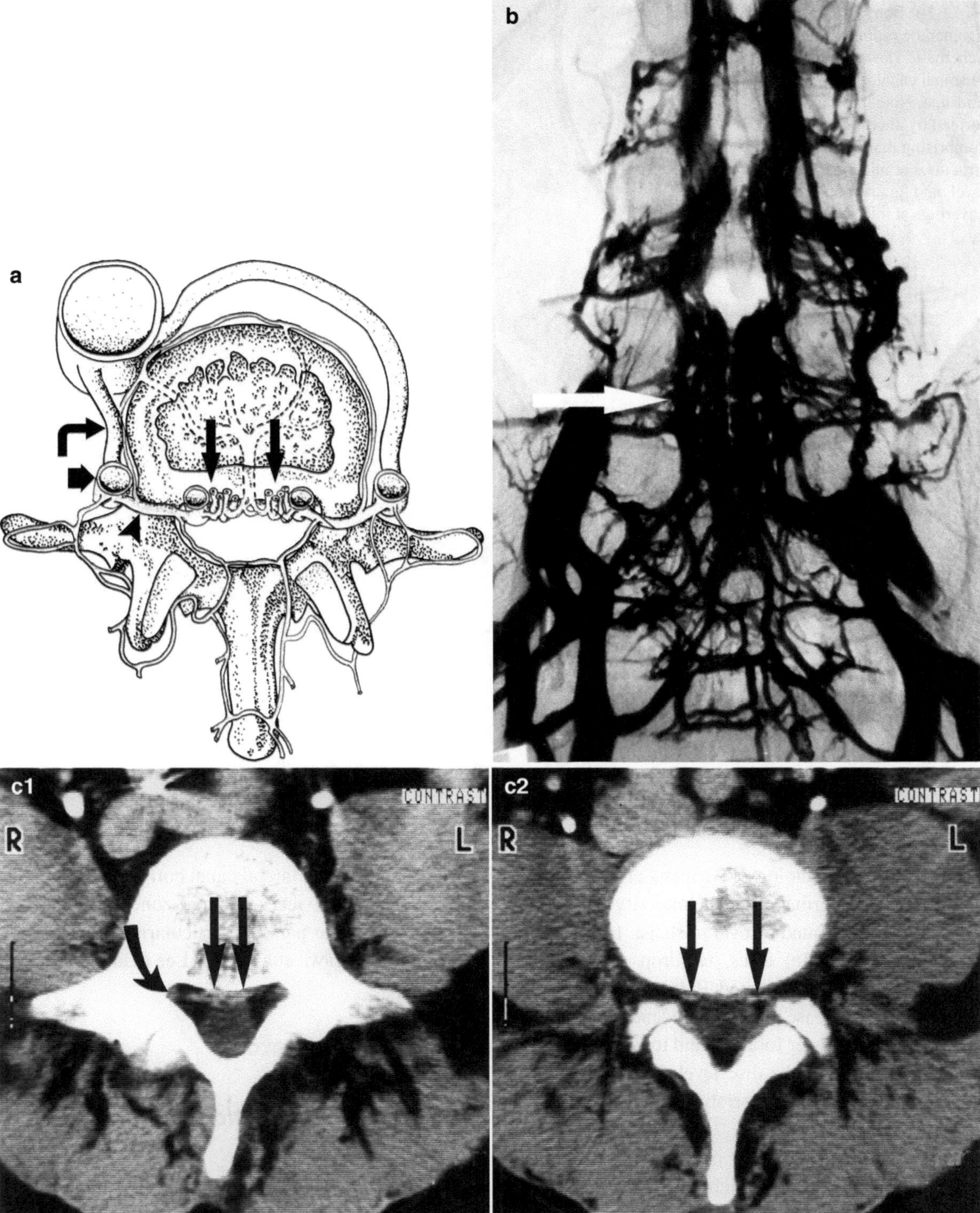

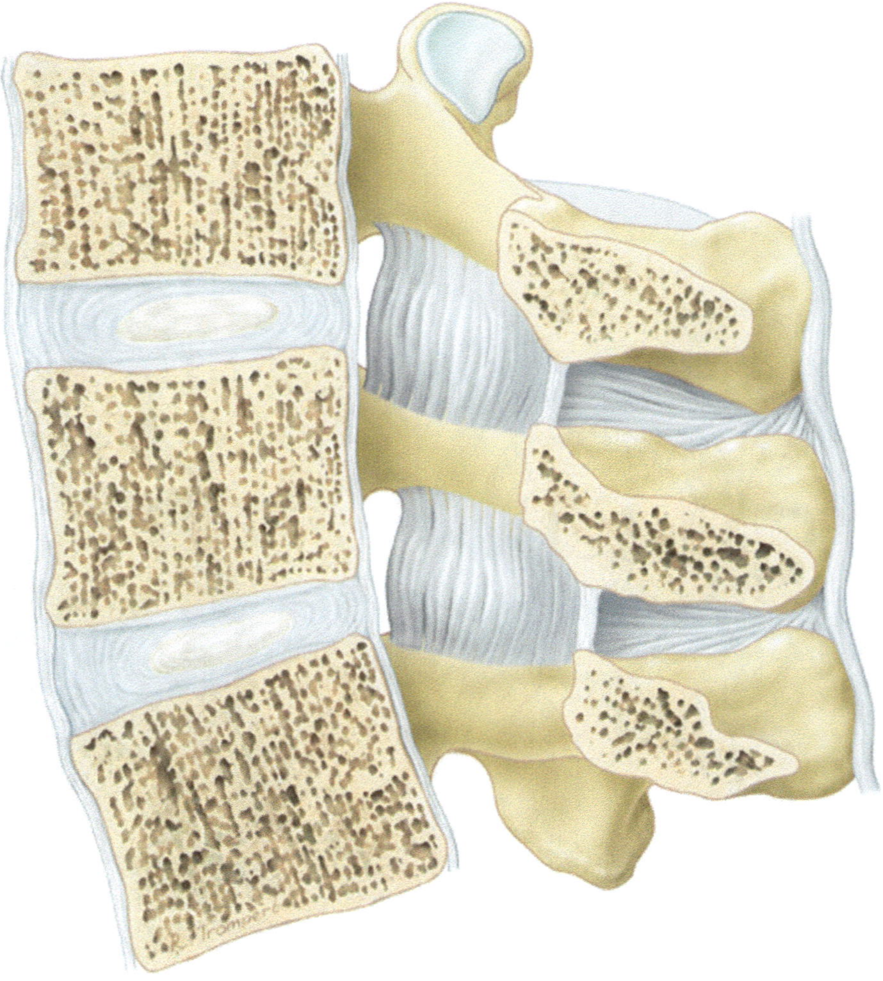

Fig. 3.10 Bony and ligamentous spinal canal. Schematic view of right half of spinal canal seen from mid-line. Note that canal is formed by alternating rings comprising mainly bony structures at mid-vertebral level, and ligamentous coverings at intervertebral level

presence of disc pathology (Stephens et al. 1991). In individuals with normal discs, the majority of foramina were found to be round or oval in shape. In those with abnormal (degenerate) discs, teardrop- or auricular-shaped foramina predominated. Putting this differently: in degenerative disease there is a tendency towards A-P narrowing of the lower foramen and towards formation of a lateral recess at the disc level, by bulging of the annulus fibrosus and degenerative enlargement of the superior articular process.

In the literature mention is made of a *radicular canal or nerve root canal* which is formed in the lateral part of the spinal canal of the lower lumbar vertebrae. This canal has been confusingly subdivided: by some into three parts: retrodiscal, corresponding to the ligamentous lateral recess mentioned above; parapedicular, corresponding to the bony lateral recess; and foraminal (Vital et al. 1983); while others refer to an

entrance zone of the lateral canal corresponding to the upper bony lateral recess; a mid-zone located more caudally under the pars interarticularis, and a foraminal zone (Hasegawa et al. 1993; Lee et al. 1988).

3.2 Sectional Anatomy

3.2.1 Transverse Sectional Anatomy

Good working knowledge of sectional anatomy is essential if one is not to lose one's way in CT or MRI studies of the spine. Beside the morphological differences between various levels within a single segment which will be described below, there are also variations when passing from the thoracolumbar to the lumbosacral transition (Panjabi et al. 1992). As Fig. 3.12

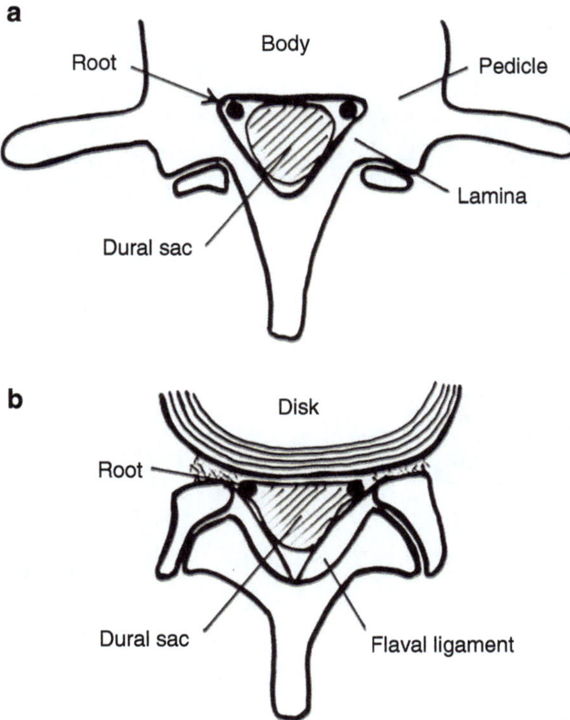

Fig. 3.11 Bony and ligamentous lateral recesses. Diagrams of lateral regions of spinal canal at pedicular level (**a**) and disc level cranial to pedicles (**b**).

shows, the cross-sectional shape of the spinal canal gradually changes from oval at L1 to triangular at L5 and S1 as the posterior surface of the vertebral bodies changes from posterior concavity to convexity (Larsen 1985). The orientation of the facets which mainly sagittal at L1 becomes much more oblique and inward-pointing at L5, while at the same time the superior articular processes shift forward on the pedicle with respect to the posterior surface of the vertebral body and the disc (Pfaundler et al. 1989).

These factors combine to create the lateral recess which has been described in the section above on topographic anatomy. Such lateral recesses are present only in the lower lumbar vertebrae and at the lumbosacral transition L4 to S1, and not in the higher lumbar region (Lassale et al. 1984). As discussed in Chapter 4 the lack of a lateral recess can explain the smaller likelihood of nerve root compression at upper lumbar as opposed to lower lumbar levels.

For practical purposes three levels can be distinguished within one spinal motion segment, which centres around the intervertebral disc and further comprises portions of the adjacent vertebrae above and below (Figs. 3.13 and 3.14).

- *The disc level syn. lower foraminal level*: This section passes through the disc and the facets with their joint capsules. At this level the spinal canal is entirely bordered by ligamentous structures (Fig. 3.13).

Bony landmarks: Parts of two adjacent vertebrae are seen in this section. The facet or intervertebral joint is best seen here, with the superior articular process of the lower vertebra forming the anterior part of the joint, and the inferior articular process of the upper vertebra forming the posterior part. The axial section at this level usually includes also a part of the lamina and the spinous process of the upper vertebra.

Ligaments: The flaval ligaments are most prominent at this level and, together with facet joint capsule and the posterior disc surface, form a ligamentous lining of the spinal canal interposed between the two bony rings formed by laminae and vertebral bodies. The lower half of the intervertebral foramen which is seen at this level may be roomy as shown in Fig. 3.13, or may be narrowed in degenerative conditions so that a ligamentous lateral recess is formed (see Fig. 3.11).

Dural sac and root sleeves: Above the level of detachment of the root sleeves the dural sac has a rounded shape (Fig. 3.13) (upper section). At the L4–5 disc level the shape of the dural sac is usually more or less triangular, as root sleeves begin to form at its ventrolateral angles (centre section). When the root sleeves have detached the dural sac is again round (lower section).

Epidural fat and veins: The retrodural fat pad is very prominent at the disc level, although there is also fat ventrolateral to the dural sac extending into the lower foramen.

Epidural veins may be identified at this level, most prominently between the disc and the dural sac at L5-S1; less conspicuously and grouped biventrolaterally at higher lumbar levels (see Figs. 3.9 and 3.18).

- *The pedicular level*. This section lies directly *below* the disc level. At this level the spinal canal is usually bordered entirely by bony structures, depending on the angulation of the section (Fig. 3.13).

Bony landmarks: These include the upper half of the vertebral body and the lamina, the pedicles, transverse processes and base of superior articular processes. A bony ring appears to surround the dural sac at this level

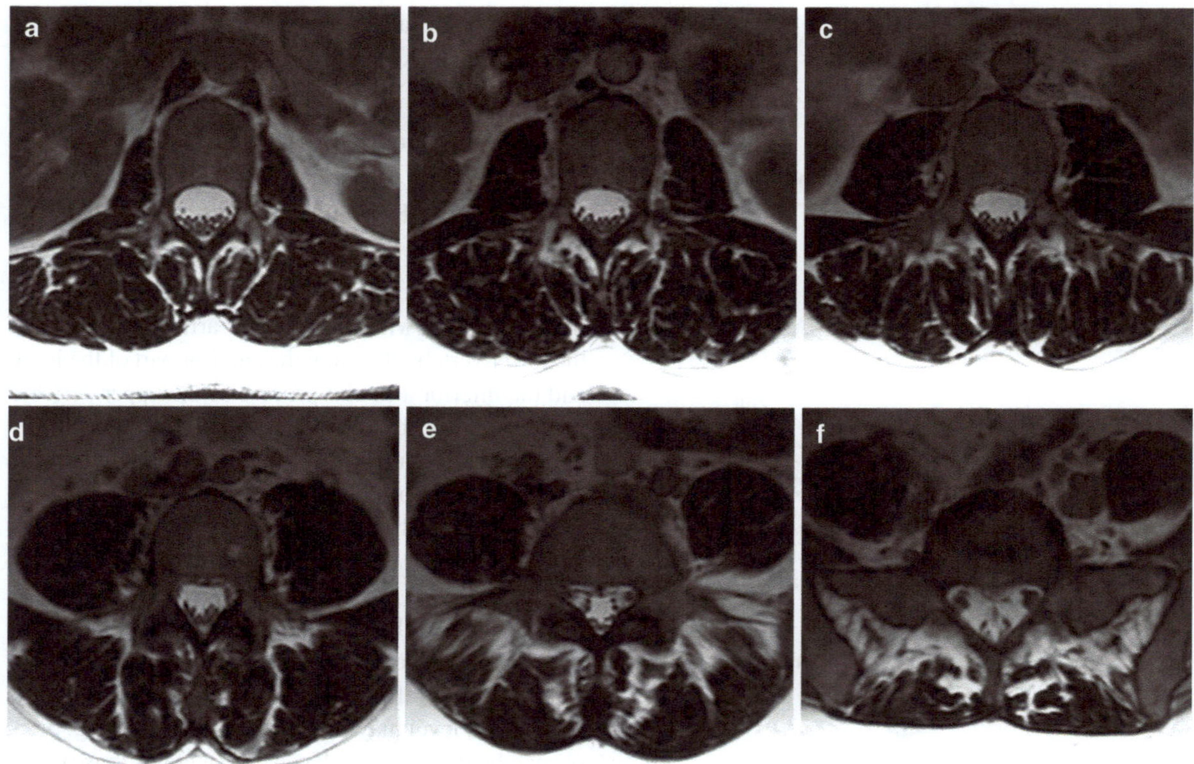

Fig. 3.12 Shape of spinal canal at higher compared to lower lumbar levels. Axial T2W MR images at pedicular levels of L1 (**a**); L2 (**b**); L3 (**c**); L4 (**d**); L5 (**e**) and S1 (**f**). Note gradual change in shape of spinal canal, from oval to triangular with lateral recesses at lower levels; also changes in orientation and thickness of pedicles

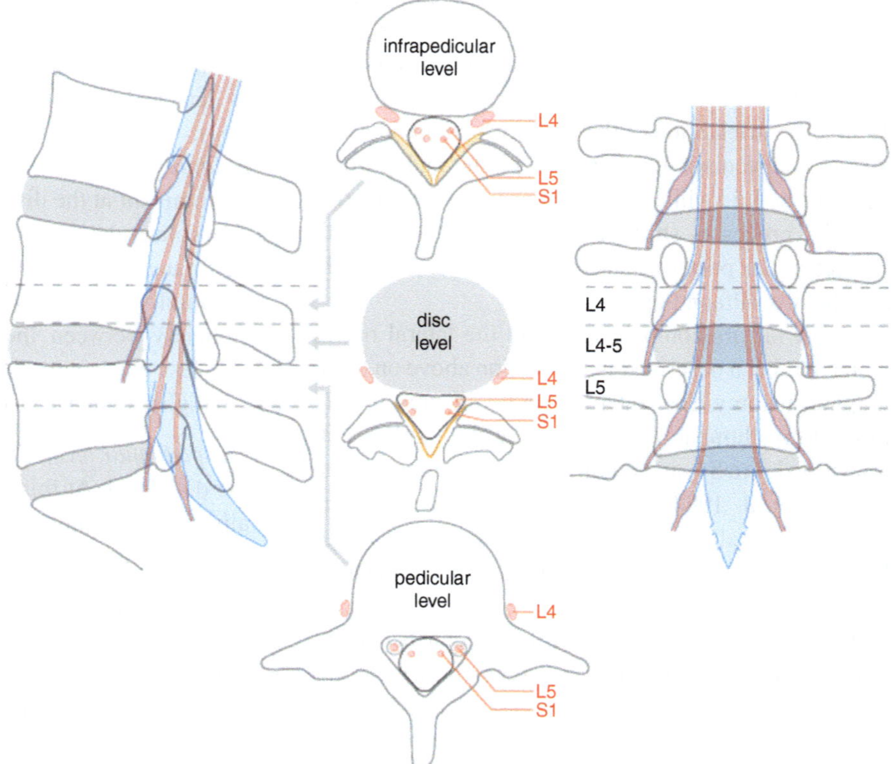

Fig. 3.13 Diagram of sectional anatomy. Axial images at centre showing L4 infrapedicular level *syn.* upper foraminal level (*upper image*), L4–5 disc level *syn.* lower foraminal level (*centre*) and L5 pedicular level (*lower image*). Proceeding craniocaudally in this slice set, note ventrolateral shift of L5 intradural root passing from L4 infrapedicular level to L4–5 disc level and then at L5 pedicular level into L5 root sleeve which later curves laterally under L5 pedicle. Similarly, L4 dorsal root ganglion at infrapedicular L4 level continues laterally and caudally as L4 spinal nerve past L4–5 disc level

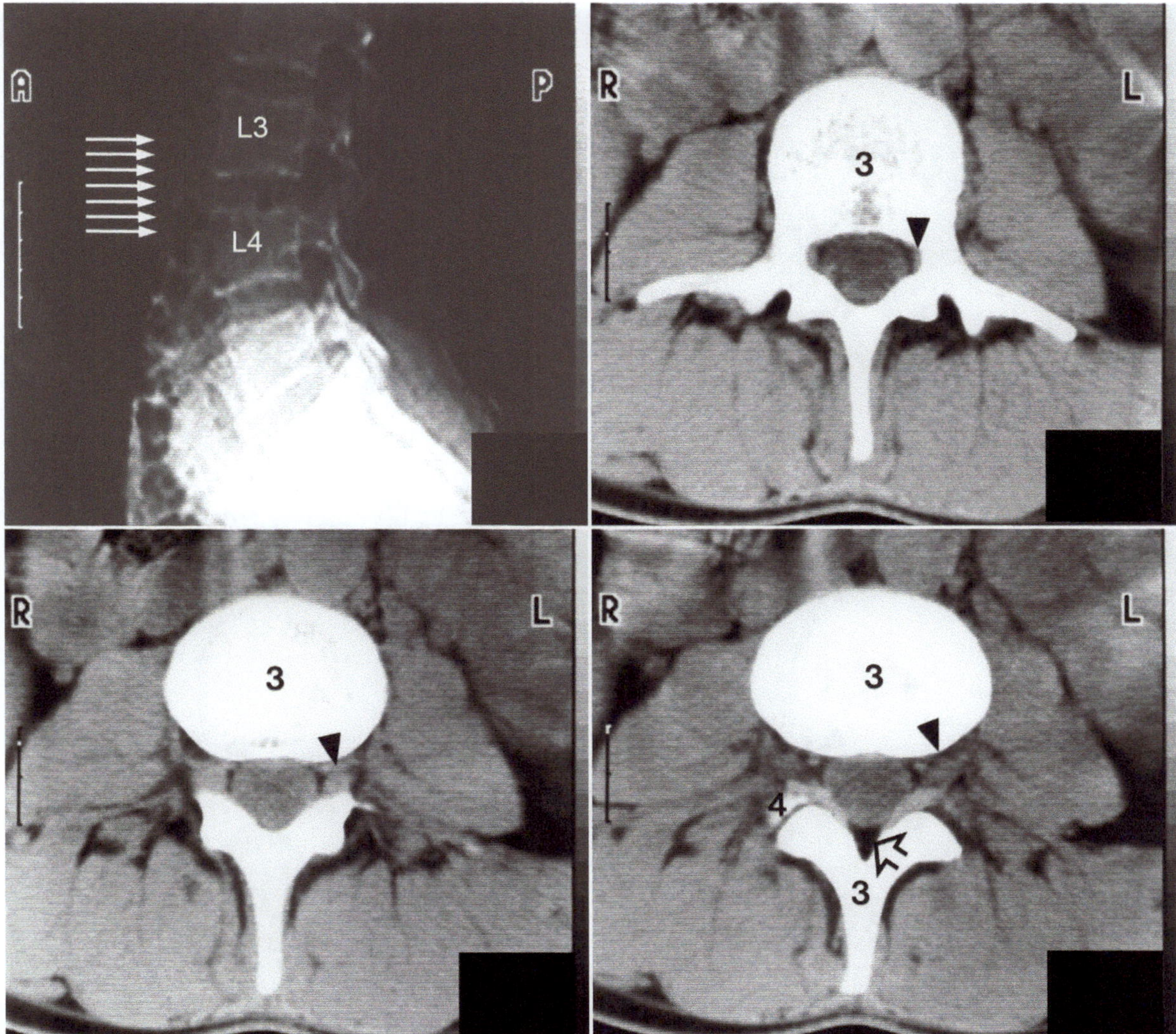

Fig. 3.14 Sectional CT anatomy. *Top row left*: Lateral scout view indicating levels of sections: 4.5 mm consecutive axial CT cuts centred around L3–4 disc. Note that three basic levels as mentioned in text can be distinguished, but there are also intervening and transitional images. *Top row right*: At low L3 pedicular level spinal canal forms a bony ring enclosing dural sac. Emerging L3 root sleeve (*arrowhead*) outlined by small band of epidural fat. *Second row left*: At high L3 upper foraminal (infrapedicular) level L3 dorsal root ganglion has formed (*arrowhead*). Note small foraminal veins outlined by fat, between *arrowhead* and *ganglion*. Still no dorsal epidural fat pad present at this transitional level. *Second row right*: At L3 upper–foraminal/endplate level *arrowhead* shows L3 dorsal root ganglion in foramen. *Open arrow* shows retrodural fat pad now formed as lamina recedes backward. Flaval ligaments coming into view, also tip of right L4 superior articular process (4). Epidural veins ventrolateral to dural sac.

although the upper edge of the lamina in the mid-line may dip to almost halfway down the vertebral body. The bony mid-sagittal diameter is at its smallest here (see Fig. 3.10). In the upper lumbar region the canal is rounded to oval in shape, becoming triangular farther caudally toward the lumbosacral transition (see Fig. 3.12). This results in bony lateral recesses being formed in the L4–5-S1 region. These recesses are bordered by the vertebral body anteriorly, the pedicle laterally and the base of the articular process dorsally. An additional suprapedicular level has been defined; this is a thin section comprising the upper few

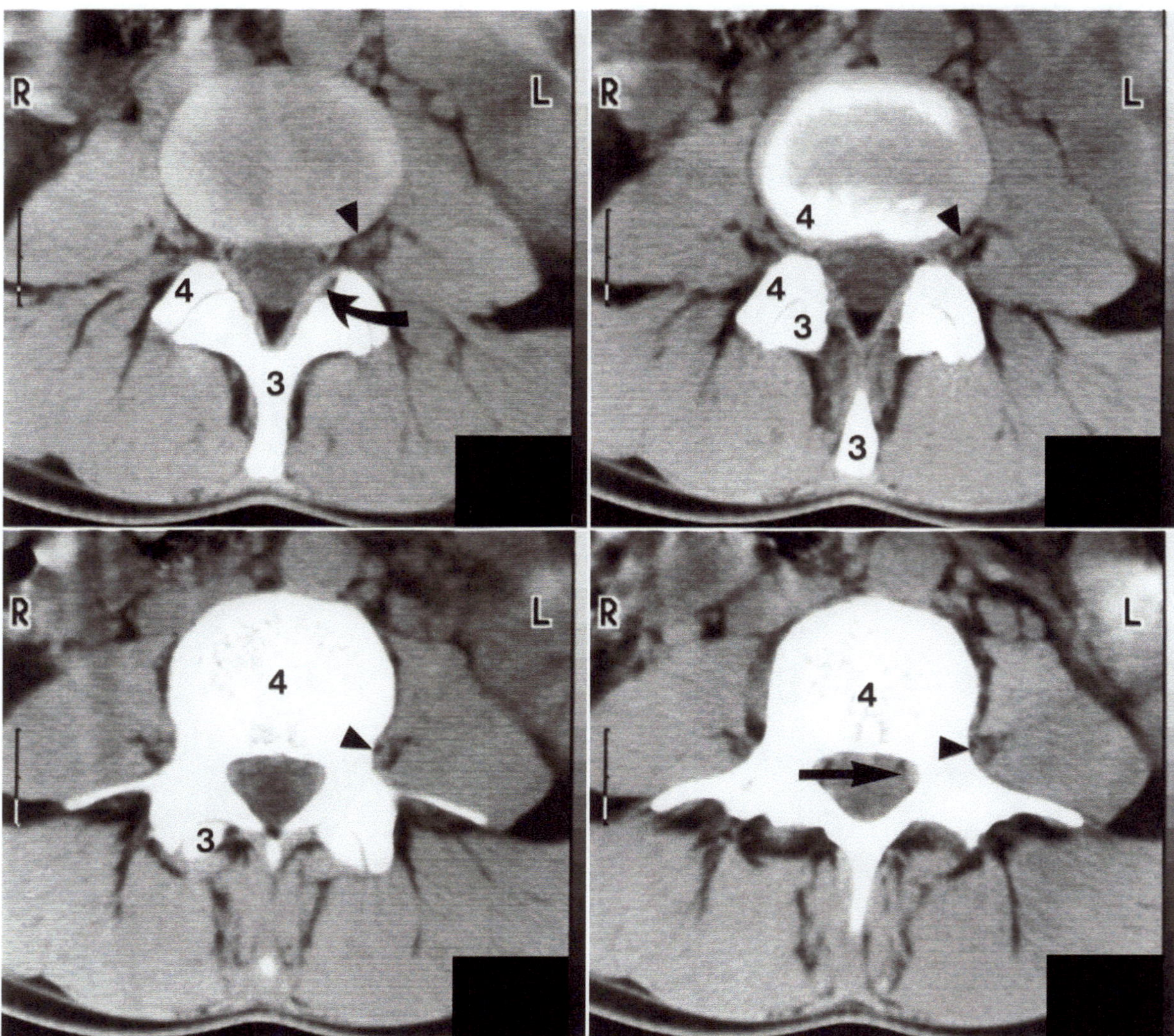

Fig. 3.14 (continued) *Top row left*: At L3–4 disc level L3 spinal nerve (*arrowhead*) is now outside foramen. L3–4 facet now fully formed, with covering joint capsule (*curved arrow*) merging dorsally into flaval ligament. *Top row right*: At L4 disc/upper endplate level, L3 inferior articular process (3) and L4 superior articular process (4) well seen, flaval ligament merging dorsally into interspinous ligament, lower tip of L3 spinous process visible (3). *Arrowhead* indicates extraforaminal L3 spinal nerve. *Bottom row left*: At L4 high pedicular level tip of L3 inferior articular processes (3) still just visible. *Arrowhead* indicates L3 spinal nerve. *Bottom row right*: At L4 low pedicular level; emerging L4 root sleeve just visible (*arrow*), medial to pedicle

millimetres of the pedicular level, from the cranial endplate of the vertebra to the upper border of the pedicle, at the transition between the ligamentous and bony lateral recesses (Wiltse et al. 1997; Ross 2004). Specifying such a separate sub-level does not appear to have much anatomical or biomechanical significance.

Dural sac and root sleeves: In the upper lumbar region the dural sac is seen as a round tube conforming to the inner surface of the rounded spinal canal, as the root sleeves usually depart below pedicular level. In the lower lumbar region the root sleeves depart from the dural sac at the pedicular level or even higher: at or above the disc level. The dural sac then presents itself as a round tube flanked by two root sleeves ("teddy bear" or "mickey mouse" appearance, see Fig. 3.5 middle row left; and Fig. 3.8c).

Ligaments: There are no ligamentous structures visible at this level.

Epidural fat and veins: There is no retrodural fat pad at this level. Small amounts of epidural fat may be seen around emerging root sleeves if these have detached in the lower lumbar region.

Epidural veins are present but usually not visualised at this level.

- *The upper foraminal syn infrapedicular level*: This section lies directly *above* the disc level. As Fig. 3.13 shows, the foramen extends over two levels; the infrapedicular and disc levels. The upper or infrapedicular part of the foramen has greater clinical significance, as it contains the dorsal root ganglion.

Bony landmarks: These include the lower half of the vertebral body, lamina and spinous process, as well as the inferior articular process and frequently the tip of the superior articular process of the vertebra below. There are no lateral recesses at this level: the foramina form bilateral openings in the walls of the bony spinal canal, and the upper portion of the foramen contains the dorsal root ganglion of the spinal nerve.

Dural sac and root sleeves: The dural sac at this level usually has a rounded aspect. There are no root sleeves to be seen here except sometimes at L5-S1.

Ligaments: As the upper part of the facet is frequently included in this section, the joint capsule and adjacent flaval ligament will also be partly seen.

Epidural fat and veins: The retrodural fat pad here is not as deep as at the disc level. There is usually quite abundant fat ventrolateral to the dural sac extending laterally into the intervertebral foramen and surrounding the dorsal root ganglion. Within this fat anterior epidural veins and small foraminal veins may be seen.

To recapitulate: The *disc (lower foraminal) level* in a transverse sectional study is recognised by the presence of the disc. When the plane of section is not parallel to the plane of the disc, look for the slice in which the posterior disc contour is visible. The *pedicular level* is recognised by the presence of pedicles and transverse processes, although the bony ring of the spinal canal may be incomplete posteriorly especially when the section is high or not parallel to the vertebral end-plate. To reach the disc from here one should proceed *cranially*. The *upper foraminal (infrapedicular) level* is recognised by the presence of intervertebral foramina containing dorsal root ganglia on either side of the dural sac. To reach the adjacent disc level one should proceed *caudally*. Transitional images may be seen at partially intervening levels as illustrated in Fig. 3.14.

The *intervertebral foramen* spans two levels: upper foraminal (infrapedicular) and lower foraminal (disc level). It is important to bear in mind that the dorsal nerve root ganglion lies at the upper foraminal level in the superior half of the intervertebral foramen, while the intervertebral disc is located below this level. This can be of relevance when assessing root compression by foraminal disc herniations (see Chap. 4).

Depending on which definition is used, the *nerve root canal* may span two levels: pedicular, and infrapedicular (upper foraminal level). Others have added an extra level, thus, making three: disc or lower foraminal level (ligamentous lateral recess), pedicular (bony lateral recess) and infrapedicular (upper foraminal). The reason for this lies in the variable level of emergence of the nerve root sleeve (Suh et al. 2005). In the upper lumbar region the axilla of the root sleeve is usually located at pedicular level and the exiting nerve root enters the foramen almost directly and the root canal is short, spanning only the pedicular and upper foraminal levels.. At the lumbosacral transition the axilla of the root sleeve lies at or above the level of the disc and the emerging nerve root follows a longer and more vertical course over three spinal levels: disc, pedicular and upper foraminal levels (see Fig. 3.6 and Fig. 4.6).

3.2.2 Sagittal and Coronal Sectional Anatomy

The advent of MRI has confronted us with sagittal and coronal images as well as the more familiar axial cuts.

The *mid-sagittal cut* shows the dural sac and retrodural fat pads to best advantage. The posterior cortical surface of the vertebral body is interrupted in the midline by the foramen of the basivertebral vein halfway down the vertebral body, and this feature can often be seen best in T2-weighted images (Fig. 3.15c, d). The dural sac usually begins to taper towards its cul-de-sac from about the L4–5 disc level. In addition, the dural sac moves dorsally, coming to lie against the posterior wall of the spinal canal at the entrance to the sacral canal. In this way a ventral epidural space of variable depth is created at the lumbosacral interspace and this space is occupied by epidural fat and a rich venous plexus.

Moving laterally the region of the *lateral recess* is entered. The sagittal imaging plane is less useful than the transverse plane for studying the lateral recess of the spinal canal because of partial-volume averaging with the adjacent pedicle, but the emerging root or root sleeve can sometimes be seen traversing this region (Fig. 3.15g, h)

Farther laterally still, the *intervertebral foramen* bordered by the pedicles above and below, the posterior vertebral body and disc surface anteriorly, and the superior and inferior articular processes posteriorly, come into view as well as the isthmus connecting the latter two structures. The dorsal root ganglion can be seen within the foramen, usually accompanied by one or two foraminal veins and well-delineated by foraminal fat (Fig. 3.15i, k).

The coronal plane is not frequently used in spinal sectional imaging. The reason for this lies in the distortion of the anatomy which occurs when the plane of imaging is not exactly coronal with respect to the vertebrae and the disc, and which may mimic the presence of pathology. In addition, the lordotic curvature of the lumbar spine makes it possible to capture only a small segment of coronal anatomy in a single, flat slice unless a curved reformatting technique is employed. Oblique spinal images are produced using specialised techniques such as MR myelography. These are, however, not sectional images but reconstructed 3D projections of the dural sac.

3.3 Functional Anatomy

When the lumbar spine moves from flexion (anteflexion, kyphosis) to extension (retroflexion, lordosis) and vice versa, measurable effects upon the spinal canal and its contents due to these postural changes can be observed in normal individuals. These effects

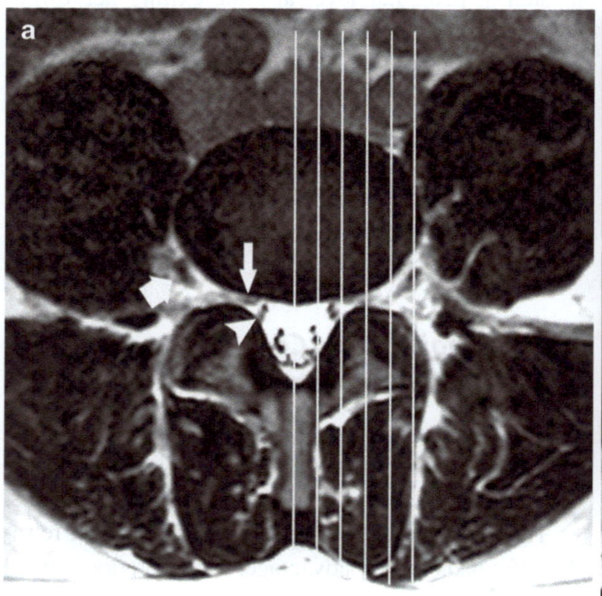
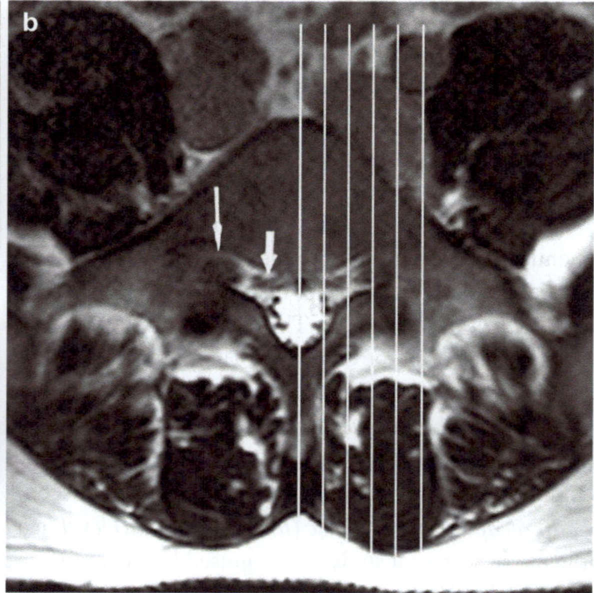
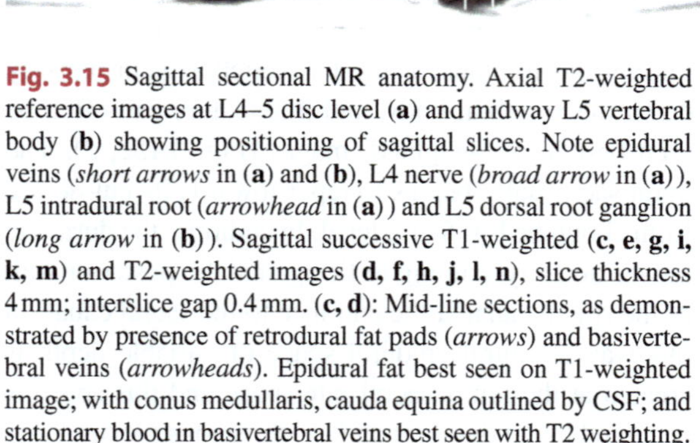

Fig. 3.15 Sagittal sectional MR anatomy. Axial T2-weighted reference images at L4–5 disc level (**a**) and midway L5 vertebral body (**b**) showing positioning of sagittal slices. Note epidural veins (*short arrows* in (**a**) and (**b**), L4 nerve (*broad arrow* in (**a**)), L5 intradural root (*arrowhead* in (**a**)) and L5 dorsal root ganglion (*long arrow* in (**b**)). Sagittal successive T1-weighted (**c, e, g, i, k, m**) and T2-weighted images (**d, f, h, j, l, n**), slice thickness 4 mm; interslice gap 0.4 mm. (**c, d**): Mid-line sections, as demonstrated by presence of retrodural fat pads (*arrows*) and basivertebral veins (*arrowheads*). Epidural fat best seen on T1-weighted image; with conus medullaris, cauda equina outlined by CSF; and stationary blood in basivertebral veins best seen with T2 weighting. (**e,f**): paramedian region. Note epidural veins behind vertebral bodies (*arrows*), best seen outlined by epidural fat with T1 weighting. (**g,h**): subarticular/lateral recess region. Epidural veins form continuous chain in lateral canal (*arrows*); roots coursing towards foramina faintly seen (*arrowheads*). (**i.j**): inner foraminal region. Inner borders of pedicles in view, with dorsal root ganglia directly underneath (*arrows*). Note also foraminal veins (*arrowheads*) best seen outlined by fat with T1 weighting. Note slight scoliotic list causing more lateral positioning of cut through pedicle in upper lumbar region. (**k,l**): outer foraminal region. (**m,n**): extraforaminal region. Note paravertebral veins: ascending lumbar vein (*arrows*) and lumbar veins (*arrowheads*).

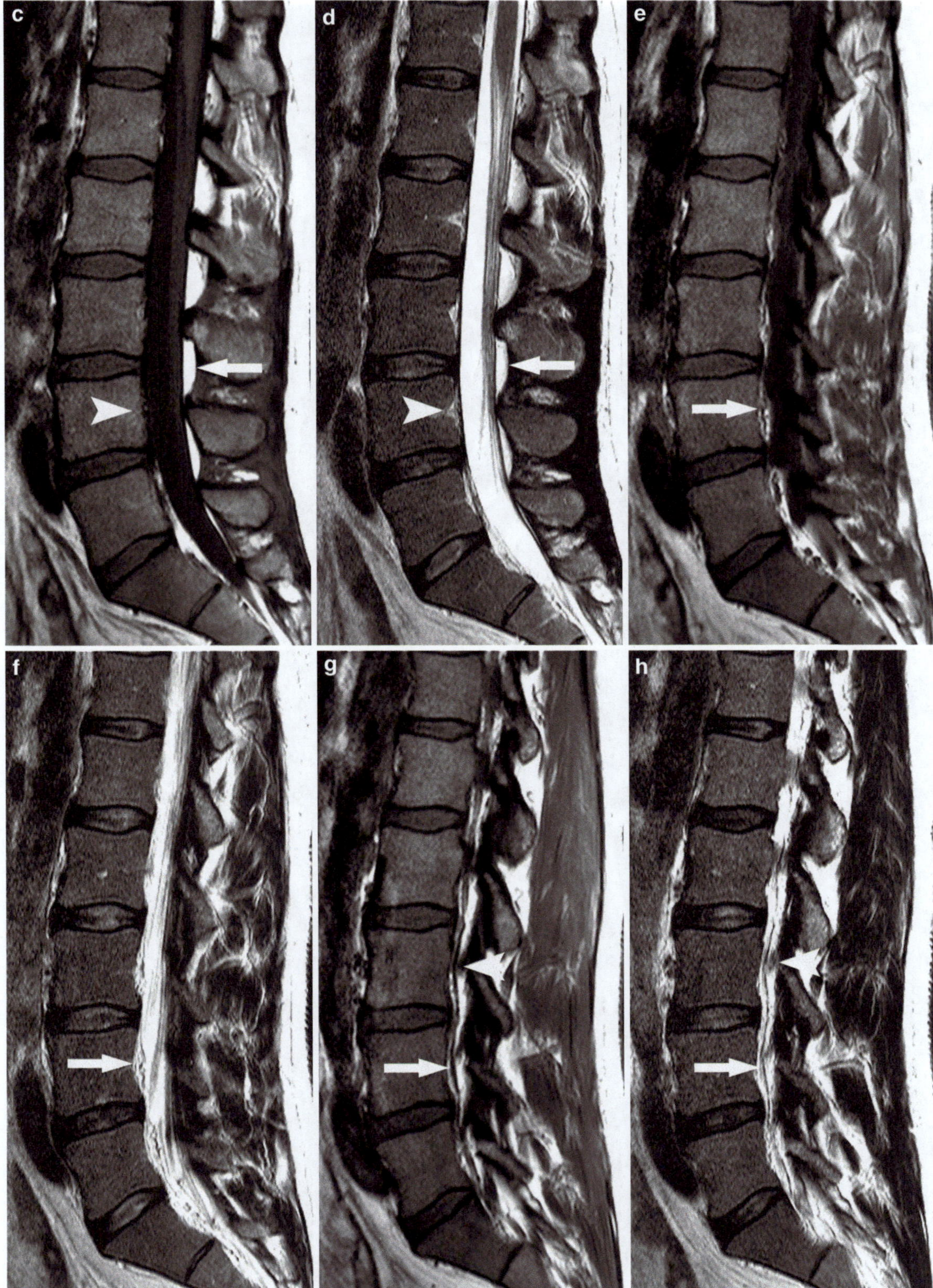

Fig. 3.15 (continued)

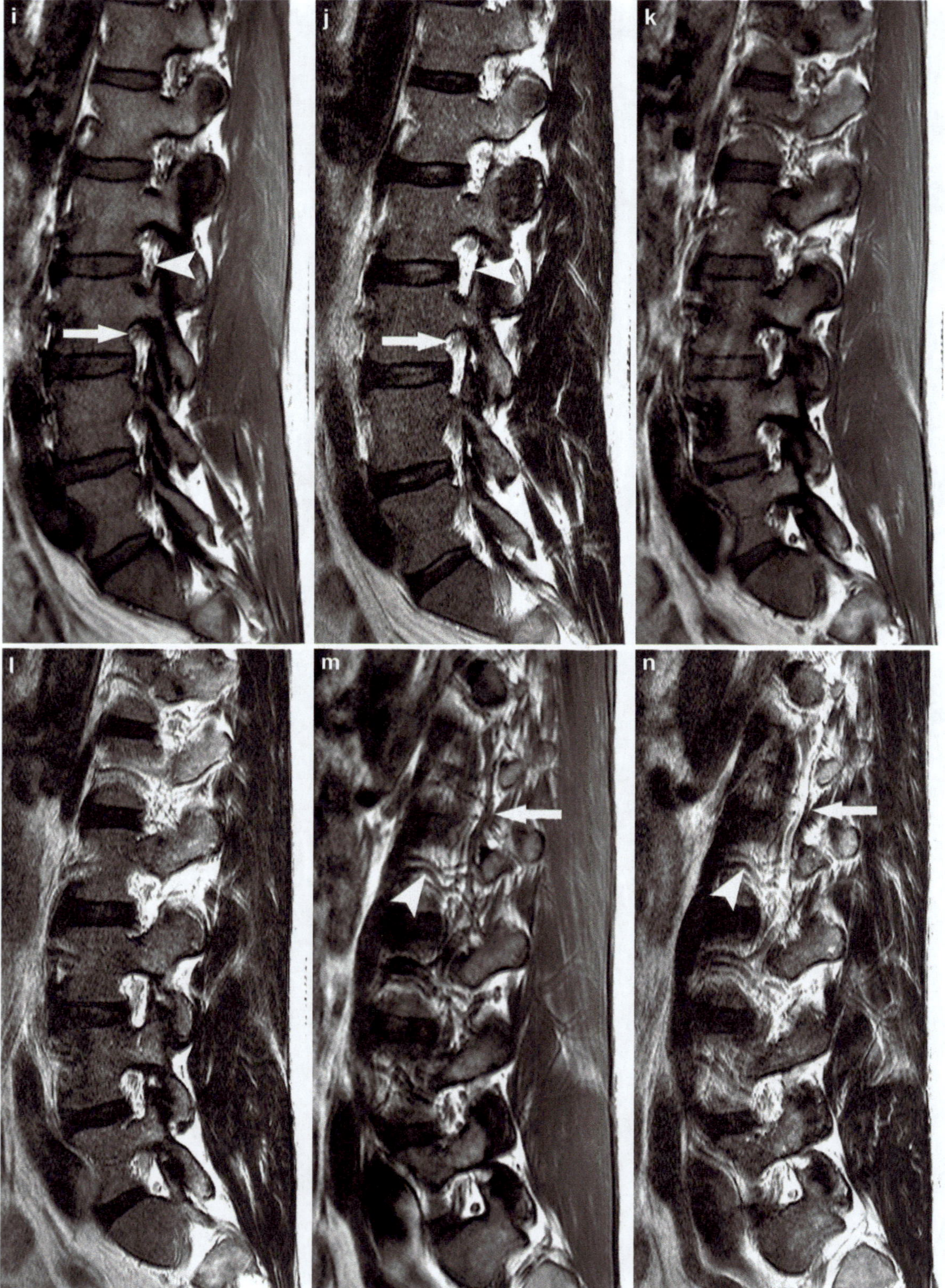

Fig. 3.15 (continued)

can become exaggerated under abnormal circumstances such as narrowing of the spinal canal, and then play a role in compression of the cauda equina or of individual nerve roots.

The study of posture-related morphologic changes within the spinal canal is not only of theoretical interest in explaining symptom production in these cases, but also has direct diagnostic relevance. In a considerable number of patients symptoms of irradiating low back pain occur in the upright posture and are relieved when the patient lies down. Most spinal imaging studies are presently performed with the patient recumbent in a CT or MRI scanner. This carries some risk of underdiagnosis especially in those with a marginally narrow spinal canal which produces nerve root compression in the upright posture but which is not visible in recumbency (Wilmink and Penning 1983). This is discussed in more detail in Chap. 4.

The effects of lumbar flexion–extension will be separately discussed for various anatomical structures mentioned earlier.

- Spinal canal: As mentioned earlier, the walls of the spinal canal consist of alternating bony vertebral and ligamentous intervertebral rings (see Fig. 3.10). The effects of flexion–extension movements manifest themselves mainly in the *ligamentous intervertebral disc region*. In the *bony vertebral region* two levels can be distinguished, as mentioned above. At the *pedicular level* the spinal canal is bordered by bony structures, and no effects of movement on the spinal canal are seen. The *infrapedicular or upper foraminal level* is a transitional zone, with little effect of flexion–extension movements on the spinal canal but with some change in the dimensions of the intervertebral foramina (see below).When the lumbar spine goes from flexion to extension, the dorsal vertebral end-plates come together and the dorsal annulus fibrosus bulges backward into the spinal canal (Fig. 3.16). This posterior disc-bulging does not usually exceed 1–2 mm. The vertebral laminae and spinous processes also come together, and this movement is of greater magnitude because these structures are farther distant from the centre of rotation, which lies within the intervertebral disc (Fig. 3.17; Penning et al. 1984). The interspinous ligaments, flaval ligaments and facet joint capsules dorsolateral to the spinal canal are normally quite elastic, but when shortened they also bulge somewhat into

the spinal canal. Under normal conditions this effect is small and the inward bulging in extension does not exceed about 1 mm. The net effect of spinal extension is therefore to cause some concentric narrowing, or decrease in cross-sectional area of the spinal canal at the ligamentous (disc) level (Inufusa et al. 1996; Knuttson 1942; Penning and Wilmink 1981, 1987). Under normal conditions this is insufficient to cause compression of the dural sac. As Fig. 3.18 shows, the reserve capacity of the spinal canal is greater at L5-S1 than at higher levels, due to the smaller dural sac and larger spinal canal, as well as the greater abundance of epidural veins.

- Lateral recess: As mentioned previously, two levels can be distinguished within the lateral recess. *The bony lateral recess* is located at the vertebral pedicular level and is not affected by flexion–extension movements. The *ligamentous lateral recess* at the intervertebral disc level on the other hand can be significantly narrowed in lumbar extension when the posterior annulus fibrosus bulges backward against the articular process and the facet joint capsule which bulge inwards, sometimes causing compression of the passing root sleeves (see Fig. 4.17; Penning and Wilmink 1987). This occurs most frequently al L4–5 and less often at L3–4. It has been reported to occur at L5-S1 in case of marked S1 facet hypertrophy, (Schlesinger 1955) but is infrequent, for anatomical reasons mentioned above (see Fig. 3.18).
- Epidural fat: In the lumbar region this is mainly present in the *retrodural fat pads* which lie dorsal to the dural sac and fill the interlaminar space between the dural sac and the dorsal interspinous ligaments (see Fig. 3.8a). This fat is semi-fluid in consistency, but is incompressible. In lumbar extension the retrodural fat pad is deformed by the laminae which come together from above and below, and must decrease in height. Being incompressible, the fat pad bulges forward against the posterior dural surface, thus further reducing the space available for the dural sac (Fig. 3.19). The deformation of the retrodural fat pad, thus, enhances the narrowing effect of lumbar spinal extension caused by inward bulging of ligamentous structures mentioned above (see Fig. 3.16). This effect becomes more marked as the amount of epidural fat, and the depth of the retrodural fat pads, increases.

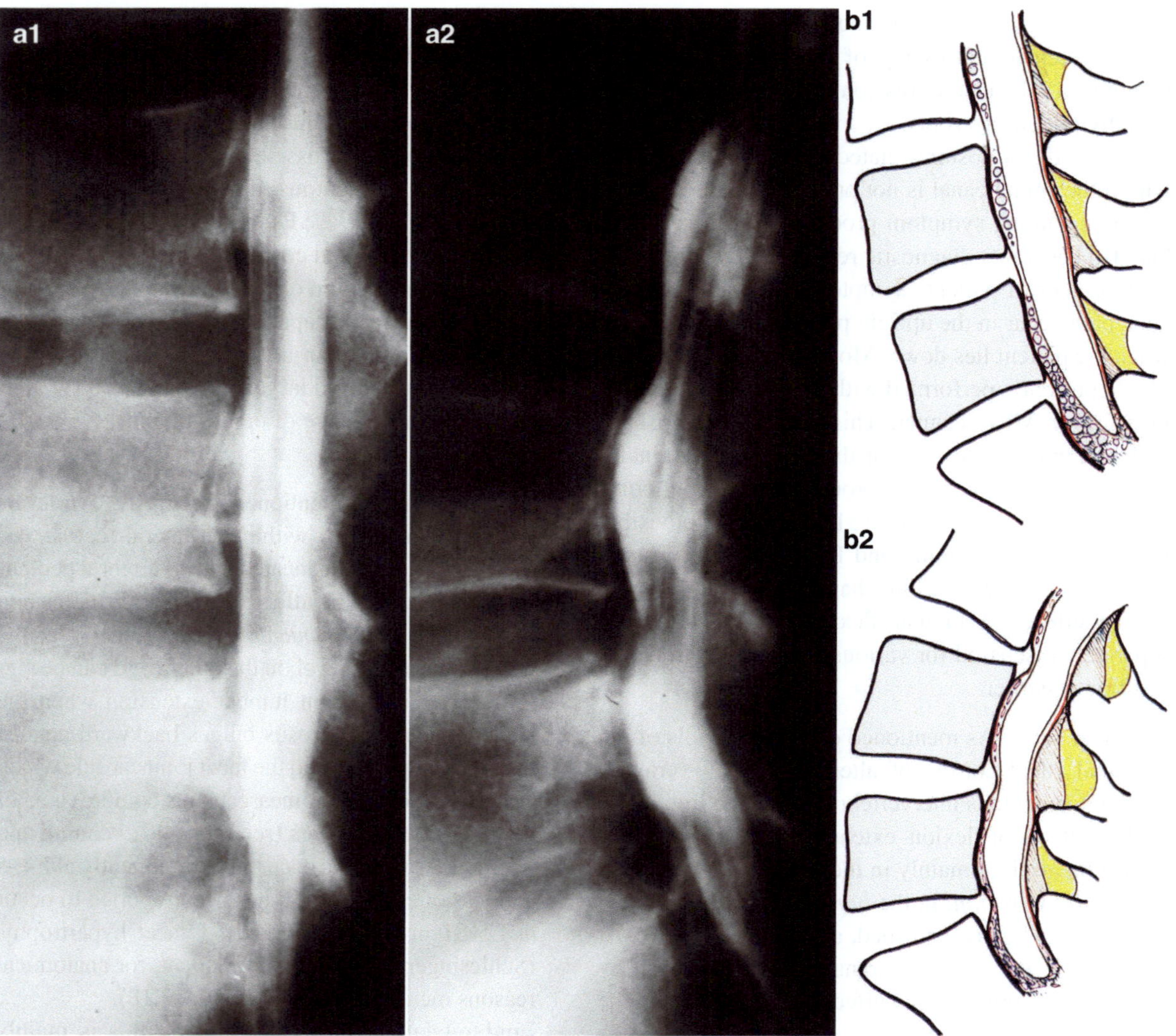

Fig. 3.16 Lumbar spine in flexion and extension. (**a1, 2**) Sitting lumbar myelogram in flexion (*left*) and extension (*right*). Note changes in shape and position in dural sac. (**b1, 2**) Diagram of effects of spinal movements. When spine moves from flexion (anteflexion, kyphosis) to extension (retroflexion, iordosis) posterior disc surfaces bulge backward into spinal canal while retrodural fat pad (*hatched*) and dorsal ligaments (*yellow*) bulge forward. Dural sac is constricted at disc level, and by way of compensation bulges forward into space behind vertebral body containing epidural venous plexus (*circles*). These veins empty into foraminal veins and paravertebral system in lumbar extension, and refill in flexion

- Dural sac and epidural veins: The combined effect of the vectors mentioned above is to cause compression and reduction of cross-sectional area of the dural sac at the ligamentous disc level. Were there to be no compensation for this, an extension movement of the lumbar spine would be accompanied by a rise in CSF pressure. Being elastic however, the dural sac can also bulge. In lumbar extension therefore the pinching of the dural sac at the disc level is compensated by bulging into a region which can accommodate this expansion: the anterior epidural space behind the concave vertebral body (Fig. 3.20, see also Fig. 3.16; Penning and Wilmink 1981). This space contains an abundant epidural venous plexus which, being valveless, is easily compressed (see Fig. 3.9). The sponge-like epidural venous plexus, thus, functions as an expansion vessel or pressure stabiliser: in extension the veins are compressed by

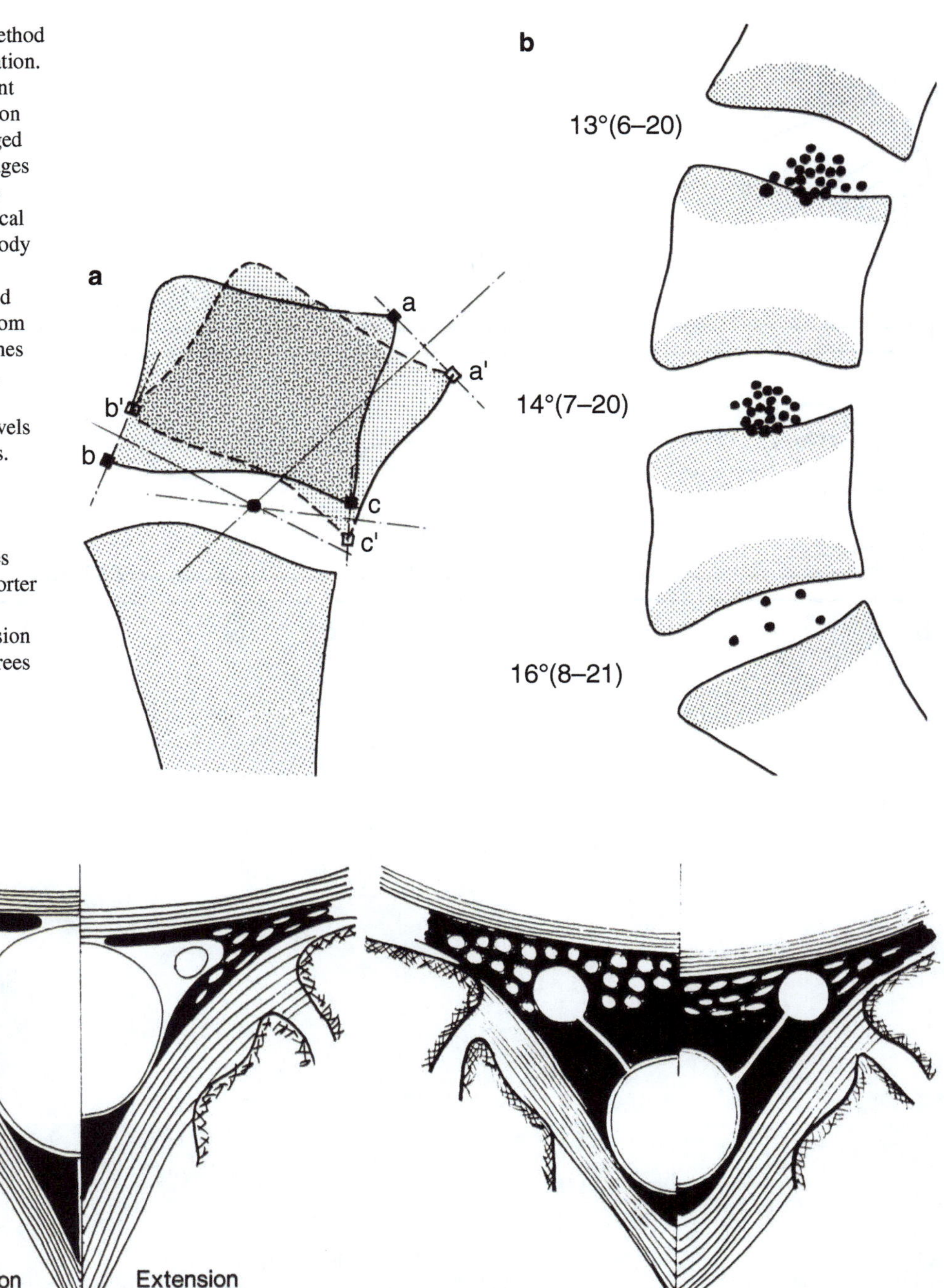

Fig. 3.17 (**a**) Euler's method to determine axis of rotation. X-ray films or transparent tracings of spine in flexion and extension are arranged with sacrum in both images superimposed. *Lines* are drawn connecting identical points on L5 vertebral body in flexion (**a, b, c**) and extension (**a', b', c'**), and perpendiculars drawn from points bisecting these lines cross in axis of rotation. (**b**) Axes of rotation determined at several levels in a group of individuals. Note that axes cluster around centre of disc, anterior to spinal canal, which therefore becomes longer in flexion and shorter in extension. Mean and spread of flexion–extension excursions given in degrees per disc level

Fig. 3.18 Spinal canal in flexion and extension at L4–5 (**a**) and L5-S1 (**b**). Narrowing of spinal canal in extension has less effect upon dural sac because of buffering effect of epidural venous plexus which is more voluminous at L5-S1 disc level and extends to mid-line. At higher disc levels the epidural veins are less voluminous and not present in the mid-line

the inward-bulging ligaments and forward-bulging dural sac, with blood being displaced to veins outside the spinal canal. In lumbar flexion the process is reversed and the volume of the epidural venous system expands as blood from outside the spinal canal is drawn in.

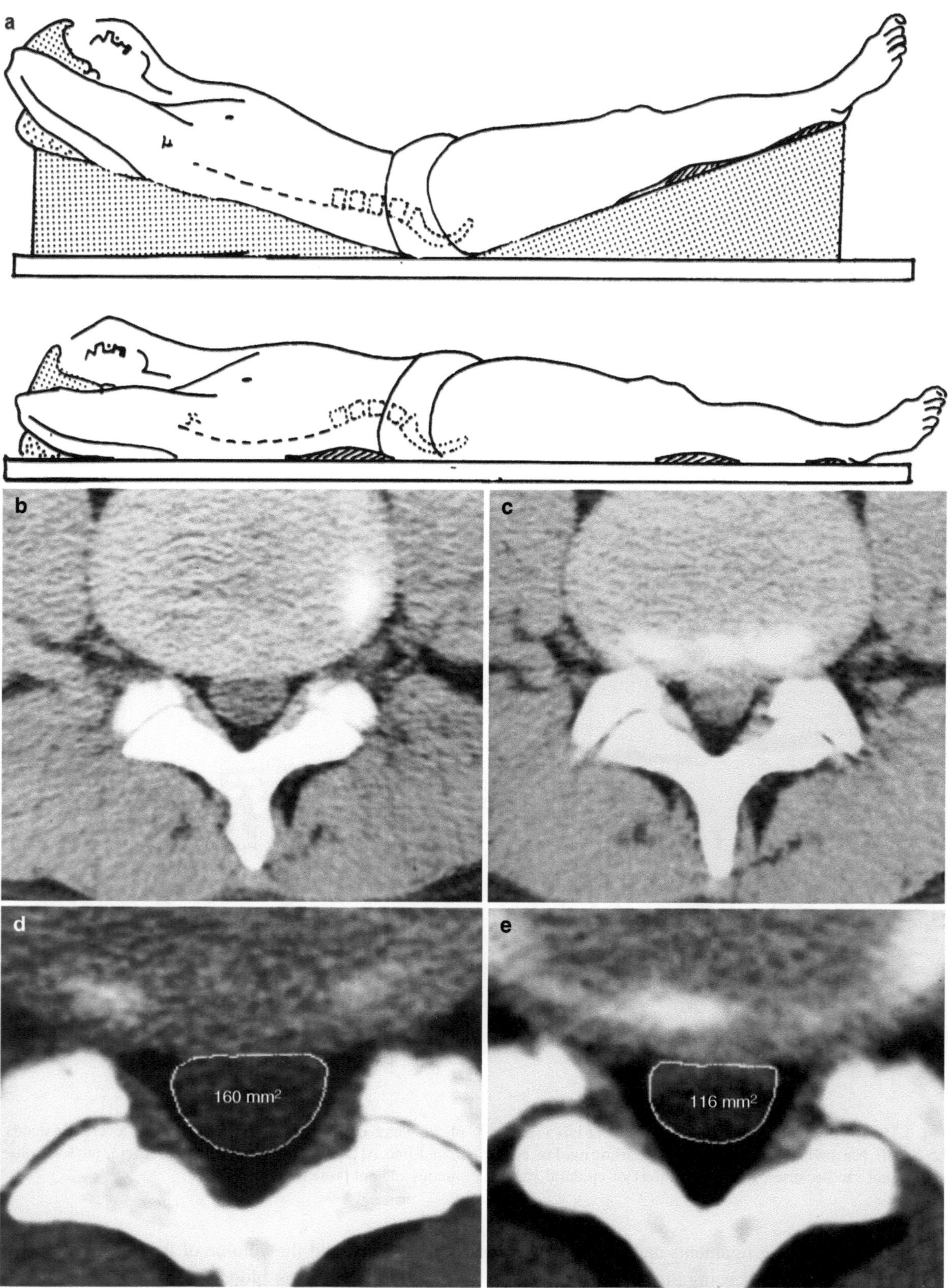

Fig. 3.19 CT study of L4–5 disc level in flexion and extension. (**a**) Positioning of subject in CT system. Lumbar extension is achieved by subject lying supine with extended legs; flexion by placing wedges under upper torso and extended legs. The pelvis is then tilted by traction via hamstrings, and lumbar lordosis reduced (Penning and Wilmink 1987). 4.5 mm slices parallel to L4–5 disc in flexion (**b**), and extension (**c**). Note backward displacement of disc surface in extension, with thickening of flaval ligaments and increase in depth of posterior epidural fat. At first sight effect does not seem great, but measured area of dural sac in extension is reduced by 27.5%, from 160 to 116 mm² (**d, e**)

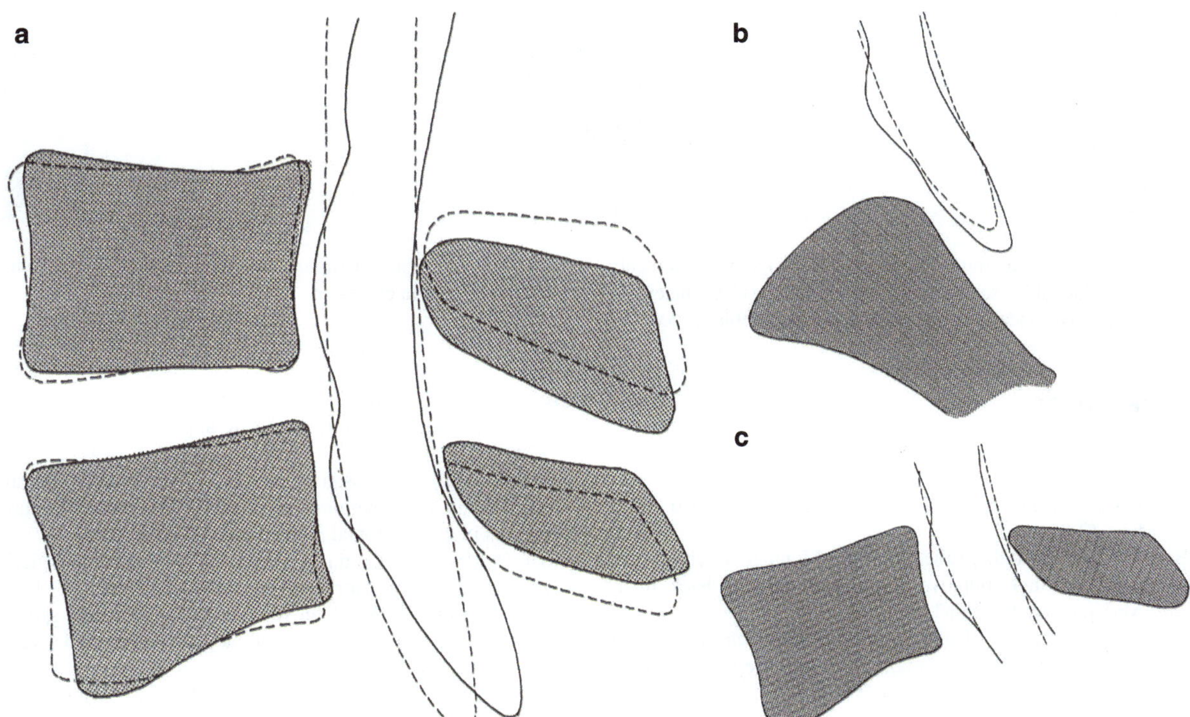

Fig. 3.20 Spinal structures in flexion and extension. Tracings from myelograms in flexion and extension, with superimposition of various structures. (**a**) L4–5 disc superimposed. Note movement of vertebrae and displacements of anterior and posterior dural borders from flexion (*dotted lines*) to extension (*drawn lines*). (**b**) *Upper diagram*: Sacrum superimposed. Note caudal movement of dural cul-de-sac by movement from flexion (*dotted line*) to extension (*drawn line*). (**c**) *Lower diagram*: L5 vertebral body superimposed. Note forward movement of anterior border of dural sac by movement from flexion to extension

Beside these effects, longitudinal movements of the dural sac can also be observed (see Fig. 3.20). A study featuring conventional myelography showed that craniocaudal movement of the dural end-sac relative to the sacral canal in lumbar flexion–extension ranged from 2 mm to 25 mm, with a mean of 7.9 mm, while the mean change in length of the bony lumbar spinal canal from L3 to S1 during the same movement was 16.5 mm (Penning and Wilmink 1981). Despite the ligamentous attachments of the dural sac and root sleeves to the walls of the spinal canal as described in Sect. 3.1 and which are presumed to limit mobility, the dural end-sac therefore appears to be relatively mobile with respect to the spinal canal.

Intervertebral foramen: In lumbar extension, the articular processes forming the facets slide over one another and the pedicles come together, and this results in decrease in foraminal dimensions (Fig. 3.21; Zamani et al. 1998). A cadaver study showed an increase in sagittal area of the lumbar foramen by 11.8% in flexion and a decrease by 15.3% in extension (Inufusa et al. 1996).

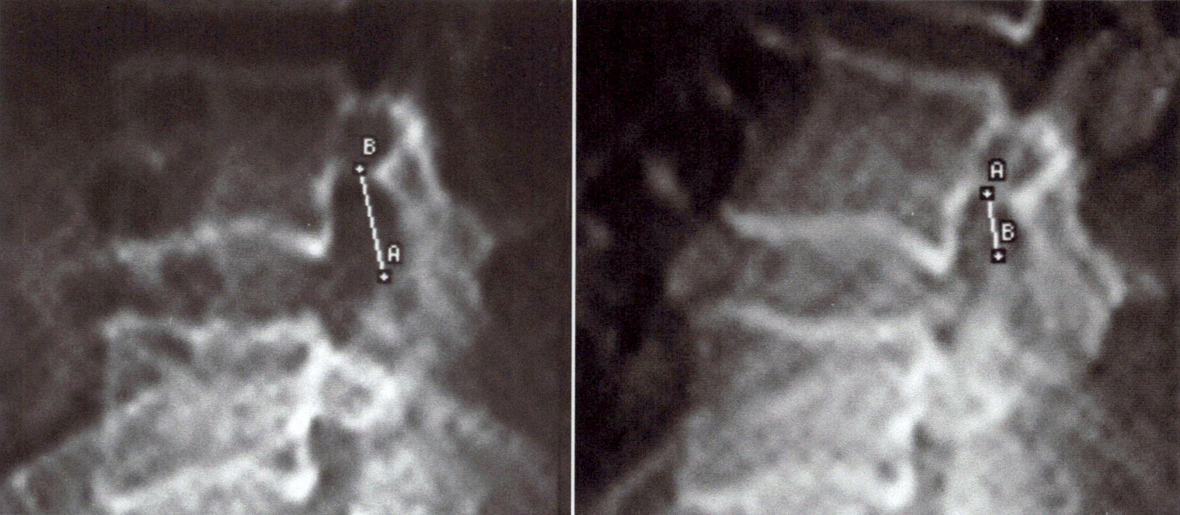

Fig.3.21 Lumbar foramina in flexion and extension. Measurements taken from lateral CT scoutviews in lumbar flexion (*left*) and extension (*right*). Distance from tip of L4 superior articular process to lower border of L3 pedicle (*dotted line AB*) decreased from 16 mm in flexion to 9 mm in extension

References

Barbaix E, Girardin MD, Hoppner JP et al (1996) Anterior sacrodural attachments – Trolard's ligaments revisited. Man Ther 1(2):88

Bashline SD, Bilott JR, Ellis JP (1996) Meningovertebral ligaments and their putative significance in low back pain. J Manipulative Physiol Ther 19(9):592

Binokay F, Akgul E, Bicakci K et al (2006) Determining the level of the dural sac tip: magnetic resonance imaging in an adult population. Acta Radiol 47(4):397

Bogduk N, Twomey LT (1991) Clinical anatomy of the lumbar spine. Churchill Livingstone, Melbourne

Bose K, Balasubramaniam P (1984) Nerve root canals of the lumbar spine. Spine 9(1):16

Grimes PF, Massie JB, Garfin SR (2000). Anatomic and biomechanical analysis of the lower lumbar foraminal ligaments. Spine 25(16):2009

Haines DE (1991) On the question of a subdural space. Anat Rec 230(1):3

Hasegawa T, An HS, Haughton VM (1993) Imaging anatomy of the lateral lumbar spinal canal. Semin Ultrasound CT MR 14(6):404

Hasegawa T, Mikawa Y, Watanabe R et al (1996) Morphometric analysis of the lumbosacral nerve roots and dorsal root ganglia by magnetic resonance imaging. Spine 21(9):1005

Inufusa A, An HS, Lim TH et al (1996) Anatomic changes of the spinal canal and intervertebral foramen associated with flexion-extension movement. Spine 21(21):2412

Knuttson F (1942) Volum- und formvariationen des wirbelkanals bei lordosierung und kyphosierung und ihre bedeutung fur die myelographische diagnostic. Acta Radiologica: 431

Kostelic J, Haughton VM, Sether L (1992) Proximal lumbar spinal nerves in axial MR imaging, CT, and anatomic sections. Radiology 183(1):239

Kostelic JK, Haughton VM, Sether LA (1991) Lumbar spinal nerves in the neural foramen: MR appearance. Radiology 178(3):837

Larsen JL (1985) The posterior surface of the lumbar vertebral bodies. Part 2: an anatomic investigation concerning the curvatures in the horizontal plane. Spine 10(10):901

Lassale B, Morvan G, Gottin M (1984) Anatomy and radiological anatomy of the lumbar radicular canals. Anat Clin 6(3):195

Lee CK, Rauschning W, Glenn W (1988) Lateral lumbar spinal canal stenosis: classification, pathologic anatomy and surgical decompression. Spine 13(3):313

Loughenbury PR, Wadhwani S, Soames RW (2006) The posterior longitudinal ligament and peridural (epidural) membrane. Clin Anat 19(6):487

Panjabi MM, Goel V, Oxland T et al (1992) Human lumbar vertebrae. Quantitative three-dimensional anatomy. Spine 17(3):299

Parkin IG, Harrison GR (1985) The topographical anatomy of the lumbar epidural space. J Anat 141:211

Penning L, Wilmink JT (1981) Biomechanics of lumbosacral dural sac. A study of flexion-extension myelography. Spine 6(4):398

Penning L, Wilmink JT (1987) Posture-dependent bilateral compression of L4 or L5 nerve roots in facet hypertrophy. A dynamic CT-myelographic study. Spine 12(5):488

Penning L, Wilmink JT, van Woerden HH (1984) Inability to prove instability. A critical appraisal of clinical-radiological flexion-extension studies in lumbar disc degeneration. Diagn Imaging Clin Med 53(4):186

Pfaundler S, Ebeling U, Reulen HJ (1989) Pedicle origin and intervertebral compartment in the lumbar and upper sacral spine. A biometric study. Acta Neurochir (Wien) 97(3–4): 158

Rauschning W (1991) Anatomy and pathology of the lumbar spine. Raven, New York

Reina MA, De Leon Casasola O, Lopez A et al (2002) The origin of the spinal subdural space: ultrastructure findings. Anesth Analg 94(4):991

Ross J (2004) Degenerative disc disease nomenclature. AMIRSYS, Salt Lake City

Schellinger D, Manz HJ, Vidic B et al (1990) Disk fragment migration. Radiology 175(3):831

Schlesinger PT (1955) Incarceration of the first sacral nerve in a lateral bony recess of the spinal canal as a cause of sciatica. J Bone Joint Surg Am 37-A(1):115

Spencer DL, Irwin GS, Miller JA (1983) Anatomy and significance of fixation of the lumbosacral nerve roots in sciatica. Spine 8(6):672

Stephens MM, Evans JH, O'Brien JP (1991) Lumbar intervertebral foramens. An in vitro study of their shape in relation to intervertebral disc pathology. Spine 16(5):525

Suh SW, Shingade VU, Lee SH et al (2005) Origin of lumbar spinal roots and their relationship to intervertebral discs: a cadaver and radiological study. J Bone Joint Surg Br 87(4):518

Vandenabeele F, Creemers J, Lambrichts I (1996) Ultrastructure of the human spinal arachnoid mater and dura mater. J Anat 189 (Pt 2):417

Vital JM, Lavignolle B, Grenier N et al (1983) Anatomy of the lumbar radicular canal. Anat Clin 5(3):141

Wilmink JT, Penning L (1983) Influence of spinal posture on abnormalities demonstrated by lumbar myelography. AJNR Am J Neuroradiol 4(3):656

Wilmink JT, Penning L, Beks JW (1978) Techniques in transfemoral lumbar epidural phlebography. Neuroradiology 15 (5):273

Wiltse LL (2000) Anatomy of the extradural compartments of the lumbar spinal canal. Peridural membrane and circumneural sheath. Radiol Clin North Am 38(6):1177

Wiltse LL, Berger PE, McCulloch JA (1997) A system for reporting the size and location of lesions in the spine. Spine 22(13):1534

Zamani AA, Moriarty T, Hsu L et al (1998) Functional MRI of the lumbar spine in erect position in a superconducting open-configuration MR system: preliminary results. J Magn Reson Imaging 8(6):1329

In 1934, Mixter and Barr reported nineteen cases of rupture of the intervertebral disc with the involvement of the spinal canal, and so ushered in the "dynasty of the disc". Their paper described compression of the spinal cord, cauda equina or exiting nerve root by the herniated material, and included four cases with a cervical localisation, four cases in the thoracic spine, ten in the lumbar spine and lumbosacral transition, and one in the sacral region! The concept of nerve root compression by herniated disc material as a cause of low back and lower extremity pain dominated etiologic and therapeutic thinking on the subject of sciatica for several decades, and its evolution is discussed in more detail in Chap. 1. Although much about the pathogenesis of sciatica and related conditions is still unclear, it is generally accepted that simple mechanical compression of an otherwise healthy nerve root by itself does not cause radicular pain: various humoral and auto-immune inflammatory factors are also at work (see Chaps. 1 and 5).

Non-neoplastic compression of lumbar nerve roots can have many causes: besides disc herniation, various types and degrees of narrowing can occur of the spinal canal, of the lateral recesses, or the foramina. There may be deformation of the spinal canal by anterolisthesis or forward slipping of a vertebral body upon its lower neighbour; encroachment upon the spinal canal by ligamentous hypertrophy or synovial cyst formation, or reduction of space within the spinal canal due to abnormal increase in epidural fat (lipomatosis).

A disc herniation can produce compression of a single nerve root, while severe stenosis of the spinal canal or spinal lipomatosis can involve the entire cauda equina (Fig. 4.1a–c). Combinations of these factors are common, and in fact such combinations occur more frequently than radicular compression due to a single cause. A study in 227 patients operated for lumbar disc syndrome revealed disc herniations in 70 (31%); spondylosis with segmental canal narrowing in 65 (27%); developmental stenosis in 5 (2%); and combined lesions in the majority 87 patients (39%) (Paine and Haung 1972) (Fig. 4.1d).

4.1 Herniated Disc

Classification and terminology of intervertebral disc disease is a source of some confusion and debate. A disc herniation can be defined (Fardon and Milette 2001) as a localised displacement of disc material beyond the margins of the intervertebral disc space. The term generally refers to the displacement of disc tissue through a defect or opening in the annulus fibrosus which is due to degenerative causes. The displaced material may consist of nucleus pulposus, fragmented annular tissue, cartilage, and even apophyseal bone, and for this reason the term "herniated nucleus pulposus" is considered less appropriate, as is "ruptured disc", which may be confused with violent traumatic rupture of the annulus or vertebral end-plate. The term "disc prolapse" is used infrequently.

Diffuse bulging of the disc may occur over 50–100% (180–360°) of the disc circumference, usually over a distance not exceeding 3 mm (Fig. 4.2a, b). Disc bulging is not regarded as a form of herniation but is certainly not always without a clinical significance: a bulging disc may contribute to compression of the nerve root in, for instance, lateral recess narrowing. Also, a coexisting bulge and herniation may be present within one disc.

The term "localised" in the definition of a herniated disc implies that the extent of the displacement in the axial plane takes place over less than 50% (180°) of the circumference of the disc (Fig. 4.2c–e).

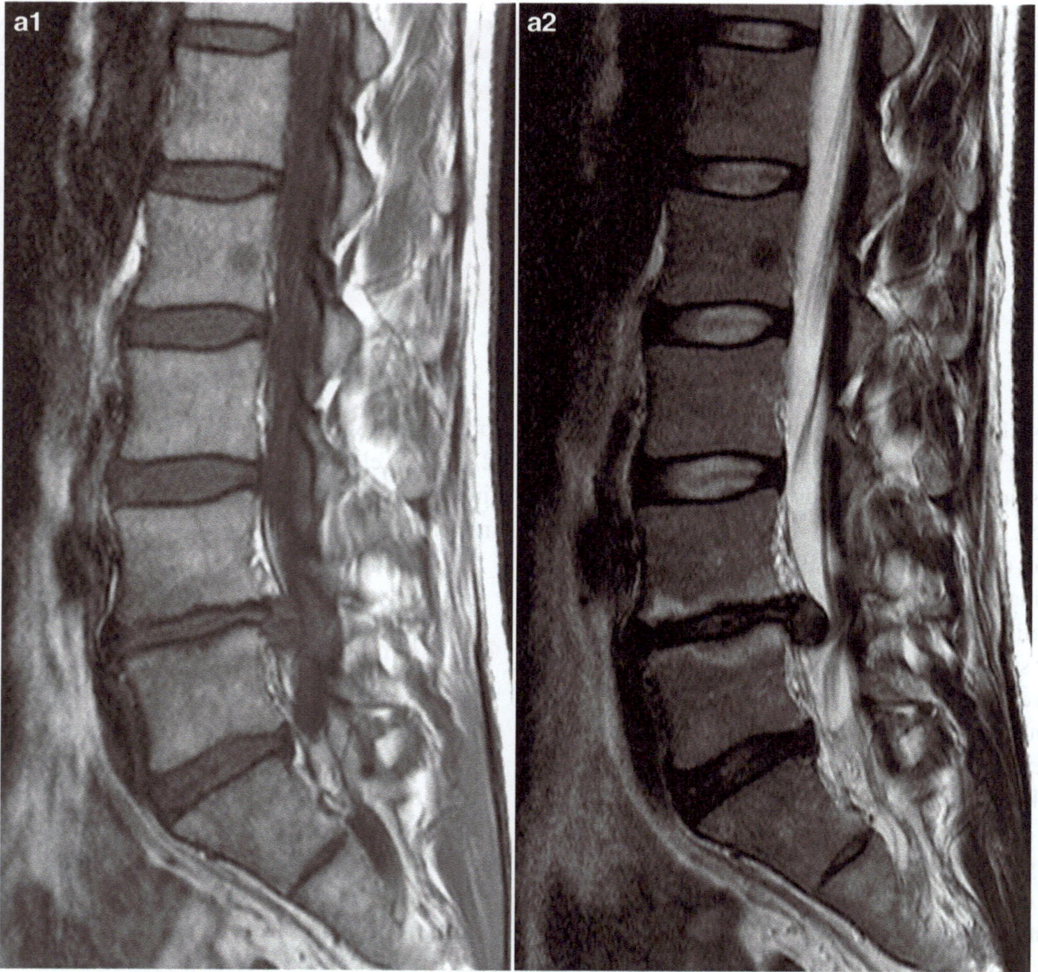

Fig. 4.1 Causes of intraspinal nerve root compression: (**a**) L4–5 disc herniation causing left L5 nerve root compression. *Presentation*: patient, male, 34 years, had left L5 sciatica with L5 sensory loss and foot drop, limitation of straight-leg-raising at left. *MRI*: sagittal T1- (**a1**) and T2-weighted images (**a2**) show disc extrusion migrating caudally. Axial T2-weighted image (**a3**) shows flattening of left ventrolateral angle of dural sac and obliteration of left L5 root image. MR myelogram (**a4**) confirms left L5 root compression, with cut-off of root sleeve filling at left (*arrow*), normal filling of root sleeves at right.

Fig. 4.1 (continued)

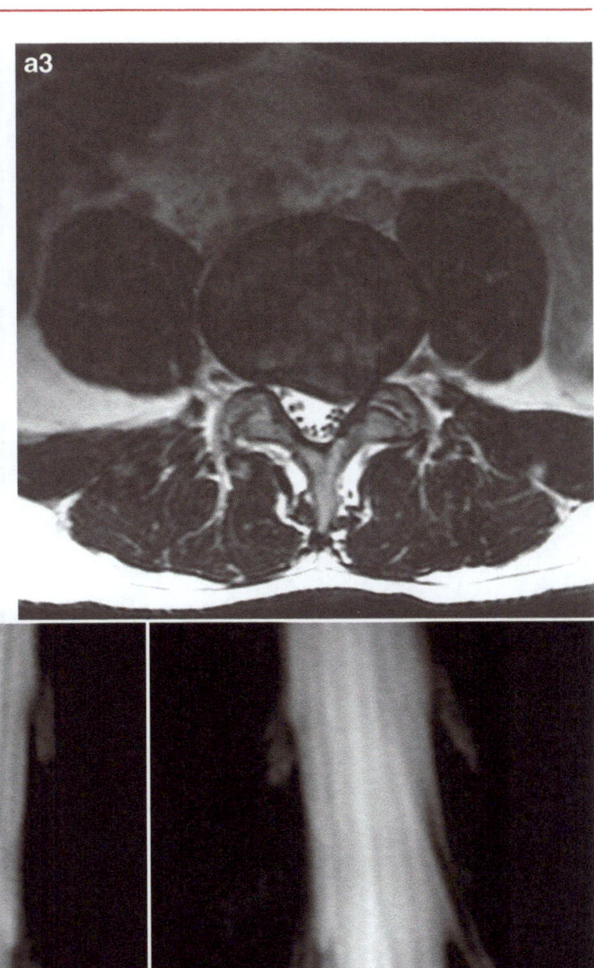

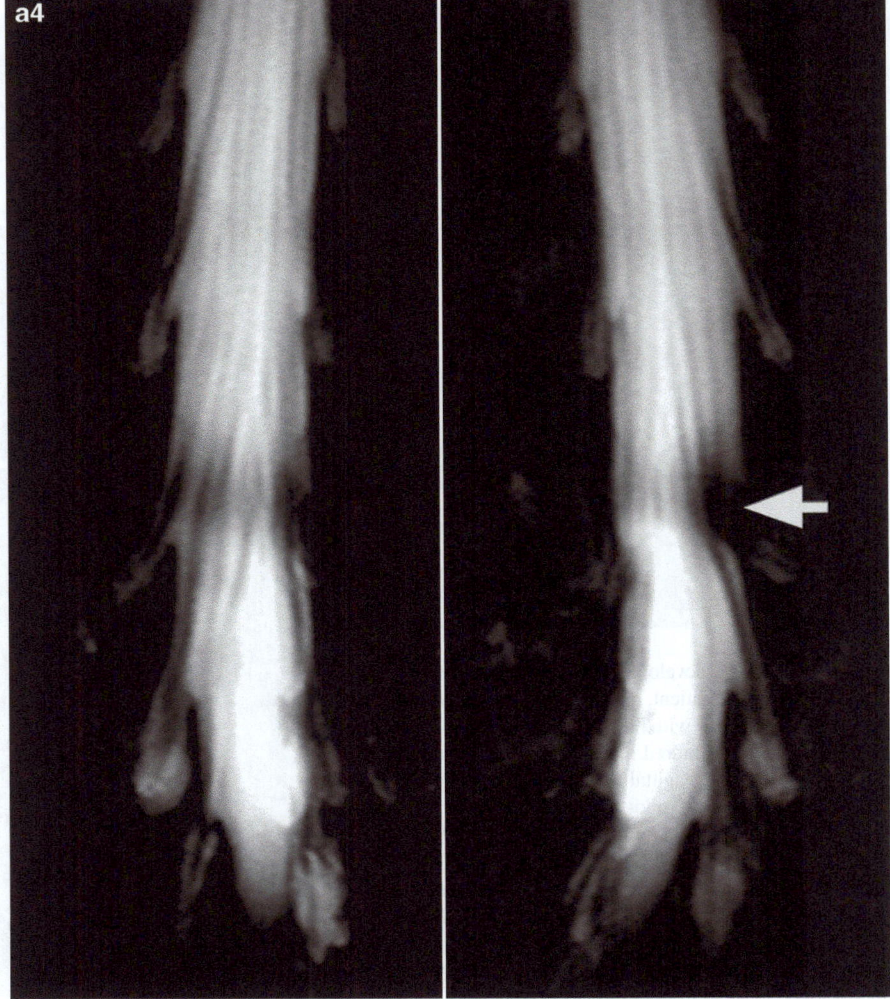

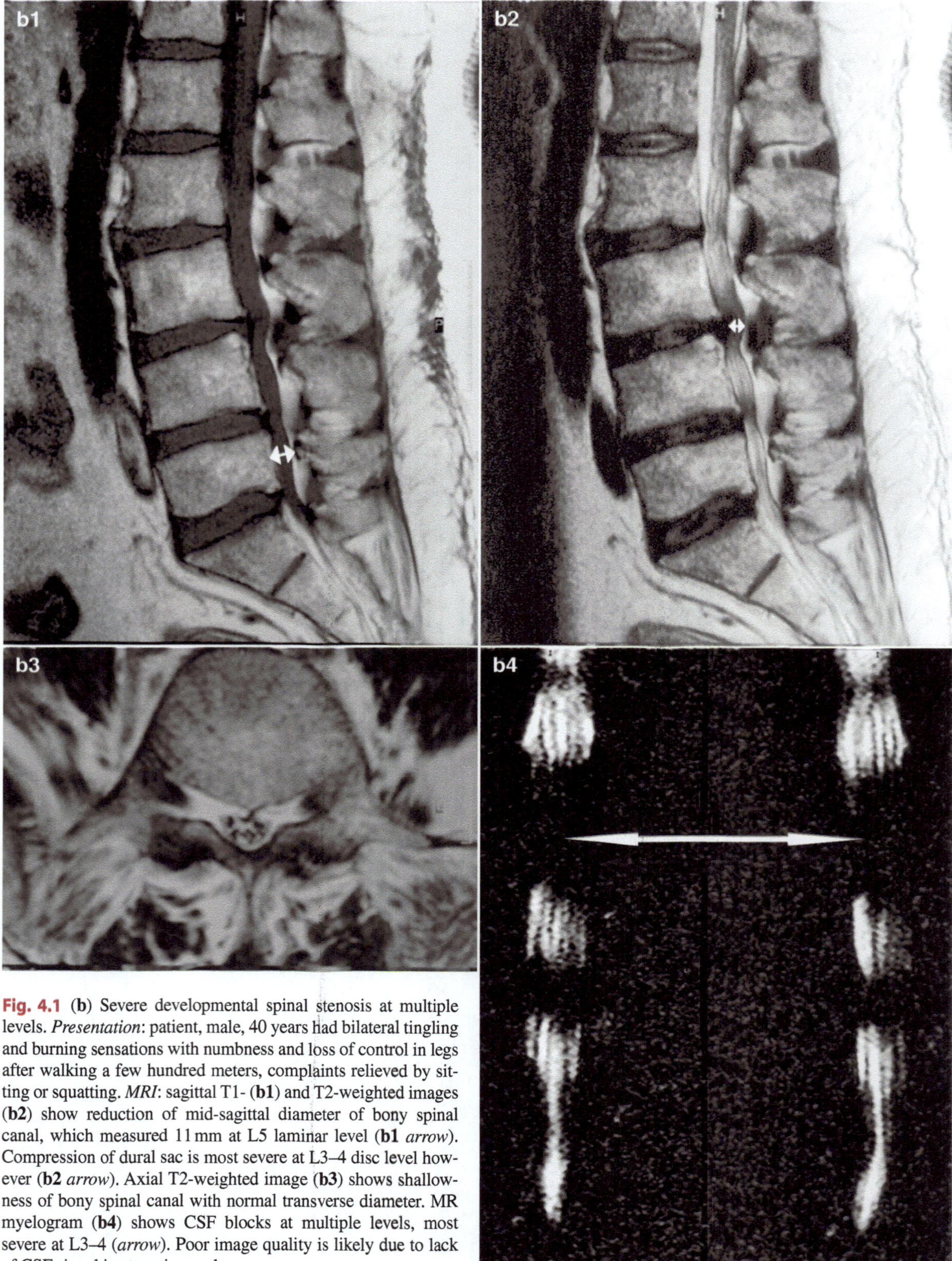

Fig. 4.1 (**b**) Severe developmental spinal stenosis at multiple levels. *Presentation*: patient, male, 40 years had bilateral tingling and burning sensations with numbness and loss of control in legs after walking a few hundred meters, complaints relieved by sitting or squatting. *MRI*: sagittal T1- (**b1**) and T2-weighted images (**b2**) show reduction of mid-sagittal diameter of bony spinal canal, which measured 11 mm at L5 laminar level (**b1** *arrow*). Compression of dural sac is most severe at L3–4 disc level however (**b2** *arrow*). Axial T2-weighted image (**b3**) shows shallowness of bony spinal canal with normal transverse diameter. MR myelogram (**b4**) shows CSF blocks at multiple levels, most severe at L3–4 (*arrow*). Poor image quality is likely due to lack of CSF signal in stenotic canal.

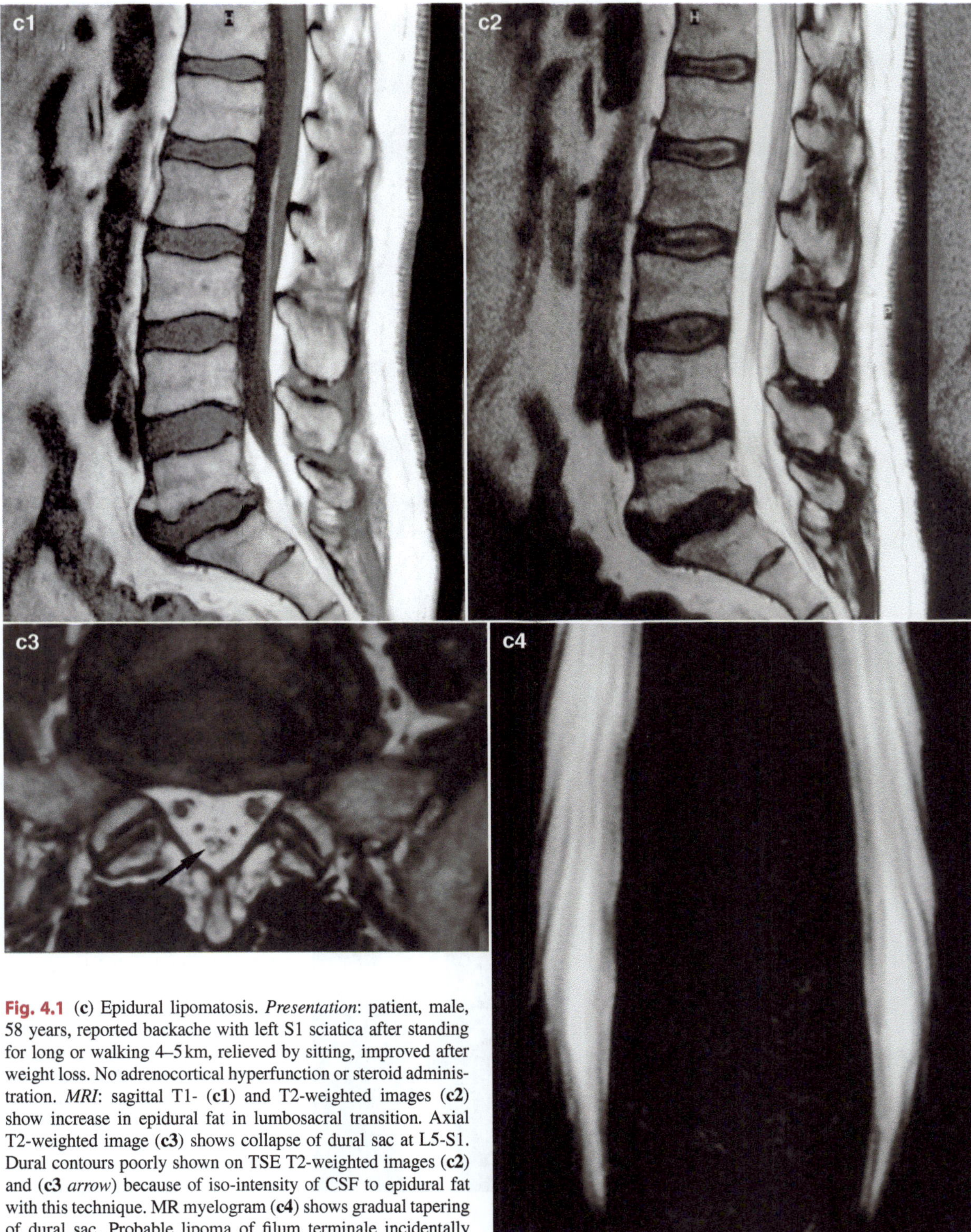

Fig. 4.1 (**c**) Epidural lipomatosis. *Presentation*: patient, male, 58 years, reported backache with left S1 sciatica after standing for long or walking 4–5 km, relieved by sitting, improved after weight loss. No adrenocortical hyperfunction or steroid administration. *MRI*: sagittal T1- (**c1**) and T2-weighted images (**c2**) show increase in epidural fat in lumbosacral transition. Axial T2-weighted image (**c3**) shows collapse of dural sac at L5-S1. Dural contours poorly shown on TSE T2-weighted images (**c2**) and (**c3** *arrow*) because of iso-intensity of CSF to epidural fat with this technique. MR myelogram (**c4**) shows gradual tapering of dural sac. Probable lipoma of filum terminale incidentally noted in (**c1**).

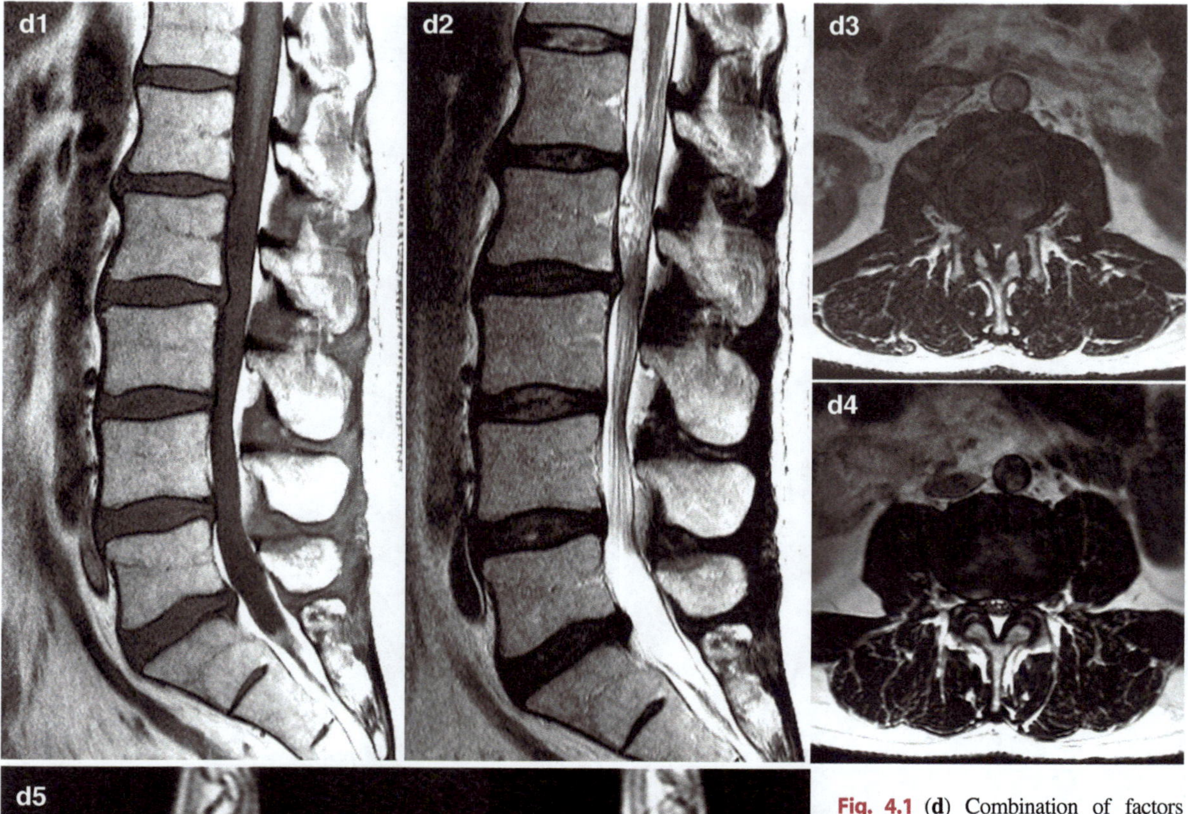

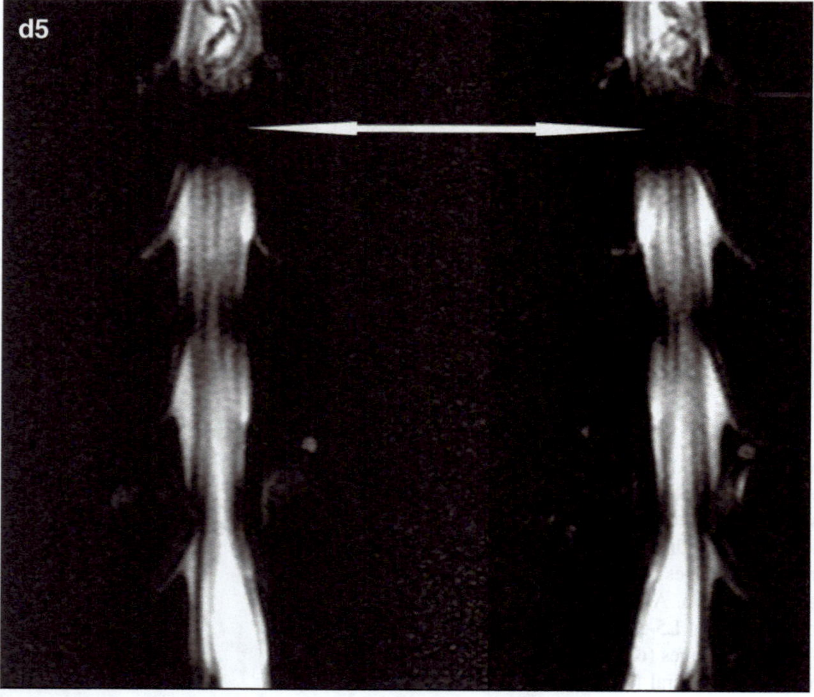

Fig. 4.1 (**d**) Combination of factors causing narrowing of spinal canal. *Presentation*: patient, male, 49 years suffered from long-standing backache irradiating to lateral and dorsal aspect of both thighs, increasing upon standing erect and walking (action radius 30 m), relieved by sitting or squatting. *MRI*: sagittal T1- (**d1**) and T2-weighted images (**d2**) show relative developmental stenosis with mid-sagittal bony diameter 12 mm at L4 and 13 mm at L3. Furthermore, some increase in retrodural fat, especially at L3–4 level, causing dorsal dural indentation. Bulging disc at L2–3, causing almost complete CSF block (**d2**). Axial T2-weighted images show collapsed dural sac at L2–3 (**d3**) and increase of retrodural fat at L3–4 (**d4**). MR myelogram (**d5**) confirms CSF block at L2–3 (*arrow*) and displacement with some swelling of nerve roots at L3–4 and L4–5. Serpentine, intradural, so-called redundant roots seen above level of CSF block in (**d2**) and (**d5**)

Localised displacements or herniations can be further sub-categorised as broad-based (25–50% of the disc circumference) (Fig. 4.2c) or focal (less than 25% of the disc circumference) (Fig. 4.2d, e).

Herniated discs can also be categorised according to the shape of the displaced material.

Protruded discs are herniated discs in which the displaced material is still contained or covered by the

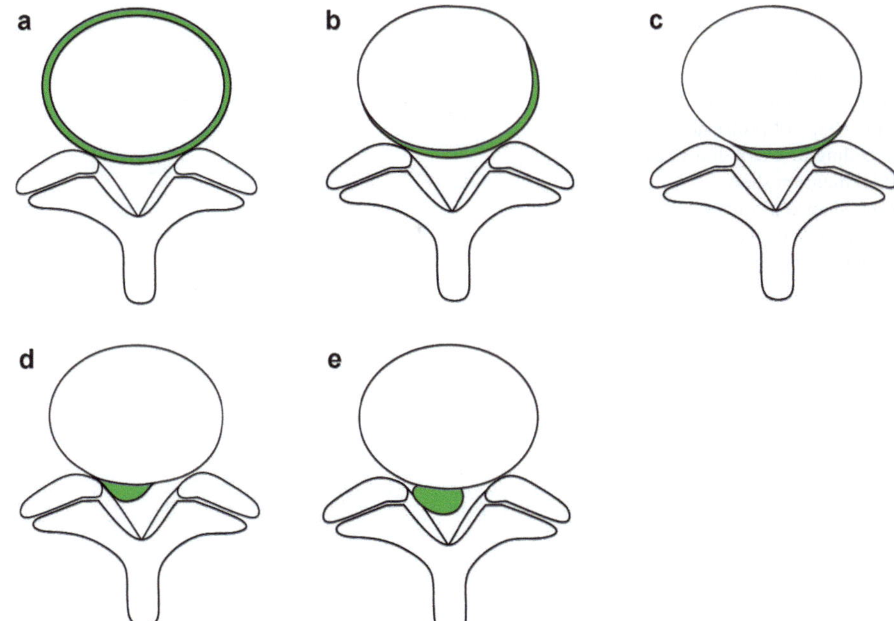

Fig. 4.2 Classification of disc displacements in the axial plane. (**a**) Concentric bulging disc: displacement over entire circumference of disc. (**b**) Diffusely bulging disc: displacement over >50% of disc circumference. (**c**) Broad-based herniation: displacement over 25–50% of disc circumference. (**d, e**) Focal herniations: displacement over <25% of disc circumference. These can be subdivided into two types: *dome-shaped or triangular* (**d**). This is seen in protrusions and also in most extrusions; *mushroom-shaped* (**e**). This is regarded as a classic sign of extrusion, but rarely seen in the axial plane

outer annulus. This is inferred from a dome-like or triangular appearance of the protrusion in the sagittal and axial imaging planes, and in which the base of the herniation is always the broadest part (Fig. 4.2d). In the sagittal plane, the height at the base of a protrusion is never greater than the distance between the endplates of the parent disc (Figs. 4.3a, 4.3b).

Extruded discs are herniated discs in which displaced material is no longer contained by the outer annulus fibrosus and has passed outside the confines of the disc. Extrusions are generally larger than protrusions (Fries et al. 1982). Sometimes, the annular rupture itself is visible, usually best on proton density-weighted MR images (see Chap. 2).

In the sagittal imaging plane, extrusion of disc material through a ruptured annulus may be deduced from the fact that the height of the herniation outside the disc is greater than the distance between the end-plates of the parent disc (Fig. 4.3c).

The appearance of the extrusion in the sagittal plane may be mushroom-shaped (Fig. 4.3d) instead of dome-shaped as in protrusions. Alternatively, an extrusion may be dome-shaped but broad-based, with the base extending above or below the end-plates bordering the disc of origin (see Fig. 4.3c).

Using the features described above, the difference between protrusions and extrusions can usually be well-established on sagittal images (MRI or reformatted CT sections), although classification may sometimes be difficult in marginal cases. In the axial imaging plane, the aspect of an extrusion, like that of a protrusion, is almost always dome-shaped or triangular, and a mushroom-shape such as presented in Fig. 4.2e is seen only in exceptional cases. The distinction between protrusion and extrusion is, therefore, more difficult to make in the axial plane, although the presence of disc material in axial sections above or below the disc level can be taken as evidence of annular disruption (Figs. 4.3c and 4.3e).

The question can be asked why it is so important to distinguish between disc protrusion and extrusion. The importance of the distinction lies in the fact that extruded discs are considered to be more frequently symptomatic compared with protruded discs, which can be seen quite often in asymptomatic individuals. An MRI study showed disc protrusions to be present in 27% and extrusions present in only 1% of 98 asyptomatic volunteers. In 27 people with back pain, protrusions were seen in 54% and extrusions in 27% (Jensen et al. 1994).

In practice, there are frequent exceptions to this rule. Figure 4.3b illustrates a case of protrusion with clear, clinical and MR myelographic signs of L5 root involvement, and Fig. 4.3d shows a case of a sizeable L5-S1 extrusion, which is apparently not causing radicular involvement.

Fig. 4.3 Protrusions and extrusions. (**a**) L4–5 protrusion shown in *green*. Sagittal diagram shows dome-shape of protrusion not exceeding levels of end-plates. Axial diagram shows dome-shaped protrusion limited to disc level, not visible in adjacent axial sections.

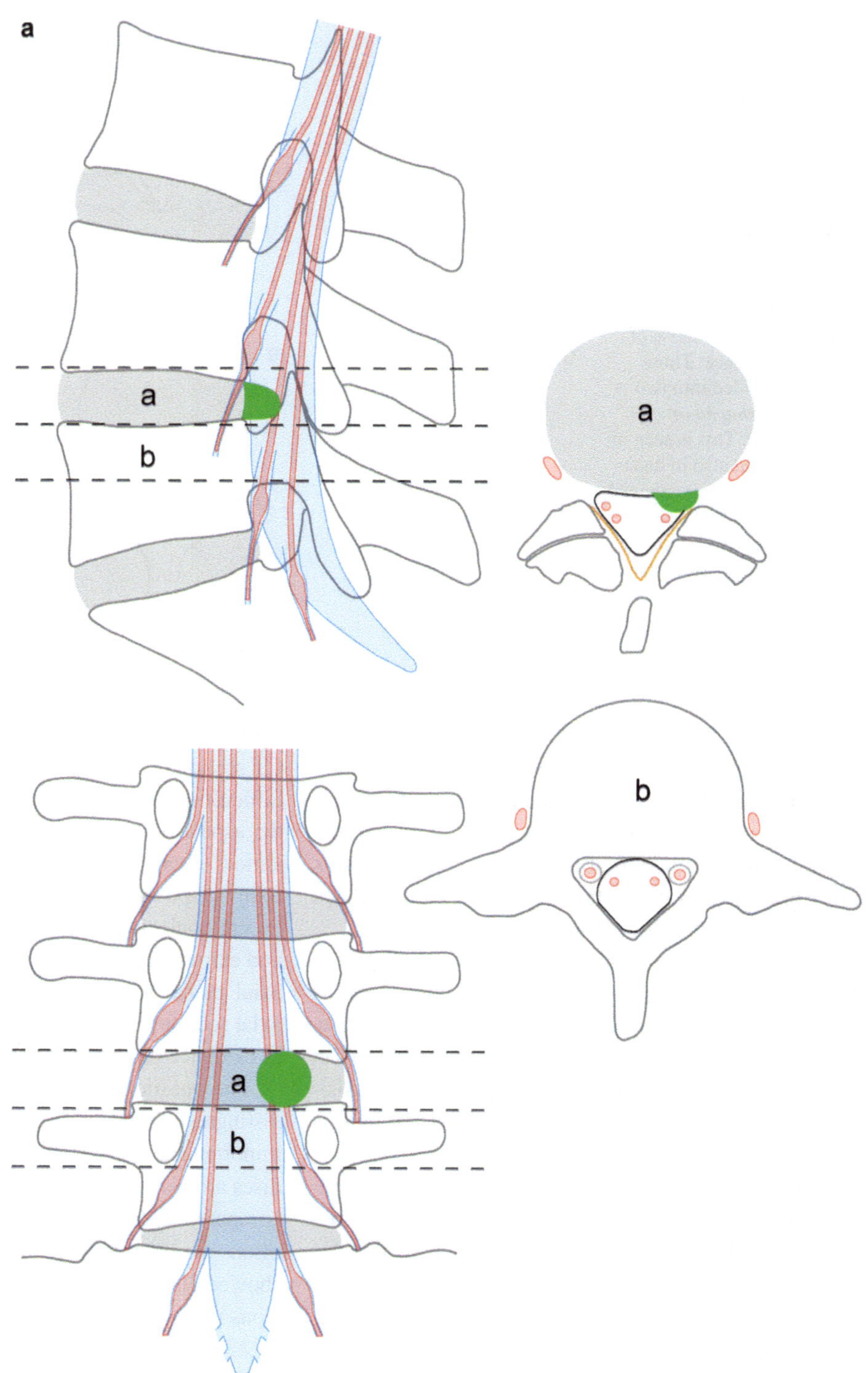

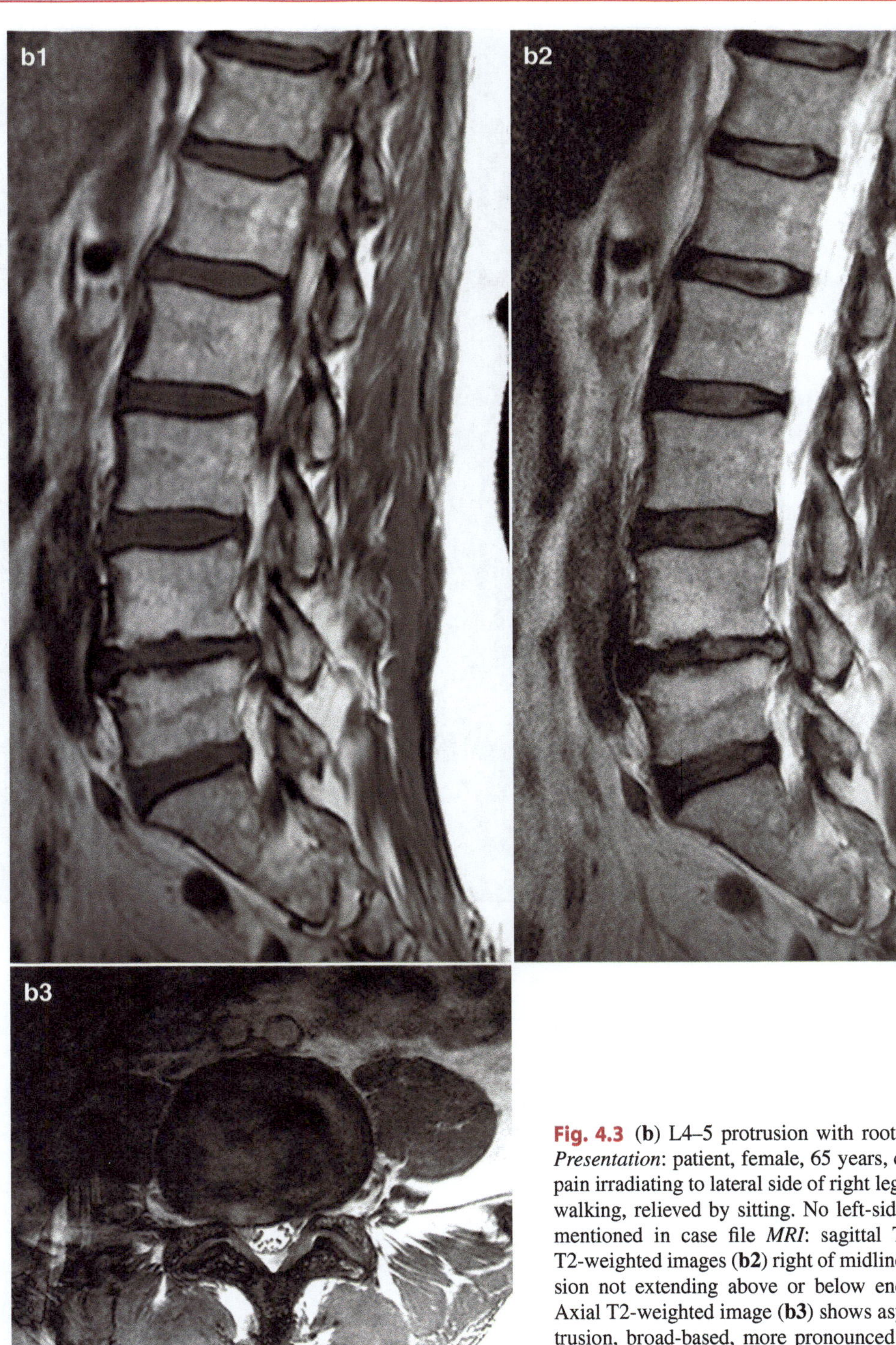

Fig. 4.3 (**b**) L4–5 protrusion with root compression. *Presentation*: patient, female, 65 years, complained of pain irradiating to lateral side of right leg, provoked by walking, relieved by sitting. No left-sided complaints mentioned in case file *MRI*: sagittal T1- (**b1**), and T2-weighted images (**b2**) right of midline show protrusion not extending above or below end-plate levels. Axial T2-weighted image (**b3**) shows asymmetric protrusion, broad-based, more pronounced at right, with flattening of ventrolateral corner of dural sac and obliteration of adjacent fat at right. MR myelographic images (**b4**) show non-filling of both L5 root sleeves, with swelling of right L5 root and adjacent dural indentation (*arrow*).

Fig. 4.3 (continued)

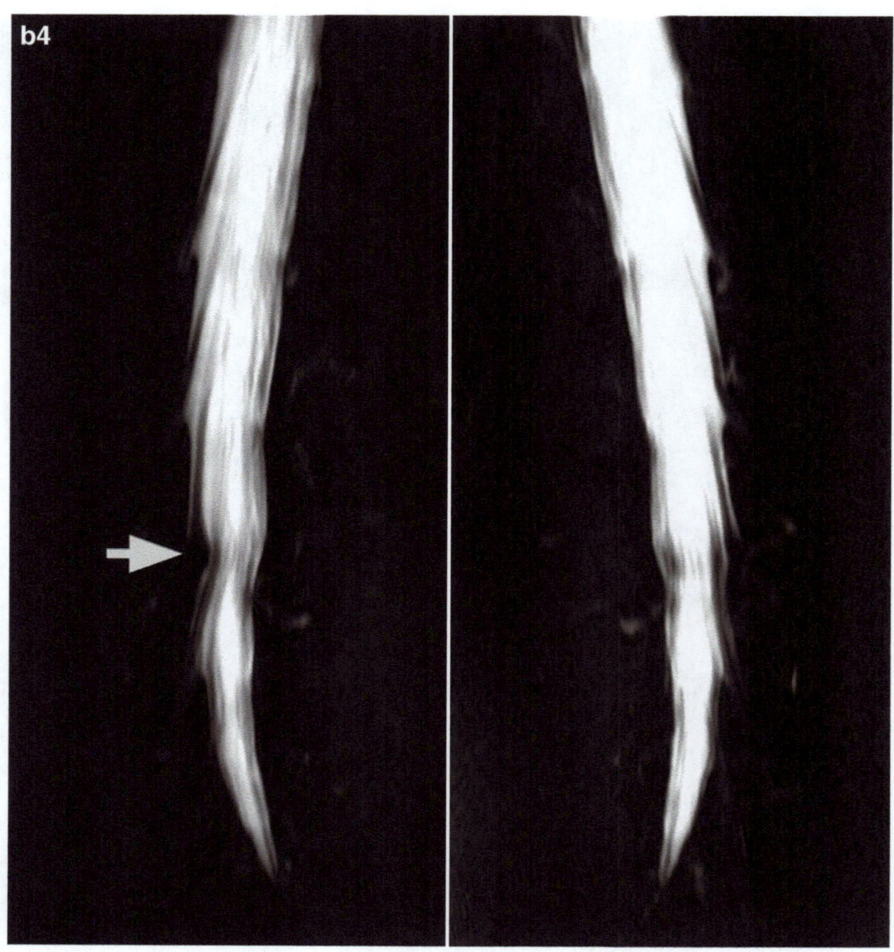

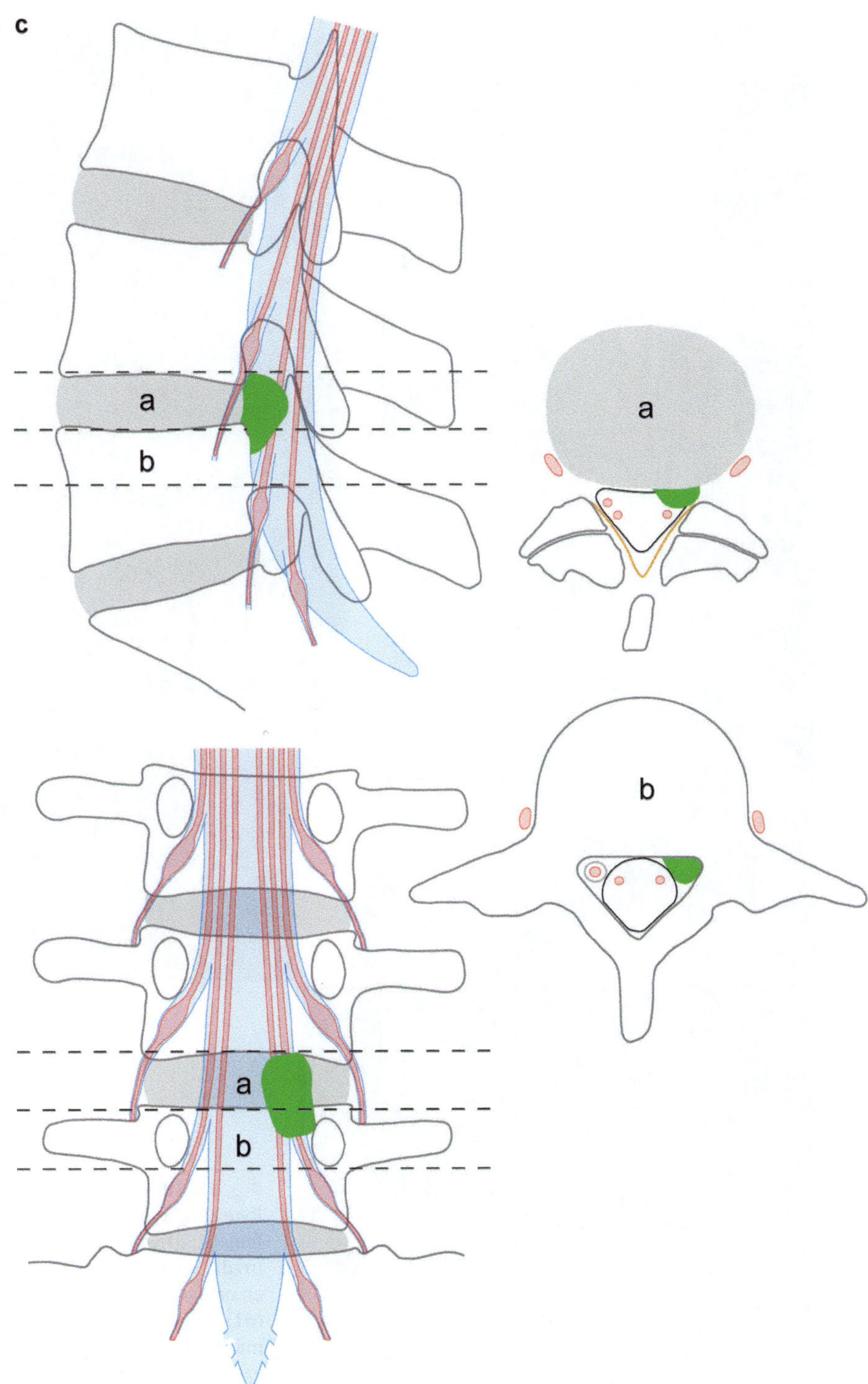

Fig. 4.3 (**c**) L4–5 extrusion shown in *green*. Sagittal diagram shows caudal migration past end-plate indicating annular rupture. Axial images show dome-shaped extrusion at disc level (**a**) extruded material visible below disc level in section through bony lateral recess (**b**).

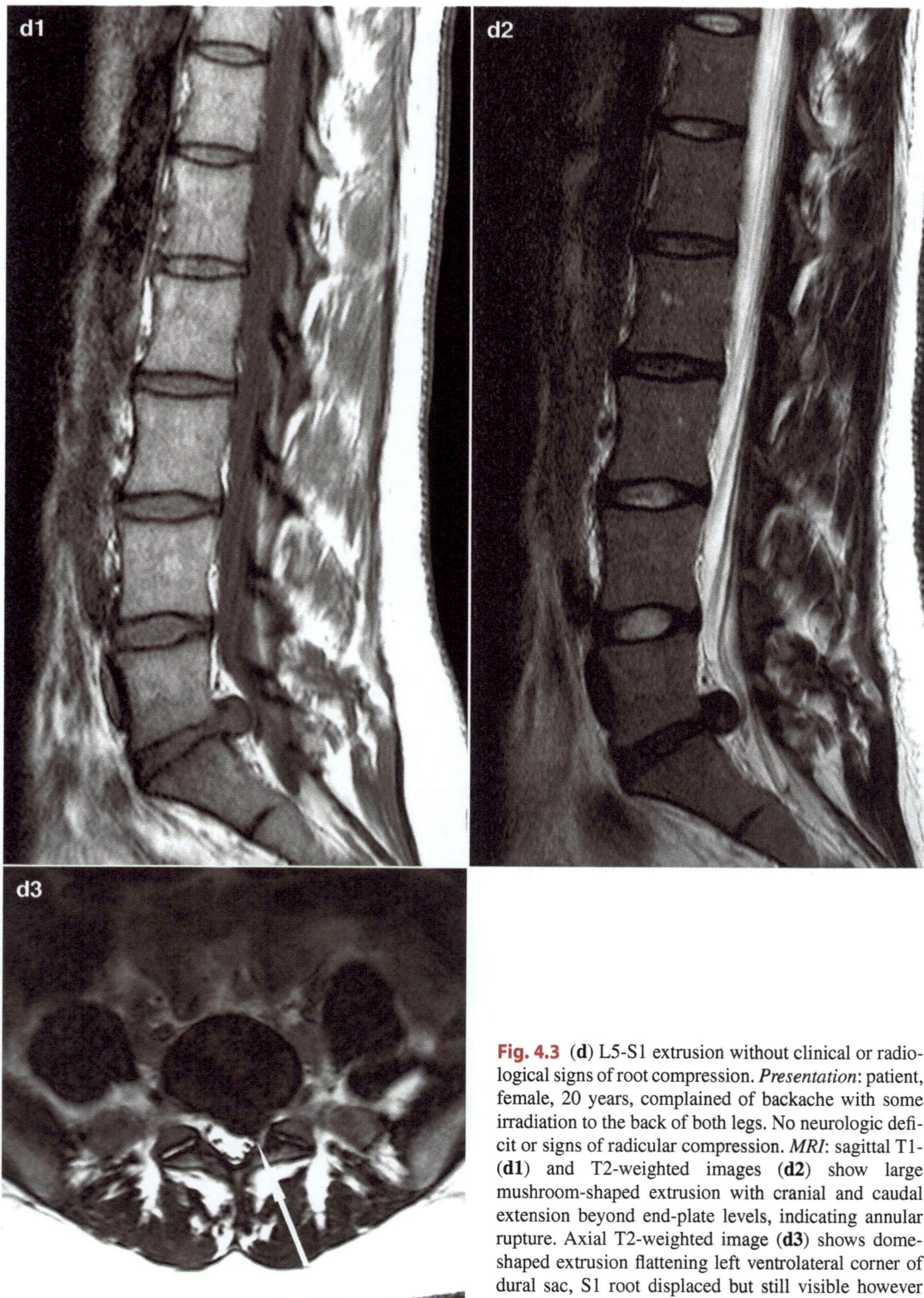

Fig. 4.3 (**d**) L5-S1 extrusion without clinical or radiological signs of root compression. *Presentation*: patient, female, 20 years, complained of backache with some irradiation to the back of both legs. No neurologic deficit or signs of radicular compression. *MRI*: sagittal T1- (**d1**) and T2-weighted images (**d2**) show large mushroom-shaped extrusion with cranial and caudal extension beyond end-plate levels, indicating annular rupture. Axial T2-weighted image (**d3**) shows dome-shaped extrusion flattening left ventrolateral corner of dural sac, S1 root displaced but still visible however (*arrow*). MR myelograms (**d4**) show some thinning of CSF around S1 root (*arrow*), but root still visible.

Fig. 4.3 (continued)

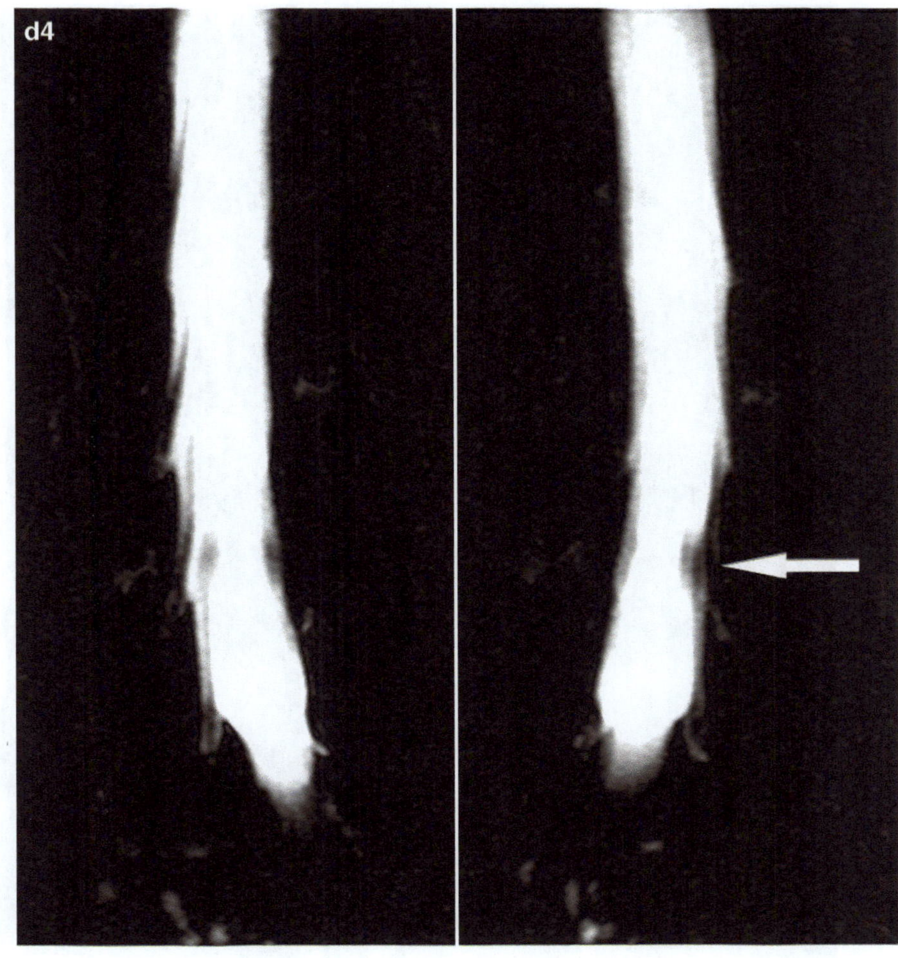

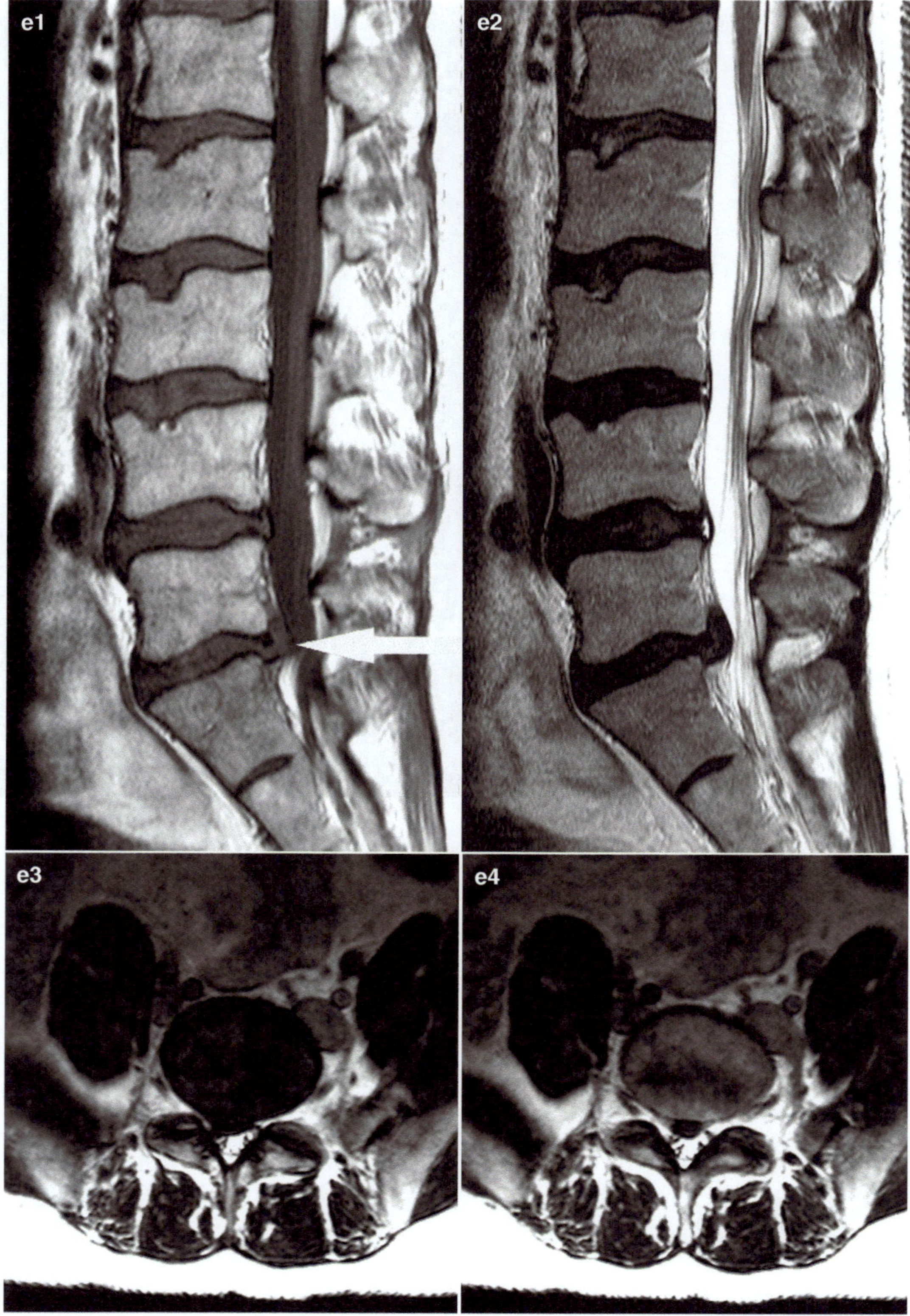

Fig. 4.3 (continued)

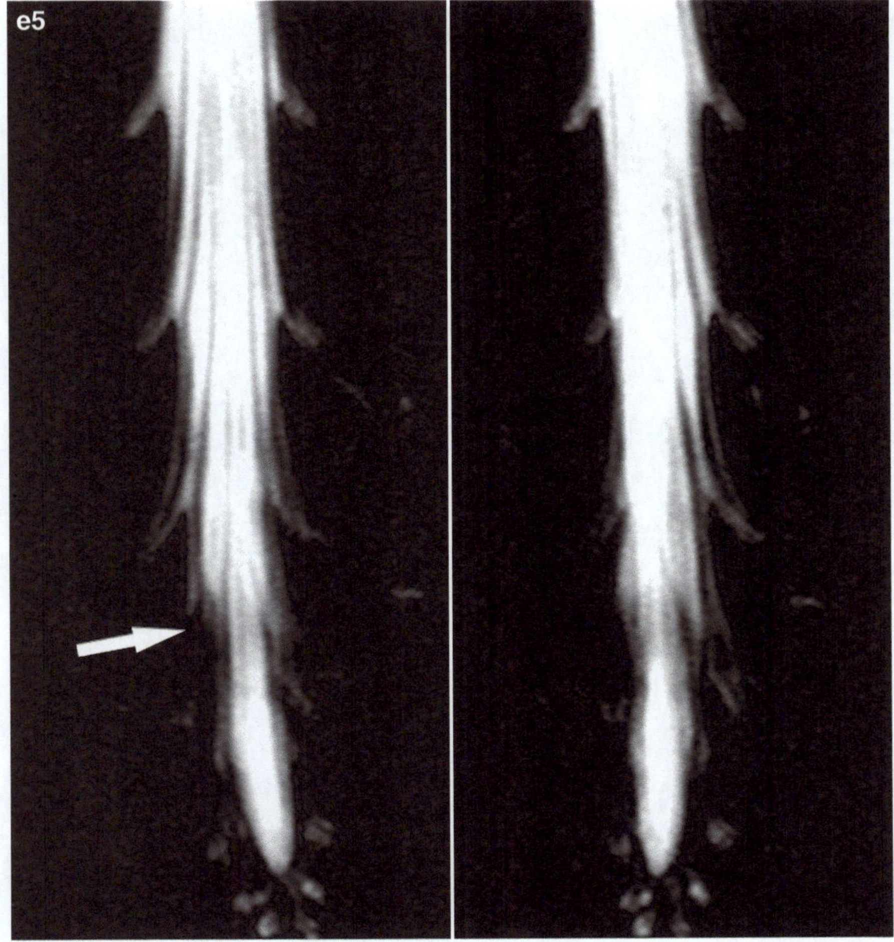

Fig. 4.3 (**e**) L5-S1 extrusion with S1 root compression. *Presentation*: patient, male, 34 years, had long-standing backache, recently irradiating to right buttock, later to posterior thigh and calf, with tingling in sole of foot. No motor or sensory deficit, slightly depressed left Achilles tendon reflex, no limitation of straight-leg-raising. *MRI*: sagittal T1- (**e1**) and T2-weighted images (**e2**) show annular rupture (*arrow*), also cranial migration of disc material above endplate level L5 also indicating rupture. In T2-weighted axial image (**e3**) extrusion is not evident from dome-shape, but annular rupture is indicated by presence of extruded disc material in section above disc level (**e4**). MR myelogram (**e5**) confirms right S1 nerve root compression (*arrow*). Annular fissures incidentally noted in (**e2**) at L3–4 and L4–5.

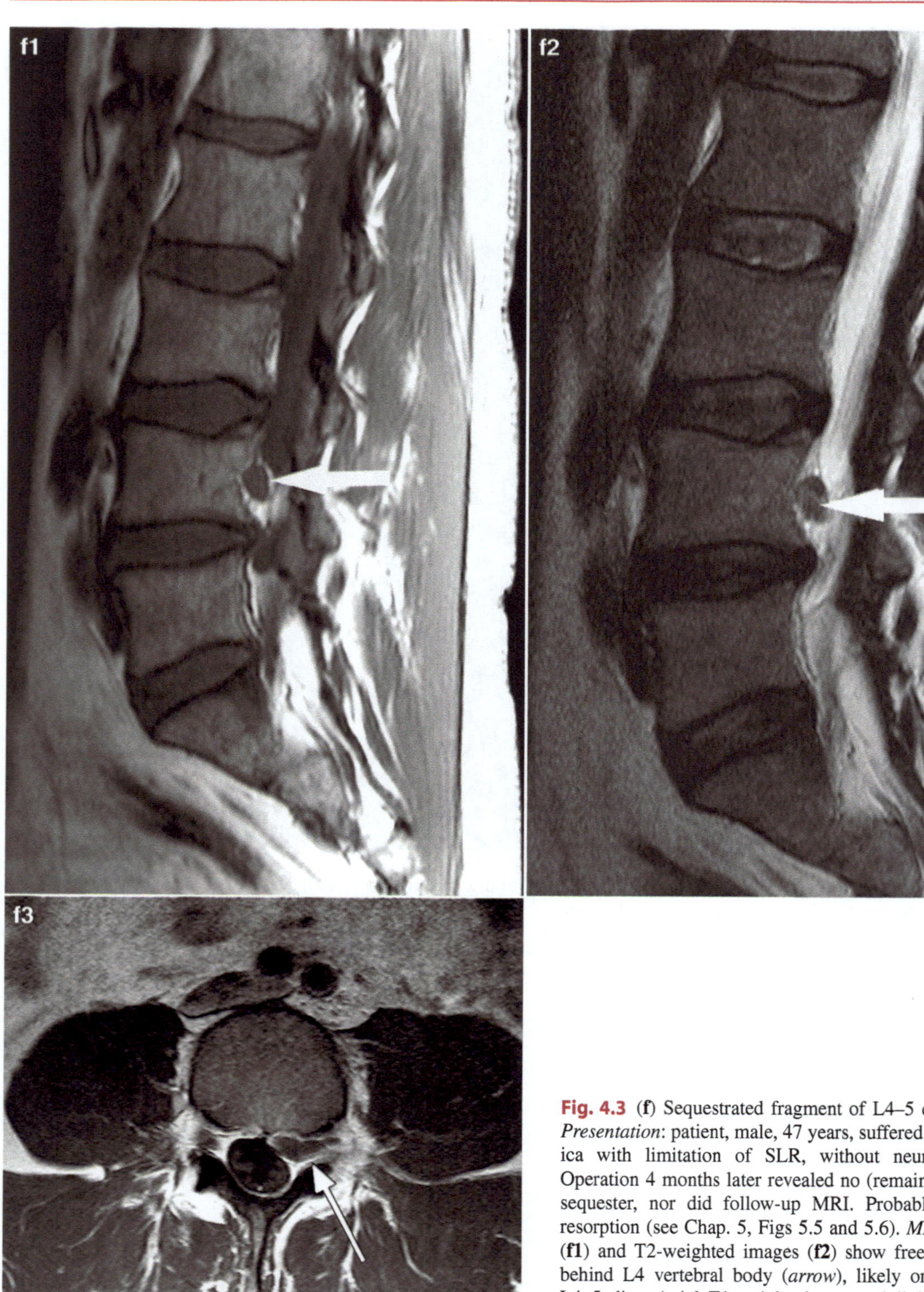

Fig. 4.3 (**f**) Sequestrated fragment of L4–5 disc herniation. *Presentation*: patient, male, 47 years, suffered from left sciatica with limitation of SLR, without neurologic deficit. Operation 4 months later revealed no (remaining) signs of a sequester, nor did follow-up MRI. Probable spontaneous resorption (see Chap. 5, Figs 5.5 and 5.6). *MRI*: sagittal T1- (**f1**) and T2-weighted images (**f2**) show free disc fragment behind L4 vertebral body (*arrow*), likely originating from L4–5 disc. Axial T1-weighted post-gadolinium image (**f3**) shows rim enhancement of sequester which is compressing left L4 dorsal root ganglion in L4–5 foramen (*arrow*). Note normal MR myelogram (**f4**): the intraforaminal root segment cannot be imaged by this technique, and there is no significant compression of the dural sac.

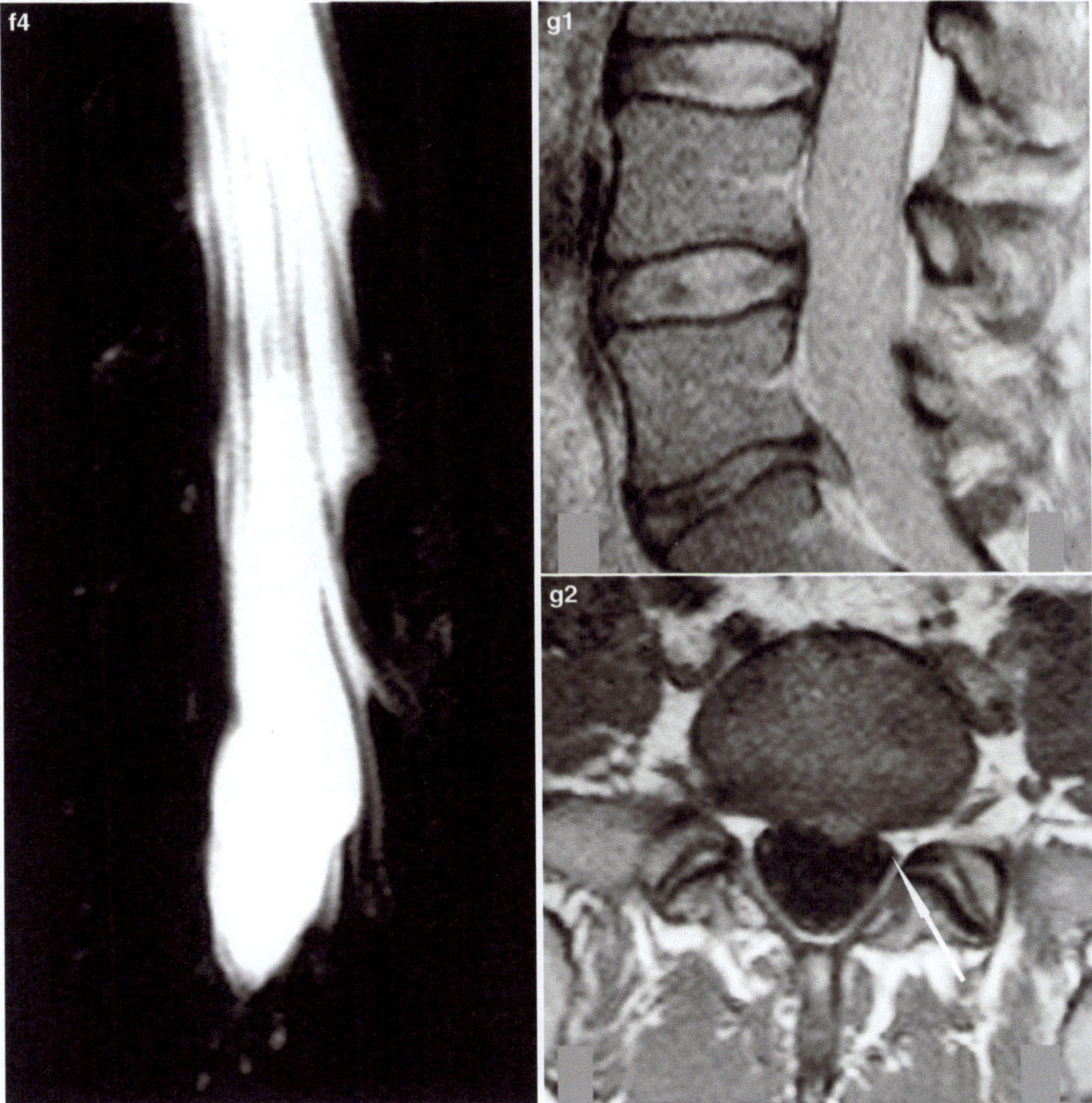

Fig. 4.3 (**g**) Small L5-S1 extrusion in roomy spinal canal, no root compression. *Presentation*: patient with right sciatica. No further clinical data available. *MRI*: sagittal proton density-weighted image (**g1**) shows annular rupture L5-S1 and caudal migration of disc material. Axial T1-weighted image (**g2**) shows relatively small size of extrusion in wide L5-S1 canal. Small left paracentral dural impression, S1 root (*arrow*) faintly seen with T1 weighting, not compressed. MR myelogram (**g3**) confirms no root involvement.

Fig. 4.3 (continued)

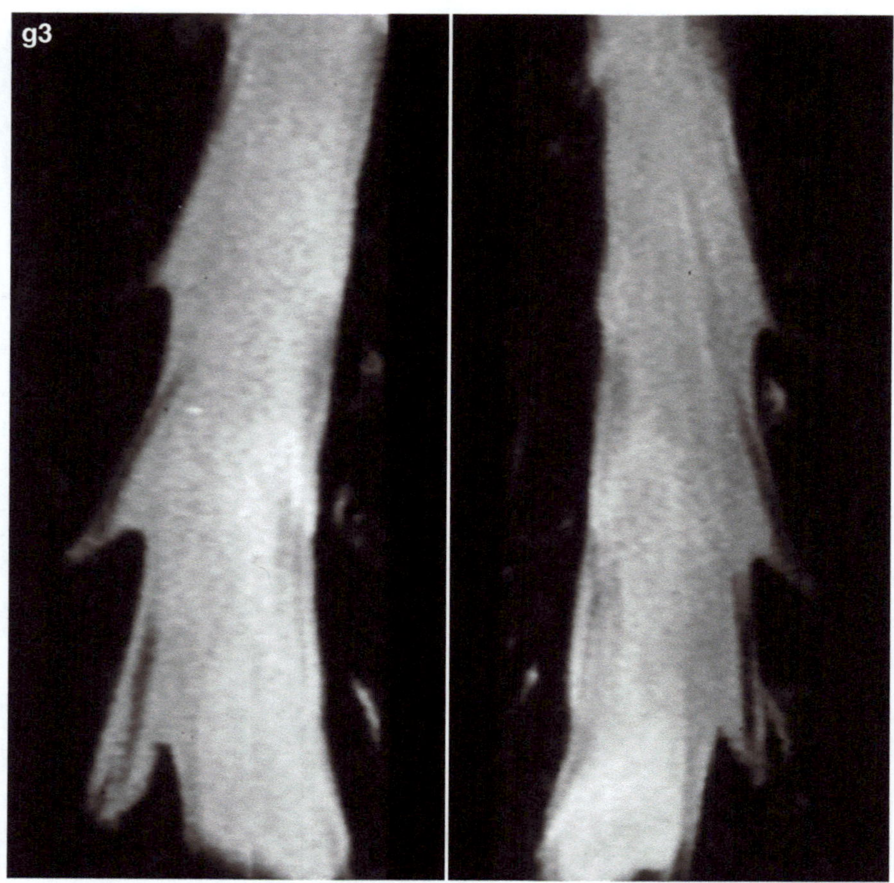

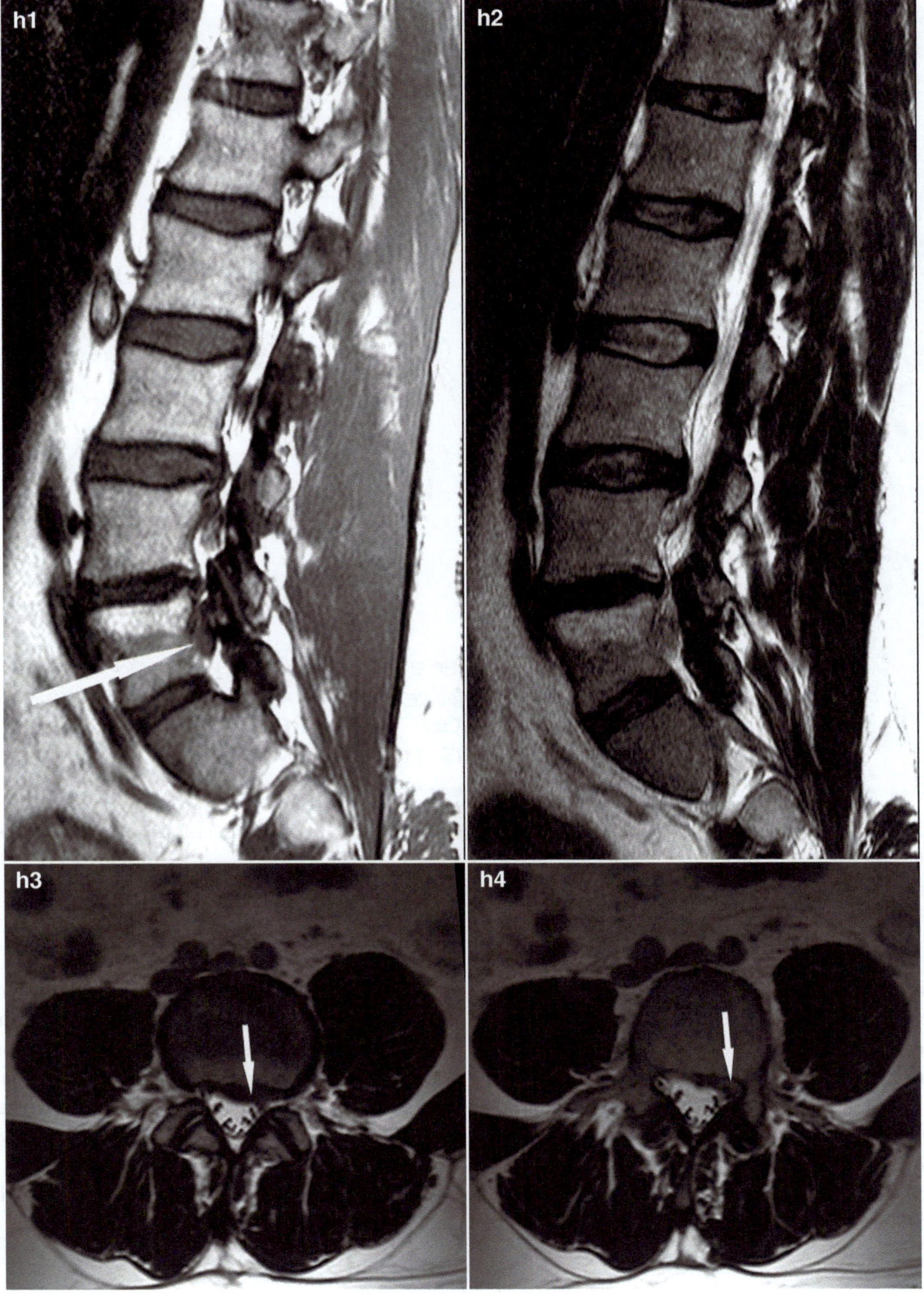

Fig. 4.3 (**h**) Small L4–5 extrusion migrating to lateral recess and compressing L5 root. *Presentation*: patient, male, 42 years, complained of left sciatica, later motor and sensory deficit, with spontaneous remission. *MRI*: sagittal T1 (**h1**) and T2-weighted images (**h2**) left of midline show small amount of extruded L4–5 disc material migrated below L4–5 disc (*arrow*). Axial T2-weighted images show shallow dome-shaped protrusion causing no root compression at disc level (**h3**, *arrow*), migrated material filling in left lateral recess and compressing L5 nerve root (**h4**, *arrow*). Coronal MR myelogram (**h5**) confirms left nerve root compression (*arrow*).

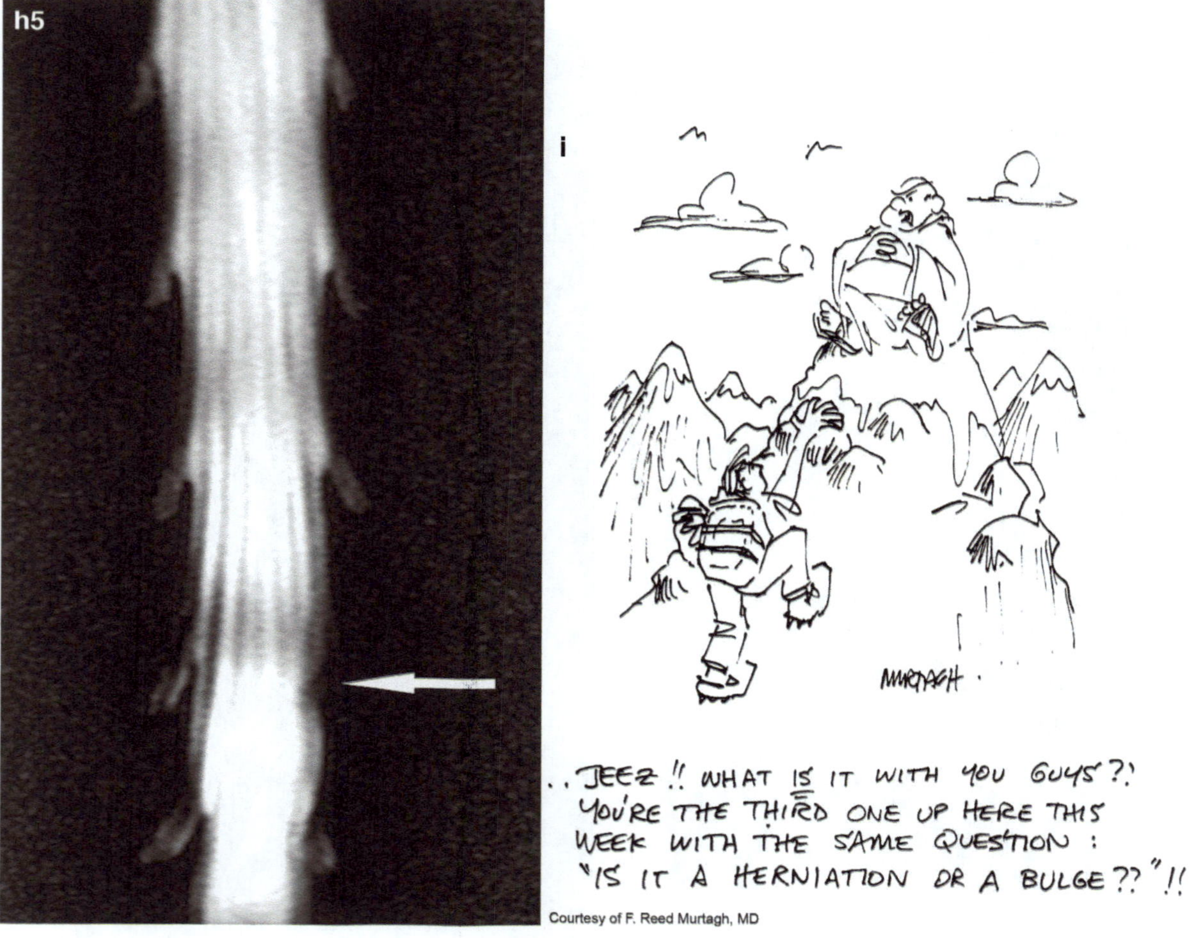

Courtesy of F. Reed Murtagh, MD

Fig. 4.3 (i) A herniation can cause symptoms of nerve root compression, but so can a bulge! (see Figs 4.9; 4.13). Cartoon reprinted by permission Radiology

Within the category of extrusions, a further distinction can be made between transligamentous and sub-ligamentous extrusions. In the first case, the extrusion has passed through the annulus fibrosus and also the posterior longitudinal ligament (PLL), and lies in, or in contact with, the epidural space behind this ligament. In the second case, the extrusion has passed through the annulus fibrosus into the anterior epidural space under the PLL but is still covered by this ligament (Herzog 1996).

Some authors regard sub-ligamentous extrusions as "contained" by the PLL, and therefore as protrusions.

Migration of extruded disc material away from its site of passage through the annulus fibrosus can take place in any direction; cranially into the space behind the adjacent vertebral body or foramen; caudally into the lateral recess or further. Sequestration is the term used to indicate complete separation of migrated disc material from the parent disc (Fig. 4.3f).

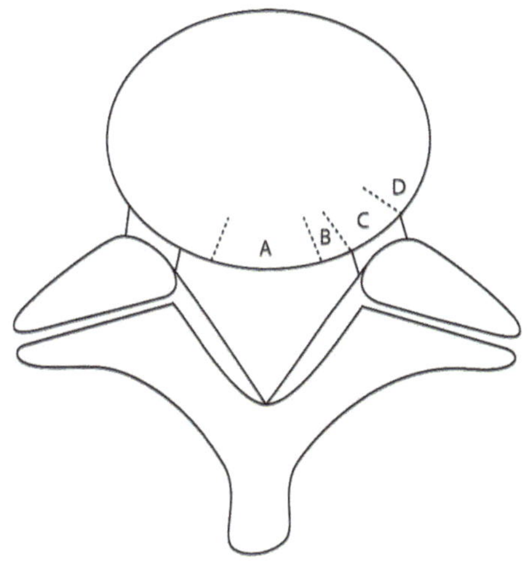

Fig. 4.4 Localisations of herniated disc in axial plane. (**a**) Central/paracentral zone (**b**) Sub-articular zone (lateral recess)(**c**) Foraminal zone (**d**) Extraforaminal zone

recess. In these cases the strict distinction between, for instance, a disc bulge and a disc herniation then becomes academic, and the discussion should not focus on this issue (Fig. 4.3i).

For the localisation of a disc herniation in the axial plane, a classification is given (Fig. 4.4) which divides the posterior disc contour into a number of regions or zones: central and paracentral; sub-articular (lateral recess); foraminal and extraforaminal.

It is useful to mention here that disc protrusions located in the lower half of the intervertebral foramen do not usually compress the dorsal root ganglion: first the annulus fibrosus must be breached so that the extruded material can migrate upward from the disc level to the infrapedicular (upper foraminal) level to compress the ganglion against the pedicle (Fig. 4.5).

Transligamentous extrusions are freer to migrate and are also more accessible to the action of macrophages, and are, therefore, considered to have a more favourable spontaneous natural history (see Chap. 5). On the other hand, the various percutaneous techniques for decompressing a disc herniation are not considered to be effective in extrusions.

In exceptional cases, the extrusion may penetrate into the dural sac, when this structure is fixed in place by adhesions to the PLL or the disc surface.

It is important to bear in mind that the aspect of the disc herniation (protruded or extruded) and its size are not the only factors determining the risk of nerve root compression. Figure 4.3g shows that a small extrusion located in the central region of a roomy canal need not cause nerve root compression. The same may even occur with a larger extrusion in a roomy canal (see Fig. 4.3d). Even a small extrusion which migrates to the confined space of the lateral recess, however, is likely to compress the traversing nerve root (Fig. 4.3h).

Even a non-herniated bulging disc can compress a root which is immobilised in a shallow canal or lateral

4.1.1 Why Are Disc Herniations Diagnosed So Rarely in the Upper Lumbar Region?

The great majority of symptomatic disc herniations are found at the lower two lumbar interspaces, 50% at L4–5 and 47% at L5-S1. The remaining 3% are found at higher lumbar levels (Spangfort 1972). This does not necessarily mean that disc herniations in the upper lumbar region occur so rarely; but it could be that they cause symptoms less frequently and are therefore not diagnosed so often in this location. A study comparing patients with upper lumbar (L1–2 and L2–3) herniations to those with herniations located at L3–4, L4–5 and L5-S1, showed that the first group appeared to form a separate category: these patients had frequently undergone previous disc surgery, and surgical outcomes were significantly poorer (Sanderson et al. 2004). This could quite possibly be due to a relatively greater prevalence of asymptomatic disc herniations in the upper lumbar region, and thus explain the poor results of operation.

Fig. 4.5 Foraminal disc herniations. (**a**) *L4–5 foraminal disc protrusion in green*. Note that an unmigrated protrusion is located at the disc level b and below the L4 dorsal root ganglion (located in level a), and does not compress this dorsal root ganglion. The protrusion also lies medial to the extraforaminal L4 root segment, and lateral to the intradural L5 root, and in this location does not cause nerve root compression.

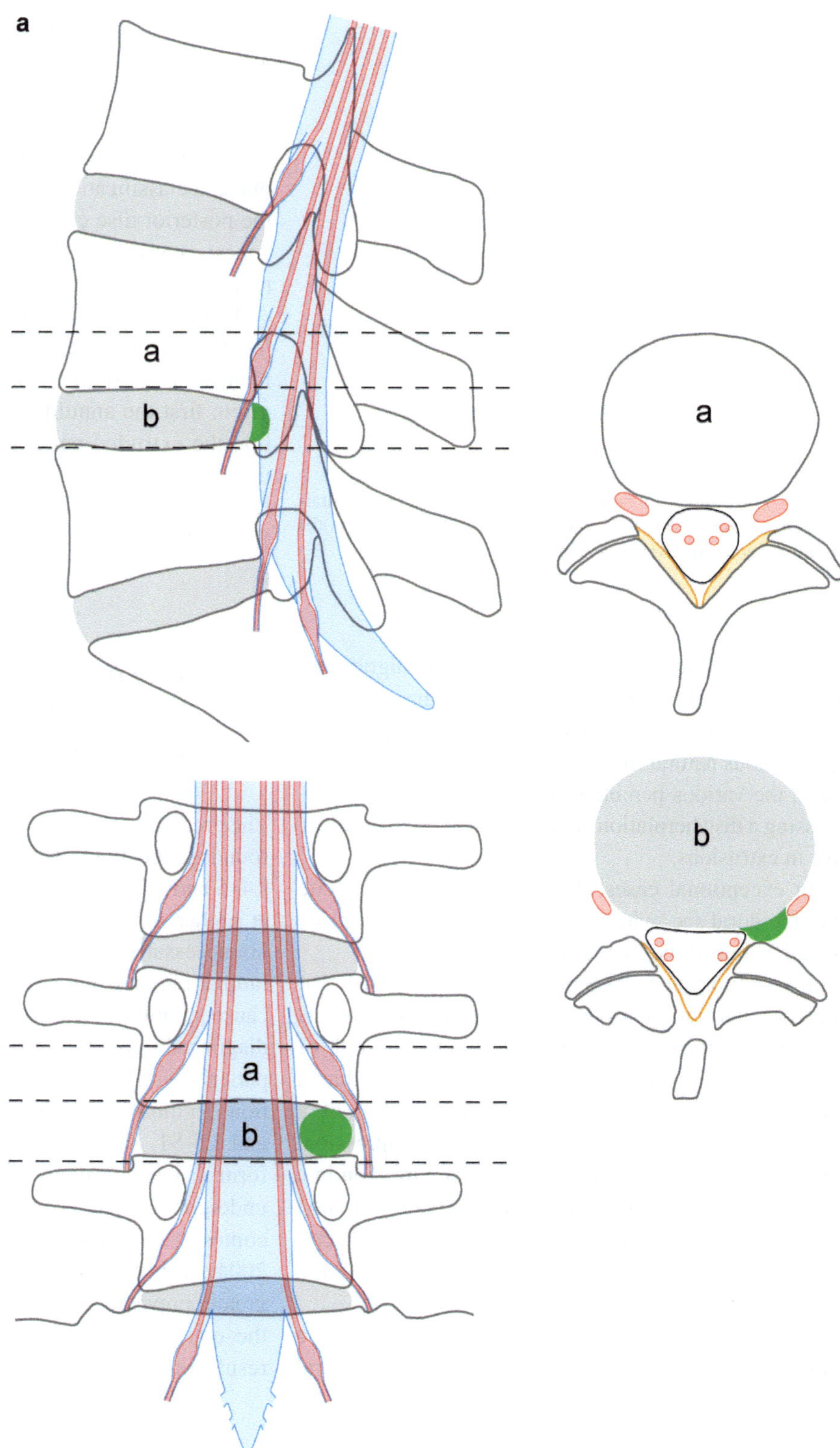

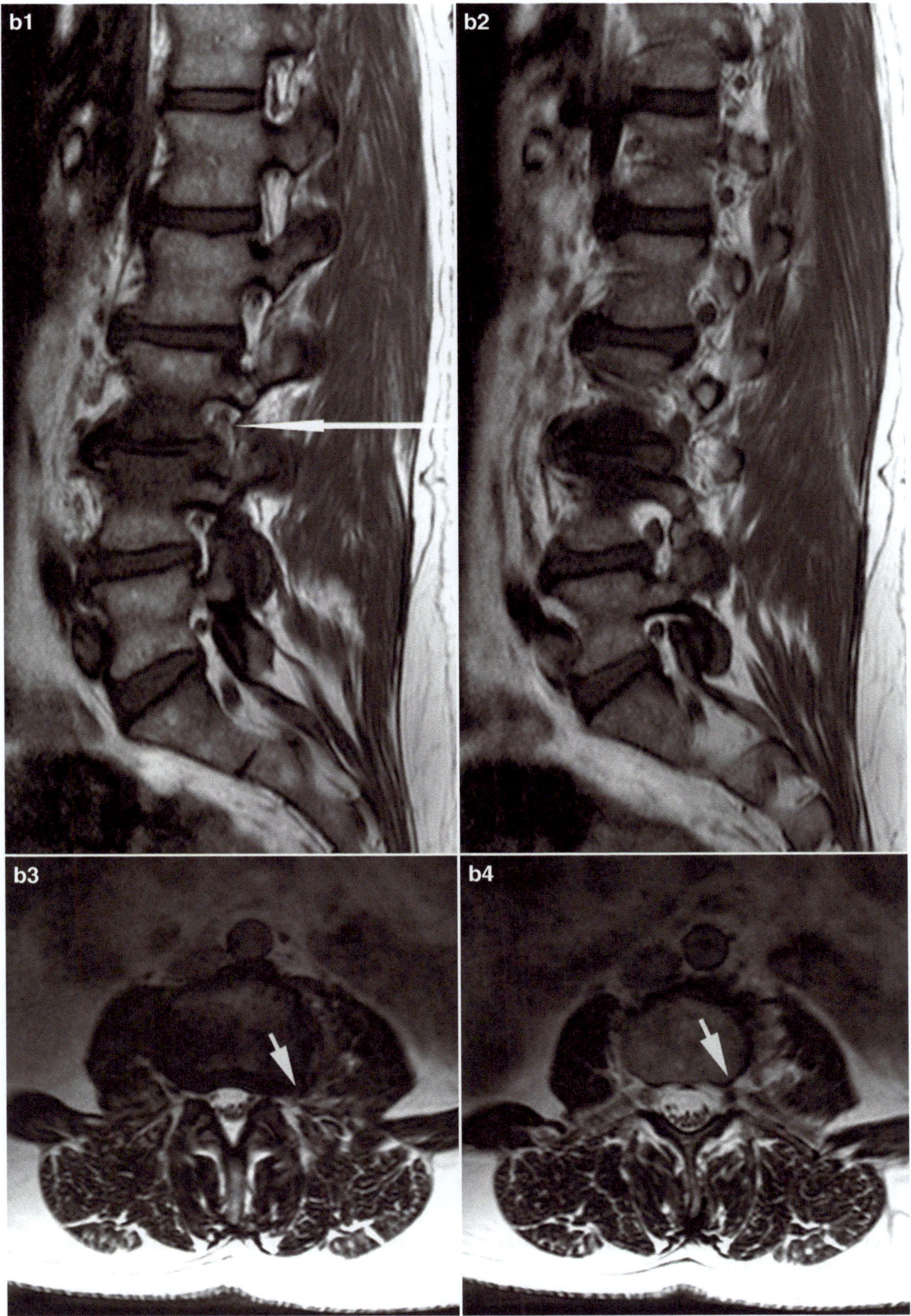

Fig. 4.5 (**b**) Left L3–4 foraminal protrusion. *Presentation*: patient, female 46 years, reported pain in lower back and left leg, had undergone several operations for left retropatellar chondropathy, no neurologic deficit. Spontaneous resolution. *MRI*: sagittal T1-weighted images (**b1** and **b2**) show L3–4 herniation extending into lower half of left foramen, but not compressing dorsal root ganglion which is still surrounded by fat (*arrow*). Axial T2-weighted images confirm some protrusion into lower part of foramen (**b3,** *arrow*), but uncompressed dorsal root ganglion in upper part (**b4,** *arrow*). Cause of pain not clear.

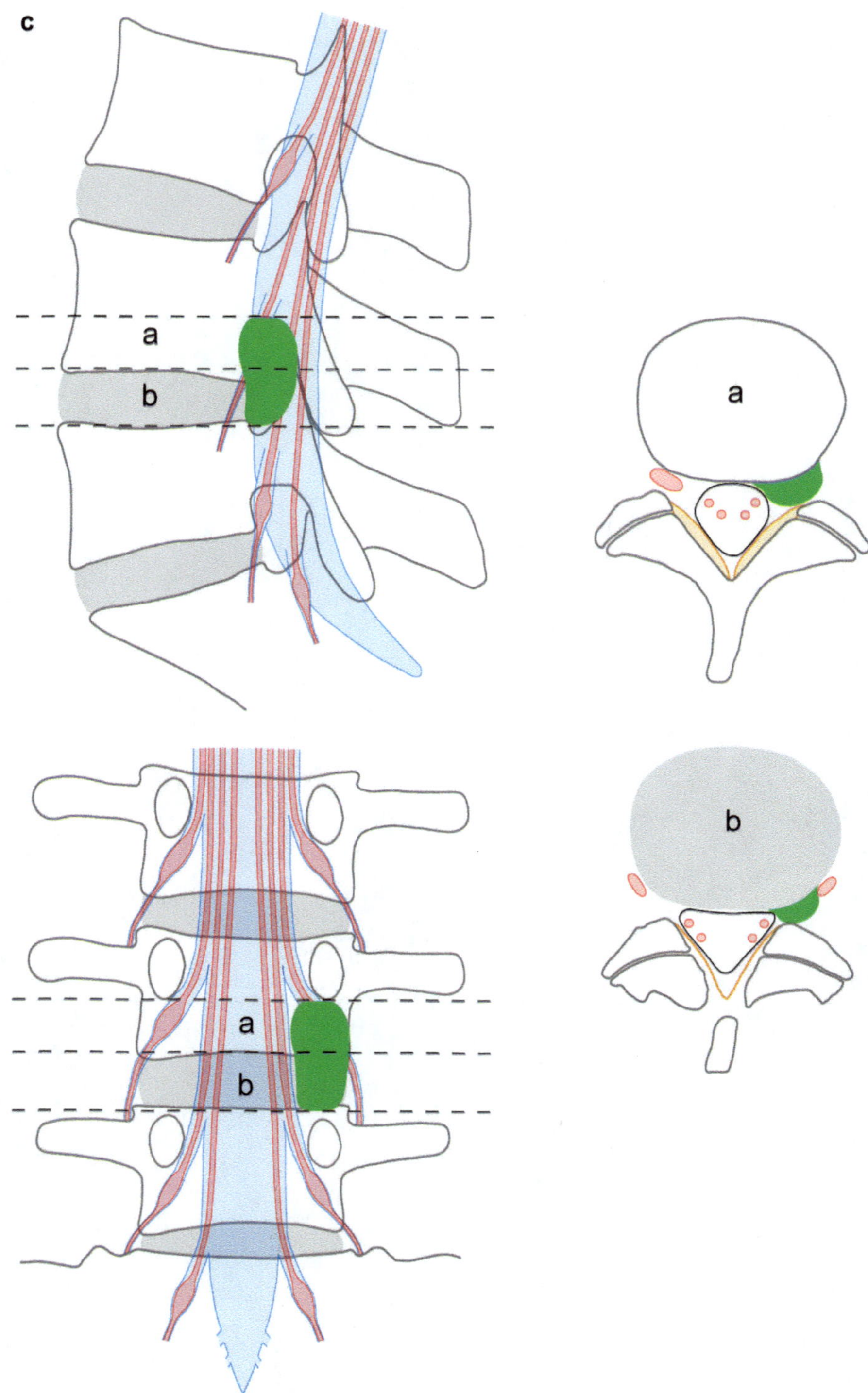

Fig. 4.5 (**c**) L4–5 foraminal disc extrusion in *green*. The extrusion has migrated cranially to level a, and is now compressing the foraminal segment of the L4 root.

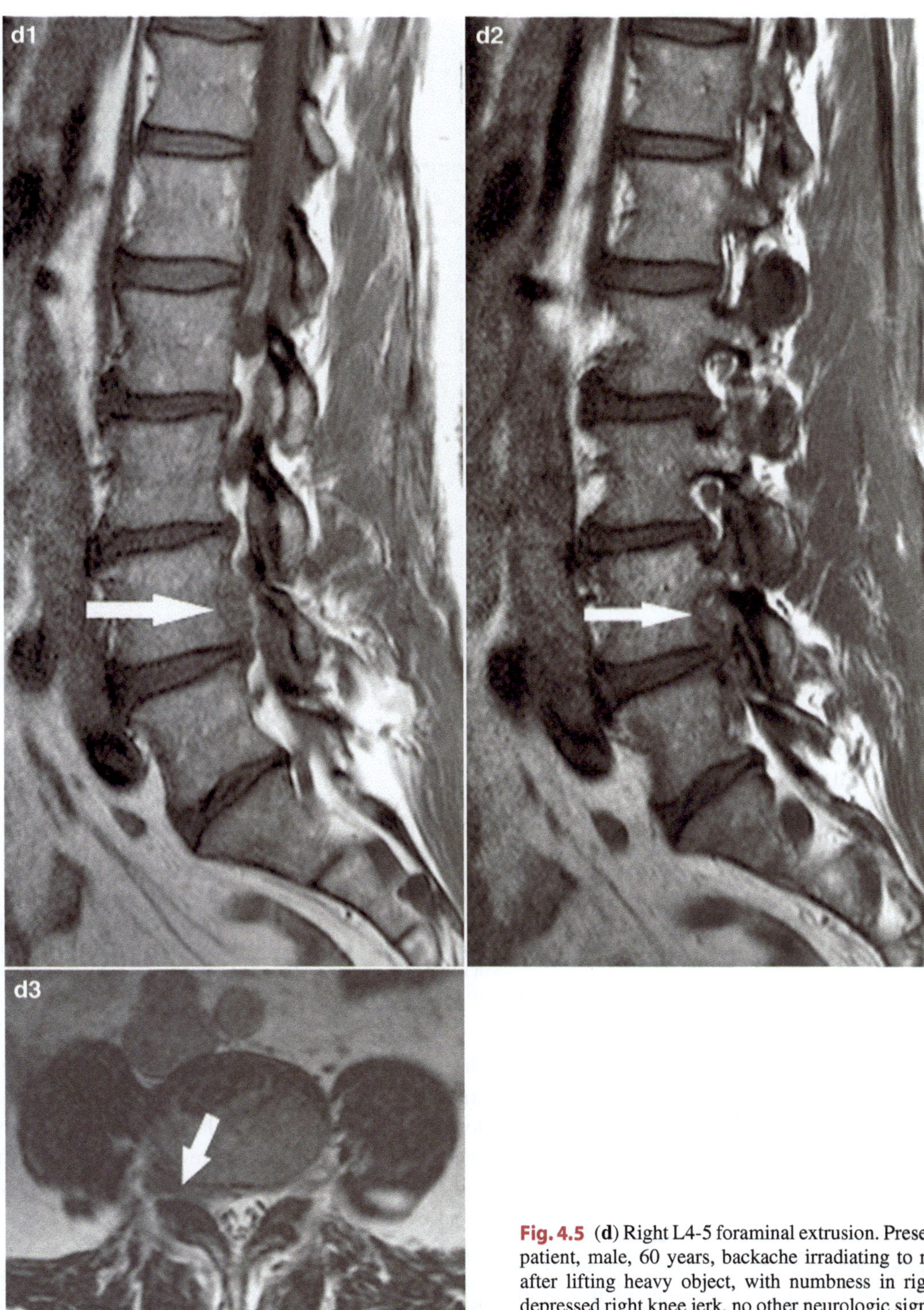

Fig. 4.5 (**d**) Right L4-5 foraminal extrusion. Presentation: patient, male, 60 years, backache irradiating to right leg after lifting heavy object, with numbness in right shin, depressed right knee jerk, no other neurologic signs. MRI: sagittal T1 weighted image (**d1**) shows migrated material behind L4 vertebral body (*arrow*), adjacent lateral section (**d2**) shows displacement of foraminal fat by extrusion (*arrow*) and nonvisualised L4 dorsal root ganglion, confirmed on axial T2-weighted image (**d3**, *arrow*)

For this supposition two possible anatomical explanations can be given, both involving the relative vulnerability of the nerve root to compression by upper and lower lumbar herniations respectively.

Within the dural sac the individual nerve roots making up the cauda equina are tethered in the longitudinal direction by their attachment to the conus medullaris cranially and the root sleeve caudally (see Fig. 3.2). In the transverse plane the roots have more freedom of movement, and when an epidural mass such as a disc herniation impinges upon the dural sac anteriorly or anterolaterally, the effect will usually be to displace the intradural nerve roots in the axial plane, unless they are compressed against an unyielding bony or ligamentous structure. A disc herniation will have to be very large and to collapse the dural sac or a major part of it in order to compress one or more of these relatively mobile roots.

As the root approaches and enters the root sleeve, its freedom to move axially is limited as it is restricted by the surrounding dural structures. The point of emergence or axilla of the root sleeve relative to the disc is therefore of significance. As mentioned in Chap. 3, the root sleeve in the upper lumbar region emerges from the dural sac well below the level of the disc, and the intradural root will be displaced rather than compressed by a disc herniation at this level (Fig. 4.6 upper). In order to impinge on the axilla of the root sleeve where the intradural nerve root is relatively immobilised and vulnerable, an L1–2 extrusion would have to migrate downward from the disc level to almost the L2 mid-vertebral level. An alternative route of compression would be for the extrusion to migrate laterally to the foramen to compress the dorsal root ganglion (see Fig. 4.5). Asquier et al. (1996) studied 100 patients with femoral neuralgia due to degenerative disease and found foraminal herniations in 71.

In the upper lumbar region therefore only very large or extensively migrated disc extrusions are likely to cause nerve root compression.

As Fig. 4.6 lower shows, in the lower lumbar region the axilla of the root sleeve is located much closer to the disc level; at L5-S1, frequently even above this level, Therefore, a lower lumbar herniation is much more likely to compress the immobilised nerve root here.

Another factor contributing to the vulnerability of the nerve root in the lower lumbar region is the presence of a lateral recess. As mentioned in Chap. 3, the shape of

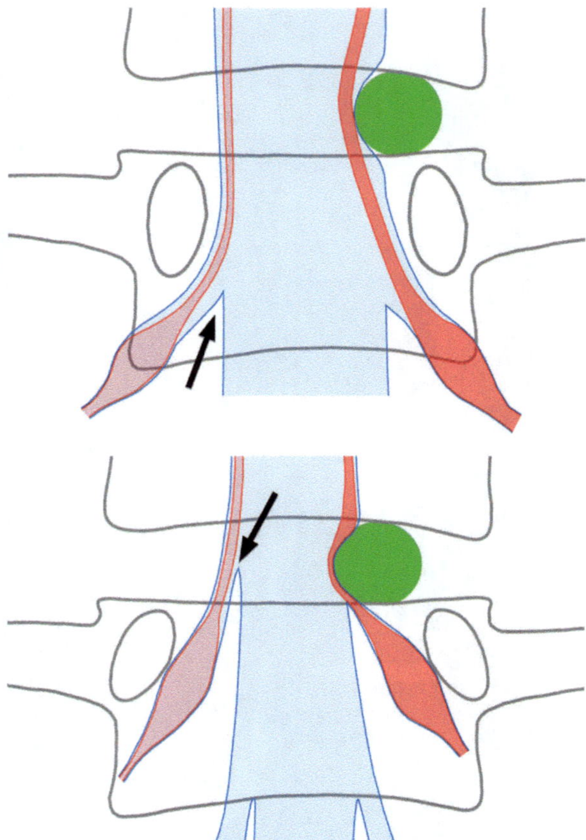

Fig. 4.6 Mobility of intradural nerve root. *Upper image*: in the upper lumbar region the axilla, or point of departure of the root sleeve (*arrow*) is located well below the disc level. An L1–2 herniation (*green*) impinging upon the dural sac will tend to displace rather than compress the L2 root. *Lower image*: in the lower lumbar region the axilla is located at or sometimes above the level of the disc. An L4–5 herniation here (*green*) encounters a nerve root which is relatively immobile and this is more likely to cause root compression

the spinal canal is oval in the upper lumbar region, and triangular with clearly defined lateral recesses in the lower lumbar region. These lateral recesses tend to fix the root sleeve in place, and prevent the nerve root from moving backward out of harm's way when encroachment by a herniated disc takes place (Fig. 4.7, see also Fig. 3.12 and Sect. 4.3).

To recapitulate: Lumbar disc herniations are most likely to compress a nerve root in areas where the root is most vulnerable to entrapment. These are:

- In the lower lumbar region: herniations located in the lateral *syn*: sub-articular zone (see Fig. 4.4), especially when these migrate caudally into the

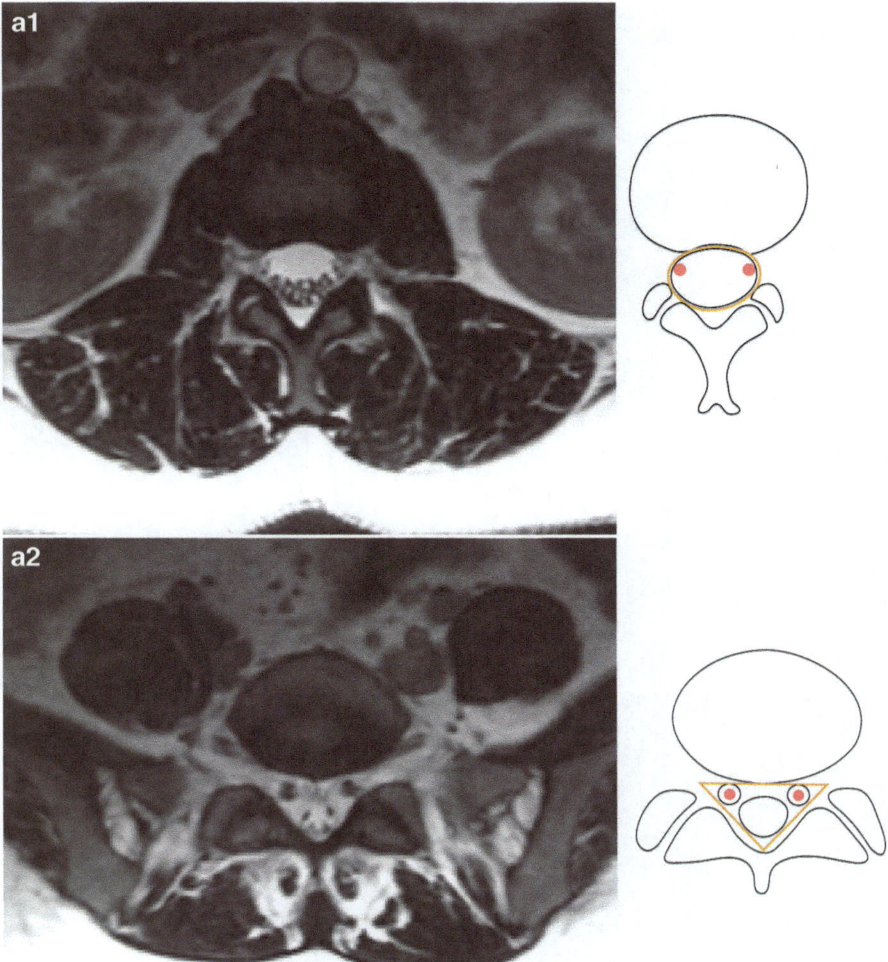

Fig. 4.7 Upper and lower lumbar spinal canal. (**a**) T2-weighted axial MR images and drawing of spinal canal, dural sac and intradural nerve roots. *At L1–2 level* (**a1**). Note *oval shape* of canal and dural sac, without lateral recesses. L2 roots in *red*; at *L5-S1 level* (**a2**). Spinal canal is *triangular in shape* at this level, with less reserve space around root sleeves. Nerve roots in red are more vulnerable to compression here.

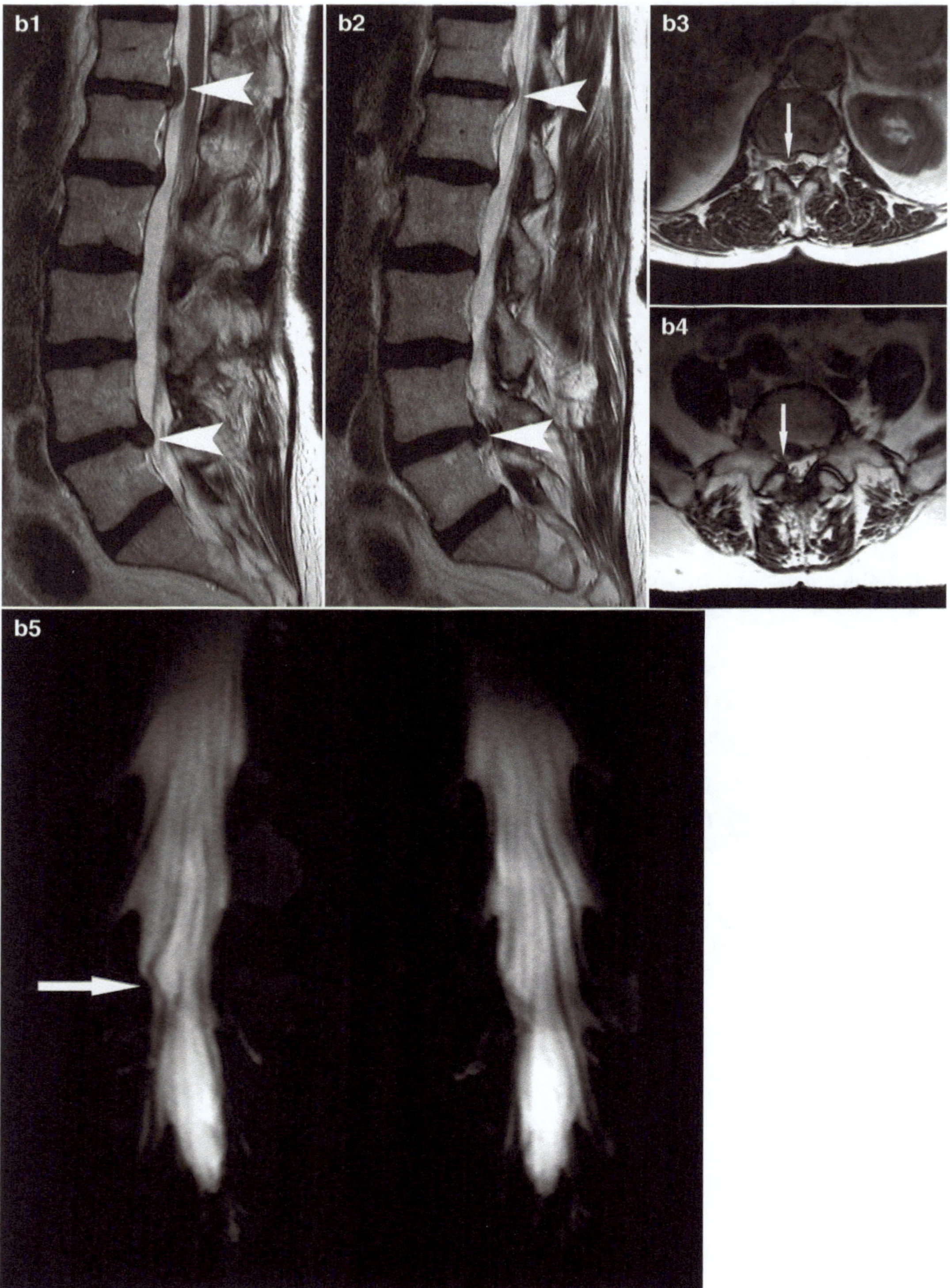

Fig. 4.7 (**b**) T12-L1 and L4–5 extrusions in same individual. Presentation: patient, female, 75 years, complained of right-leg pain, worse after walking, with foot drop after walking half hour. No neurologic deficit, no radicular signs or cord signs. MRI: T2-weighted sagittal images left of midline (**b1**), and farther lateral (**b2**). Extrusion visible at T12-L1 (upper arrowhead), migrating cranially in midline, causing minimal indentation of spinal cord and not compressing nerve roots, as axial T2-weighted image (**b3**, *arrow*) shows. Second extrusion at L4–5 (lower arrowhead), filling in L5 lateral recess and compressing right L5 root (**b4**, arrow). MR myelogram (**b5**) shows non-filling right L5 root sleeve (arrow)

lateral recess; also foraminal herniations migrating cranially against the pedicle (see Fig. 4.5c and d). Central and paracentral herniations, unless very large, are less likely to cause root compression as the spinal canal here is relatively roomy. Some degree of cranial or caudal migration does not increase significantly the likelihood of nerve root compression. In case a large central or paracentral herniation does occur here, collapse of the dural sac and compression of the entire cauda equina is more likely than entrapment of a single nerve root.

- In the upper lumbar region the risk of nerve root compression by a herniation of up to moderate size is much less than at the lower interspaces, for the anatomical reasons mentioned above. Migration to the foramen is probably most likely to cause root compression here.

Extraforaminal herniations lack an unyielding hard surface against which to compress the root. The clinical relevance of these herniations should be assessed with extra care by physical examination and, in questionable cases, by diagnostic nerve block.

4.1.2 Other Focal Mass Conditions Causing Intraspinal Compression of Nerve Roots

4.1.2.1 Tumours

Neoplasms originating from or compressing nerve roots in the spinal canal or intervertebral foramen, will not be discussed in detail here. Briefly summarised, we are dealing most frequently with metastases from distant malignancies: carcinoma of the breast and the prostate, lung and GI tract. Primary malignant tumours of the spine such as osteosarcoma and chondrosarcoma are rare, as are fibrosarcoma and Ewing's sarcoma of the spine. Bone marrow disorders such as multiple myeloma, leukaemia and lymphoma can affect the spine and the intraspinal nervous structures, and an embryologic tumour such as chordoma is occasionally encountered. Spinal intradural extramedullary tumours such as schwannomas, neurofibromas and meningiomas are benign in nature but frequently cause nerve root or spinal cord compression as do leptomeningeal metastases.

4.1.2.2 Synovial (Juxta-Articular) Cysts

These cysts classically originate from and communicate with a degenerated facet joint at its inner or outer border, have a fibrous capsule with a synovial lining and contain a clear serous fluid (Fig. 4.8), though haemorrhage may occur into the cyst, causing enlargement and inducing radicular symptoms. Intraspinal synovial cysts jutting inwards from the facet can produce dorsolateral compression of the nerve root or even the dural sac and cauda equina. Imaging method of choice is MRI (Van den Hauwe 2007).

4.1.2.3 Hypertrophic Callus Formation in Spondylolysis

Spondylolysis is a fracture through the isthmus or pars interarticularis of the vertebra, described in more detail in Sect. 4.3. In rare cases, hypertrophic and ossified callus may encroach upon the lateral recess dorsally, and compress the nerve root there.

4.2 Narrowing of Spinal Canal; General or Regional

In 1948, Van Gelderen described two patients in whom disabling lower limb pain occurred during walking (lordosis), but not during cycling (kyphosis). The symptoms were ascribed to lordotic pressure on the dural sac by hypertrophic flaval ligaments.

Verbiest (1976b) named the symptom "intermittent neurogenic claudication", caused by compression of the lumbar dural sac and cauda equina in spinal retroflexion, (extension, lordosis). This condition is distinguished from intermittent vascular claudication due to arterial disease of the lower extremities by the fact that the onset of leg pains is related to the erect, lordotic spinal posture, and not to exercise-induced ischemia of the leg muscles as in the latter condition. He described operative findings of an abnormally small AP bony diameter of the lumbar spinal canal. In these patients the pedicles are short but the interpedicular diameter is not markedly reduced. An important factor in compression of the lumbar dural sac was encroachment upon the spinal canal by hypertrophic articular processes (Verbiest 1954). In patients with a bony AP

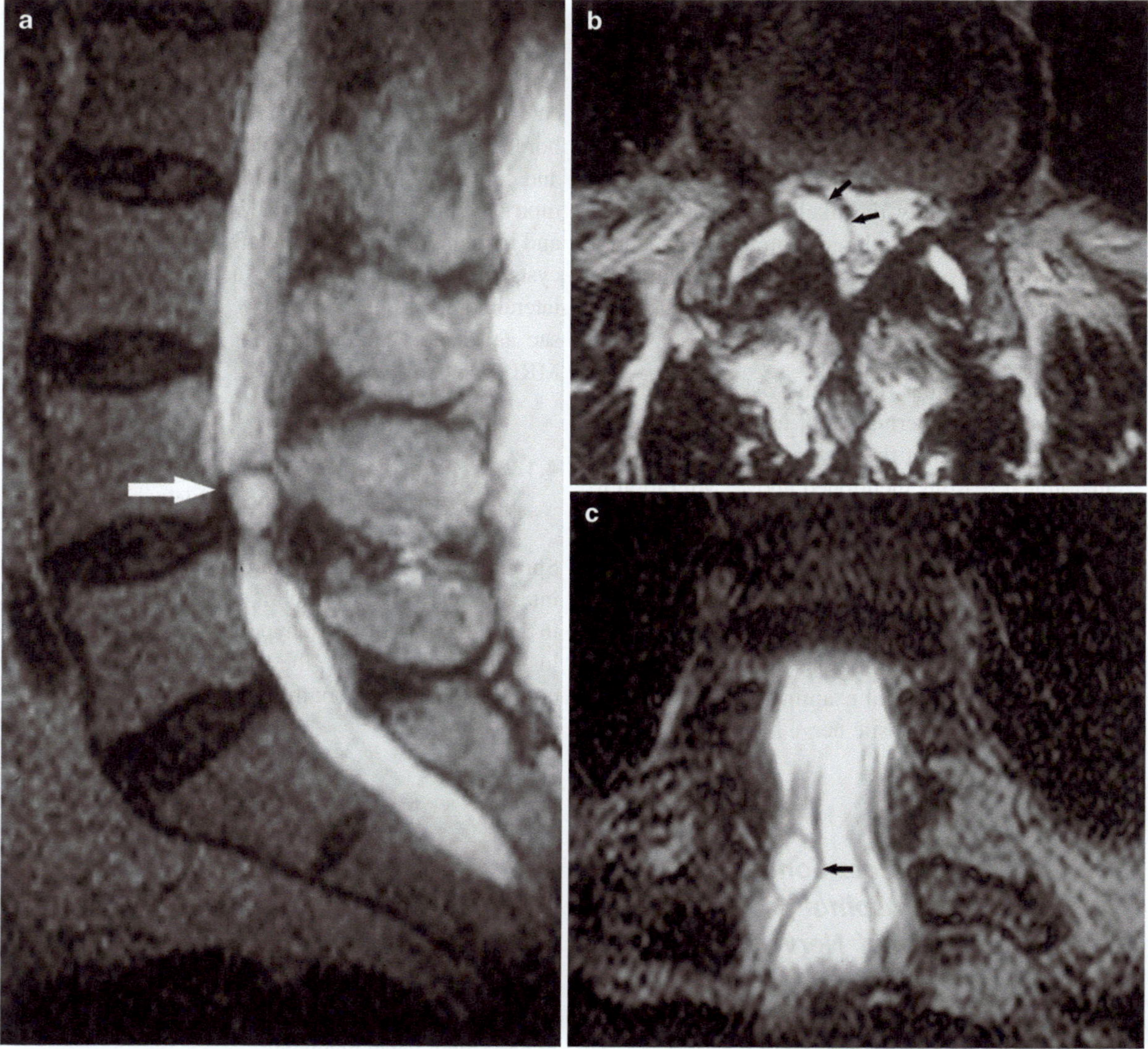

Fig. 4.8 Synovial cyst. T2-weighted sagittal (**a**) and axial images (**b**) show demarcated mass iso-intense to CSF, causing left dorsolateral impression on dural sac (*arrows*). Note facet hydrops associated with this condition. Coronal section (**c**) also shows cystic lesion. No patient data available

canal diameter less than 10 mm ("absolute stenosis") the condition was considered to be of an "idiopathic developmental" nature, capable of producing symptoms of cauda equina compression by itself. In "relative stenosis" the bony AP canal diameter measured 10–12 mm, and symptoms were caused by a combination of a developmentally shallow spinal canal with small disc protrusions or vertebral osteophytes which would have remained asymptomatic in a normal canal.

It is useful to stress the following: stenosis does not mean anything more or less than "narrowing". Giving it a separate name tends to obscure the fact that stenosis of the spinal canal, like narrowing, is a relative term, and meaningless without quantification.

Verbiest used the term stenosis in an early French-language publication (Verbiest 1949), but in later English-language reports (Verbiest 1954) the term "narrowing" was also used. In a later review (Verbiest 1976a) this author disapproved the use of the term "stenosis" in cases with narrowing of the lateral recess or the intervertebral foramen.

In the present text, the use of the term "stenosis" is limited to those cases with developmental shallowness of the spinal canal as described by Verbiest, as this term is presently in common usage. In case of encroachment upon the spinal canal by degenerative hypertrophy of the facets and flaval ligaments, foraminal encroachment by osteophyte formation and deformation of the spinal canal and foramina by degenerative anterolisthesis (see below) the term "narrowing" is preferred.

Two further points must be mentioned here:

1. Absolute and relative developmental stenosis as defined by Verbiest are rare conditions: Eisenstein (1977) saw relative bony stenosis in only 4.7% of 433 skeletons studied, and absolute stenosis in none. In a CT study of 24 patients with neurogenic claudication, Schönstrom et al. (1988) found a mean bony AP diameter of the spinal canal of 14 mm, with relative stenosis (10–12 mm) seen in only two patients and absolute stenosis (<10 mm) in none.

2. Spinal dimensions in patients with narrowing of the spinal canal are reduced most severely not at the bony pedicular/laminar level where Verbiest performed his measurements, but at the ligamentous disc level (Fig. 4.9). In Schönstrom's study, the AP dural diameter and the cross-sectional area of the dural sac at the level of the disc were always abnormally small, even though the AP diameter of the bony canal was normal in the majority (see Appendix). Even in case of severe bony narrowing, the site of maximal compression of the dural sac is never at the bony pedicular level but at the ligamentous disc level where the AP diameter of the dural sac is reduced to an average of 7 mm (spread 5–11 mm) in patients with neurogenic claudication (Penning and Wilmink 1987).

Hypertrophy of the facet joint masses and flaval ligaments further reduce the sagittal diameter and also the transverse dimensions of the spinal canal (Baddeley 1976; Penning and Wilmink 1987, see Fig. 4.9). Verbiest regarded the facet hypertrophy to be developmental rather than degenerative in nature, but a degenerative etiology better explains the fact that in all but the most severe cases of developmental stenosis, clinical symptoms do not occur during childhood or early adulthood: it is at a later age that the degenerative process superimposes an additional and different type of narrowing of the spinal canal. To a developmentally shallow bony canal with a normal interpedicular diameter as described above, is then added a further progressive transverse narrowing of the bony canal due to degenerative hypertrophy of the facets with gradual reduction of the interfacet diameter and encroachment upon the lateral regions of the spinal canal.

Degenerative hypertrophy of the facets can of course also take place without pre-existent developmental stenosis. In these cases the transverse diameter of the spinal canal between the facets is especially reduced, and the canal assumes a T-shaped or trefoil configuration (Fig. 4.10). A degree of trefoil shape of the canal can occur as a developmental variation however, and in itself is not always a consequence of degenerative processes (Eisenstein 1980, Papp et al. 1995).

Upon these bony changes degenerative ligamentous changes are additionally and progressively superimposed: hypertrophy of the facet joint capsules and flaval ligaments as mentioned above, and degenerative bulging of the annulus fibrosus (Fig. 4.11). The stenosis of the lumbar spinal canal which originally involved mainly the sagittal dimensions is in this way gradually converted into concentric narrowing with sagittal, transverse and oblique vectors.

As mentioned previously, ligamentous structures in the normal lumbar spine are influenced by changes in posture: In lumbar retroflexion or lordosis the ligaments lining the spinal canal at the disc level: annulus fibrosus, facet joint capsule and flaval ligaments, bulge inward and reduce the amount of space available for the dural sac (see Figs. 3.16 and 3.20). Under normal circumstances this concentric encroachment does not lead to symptomatic compression of the dural sac, nerve roots or root sleeves. When the spinal canal is narrow the picture changes. In the study by Sortland et al. (1977) the reduction in dural AP diameter in retroflexion amounted to about 9% in normal individuals, but in those with severe stenosis it was increased to about 67%. The absolute degree of encroachment is the same in both groups, but when the spinal canal is narrowed its effects are enhanced. We found the same phenomenon in functional myelographic and CT myelographic studies (Penning and Wilmink 1987; Wilmink et al. 1984, Fig. 4.12).

Penning (1992) formulated a "rule of progressive narrowing", which holds that "the more the spinal canal is structurally narrowed by a stenosing process, the more it will be functionally narrowed by additional retroflexion or lordosis. This means that in severe grades of stenosis even the slightest retroflexion motion or the smallest increase in axial loading may lead to compression of nervous elements".

Developmental stenosis is almost invariably only one element in a multi-factorial complex, seldom a diagnosis in itself (Fig. 4.13). Only absolute developmental stenosis with a bony AP diameter of the spinal

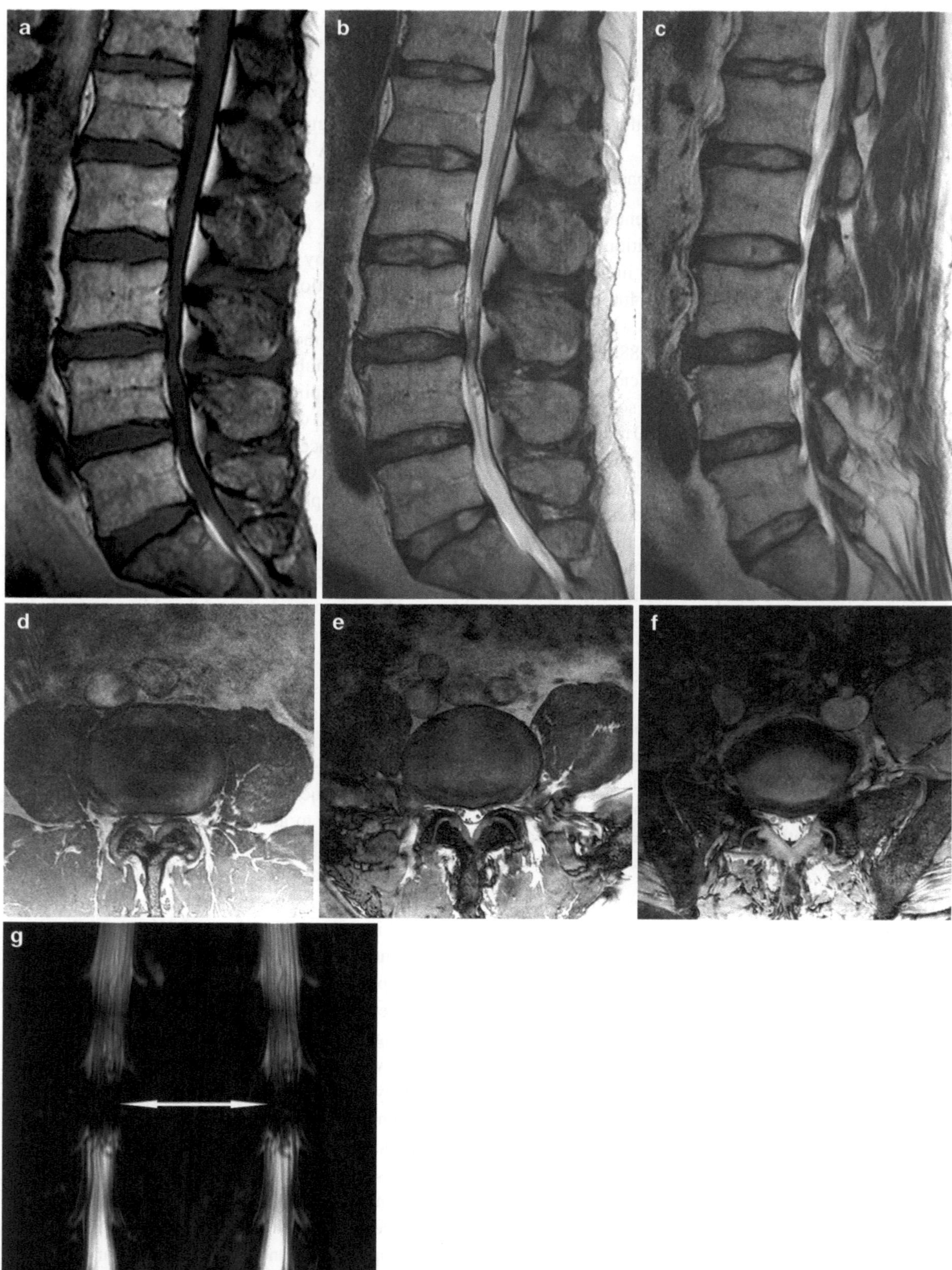

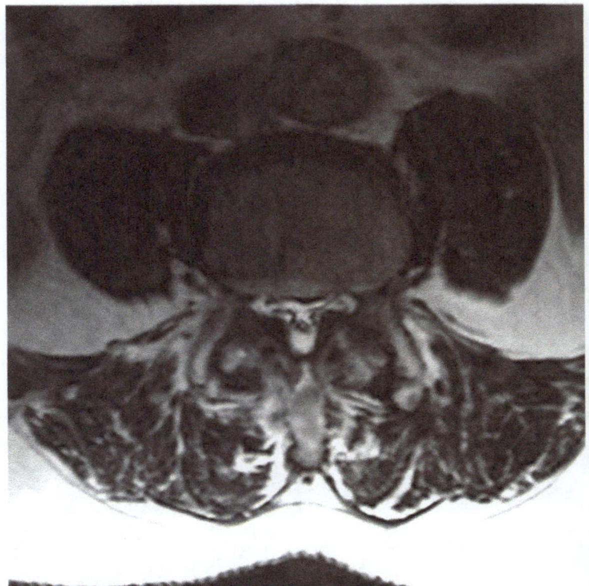

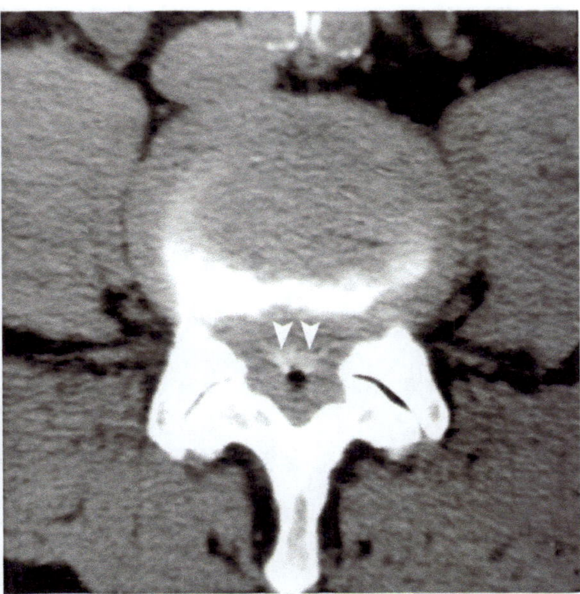

Fig. 4.10 Trefoil shape of spinal canal. *Presentation*: patient, male, 63 years, experiencing numbness in both feet, especially left, with left foot drop after lengthy standing, walking or running. *MRI*: T2-weighted axial image in supine position showing trefoil "T" shape of spinal canal due to degenerative hypertrophy of L4–5 facets jutting medially and ventrally. No cauda equina compression. Entrance to lateral recess narrowed especially at left, with L5 root possibly becoming compressed when patient moves to erect lordotic posture

Fig. 4.11 Ligamentous hypertrophy. *Presentation*: no clinical data available. *CT*: CT myelographic section at L4–5 showing hypertrophy of flaval ligaments superimposed upon bony facet hypertrophy causing severe narrowing of spinal canal and almost complete collapse of contrast-filled dural sac (*white*). Note retrodural fat pad (*black*) indenting dural sac dorsally

canal of less than 10 mm is sufficient in itself to cause cauda equina symptoms in the absence of further degenerative encroachment. As mentioned above, such a severe degree of developmental stenosis is very rare. Less severe degrees of stenosis of the spinal canal do serve to increase the likelihood of cauda equina or nerve root compression in the presence of other pathological circumstances causing reduction of space within the spinal canal (Singh et al. 2005), for instance, facet and flaval hypertrophy and degenerative anterolisthesis such as mentioned above, but also bulging or herniated disc (Ramani 1976) and increase in intraspinal fat (see Sect. 4.2.2). The greater the degree of developmental stenosis, the less severe is the additional pathology which is needed to produce compression of the cauda equina (Fig. 4.14; see also Fig. 4.9) or of individual nerve roots (see below). In this sense the upper limit for "relative" stenosis set by Verbiest at a bony mid-sagittal diameter of 12 mm, is artificial. In fact, all bony AP diameters between the normal mean value of 17 mm and the value for absolute stenosis of 10 mm could be regarded as being "relatively" stenotic to a lesser or greater degree. This makes it unwise to rely unduly on linear measurements and even area measurements of the spinal canal in diagnosis of individual patients, as the dimensions of the spinal canal are clearly not the only factors determining the occurrence of dural or neural compression. The spinal morphometric review presented in Appendix 1 is not so much intended for daily diagnostic use, as to illustrate the variability of findings encountered in different studies.

Fig. 4.9 Developmental spinal stenosis combined with bulging disc. *Presentation*: patient, male, 51 years, suffered from severe neurogenic claudication when walking >20 m, complaints relieved by spinal flexion. *MRI*: sagittal T1- (**a**) mid-sagittal and off-sagittal T2-weighted images (**b, c**) show shallow spinal canal with attenuation of CSF signal at L3–4 disc level; mid-sagittal bony diameter at L3 lamina 11 mm: relative stenosis according to Verbiest. Axial T2-weighted images show heavy facets and hypertrophic flaval ligaments especially at L3–4 (**d**), less marked at L4–5 (**e**) and L5-S1 (**f**). MR myelogram (**g**) shows CSF block at L3–4 (*arrow*) with serpentine, so-called redundant roots above and below level of block

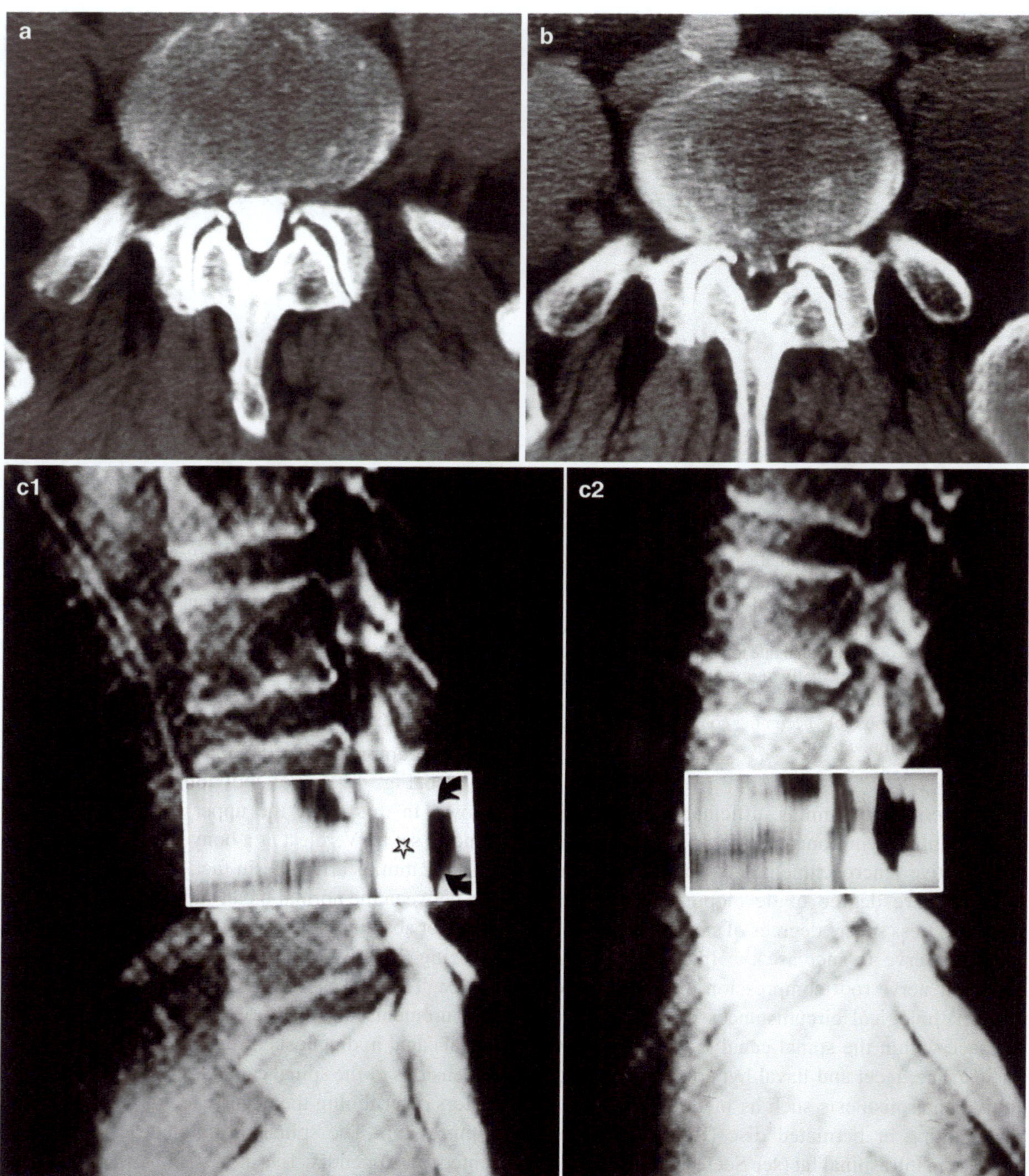

Fig. 4.12 Effects of lumbar flexion–extension in degenerative narrowing of spinal canal. *Presentation*: patient suffering from neurogenic claudication. No further clinical data available. *CT*: CT myelographic sections at L4–5 level, in supine spinal flexion (**a**) and extension (**b**) showing exaggeration of normal posture-dependent changes in case of spinal narrowing. Note bulging of disc in (**b**), with thickening of flaval ligaments, increase in depth of retrodural fat pad, collapse of contrast-filled dural sac (*white*). Compositions of sagitally reconstructed axial images upon scout views (**c**) in flexion (*left*) and extension (*right*) show same effects in sagittal plane; note how in extension, dural sac (*asterisk*) is compressed between backward-bulging L4–5 disc and retrodural fat pad (*curved arrows*) bulging forward in lordosis

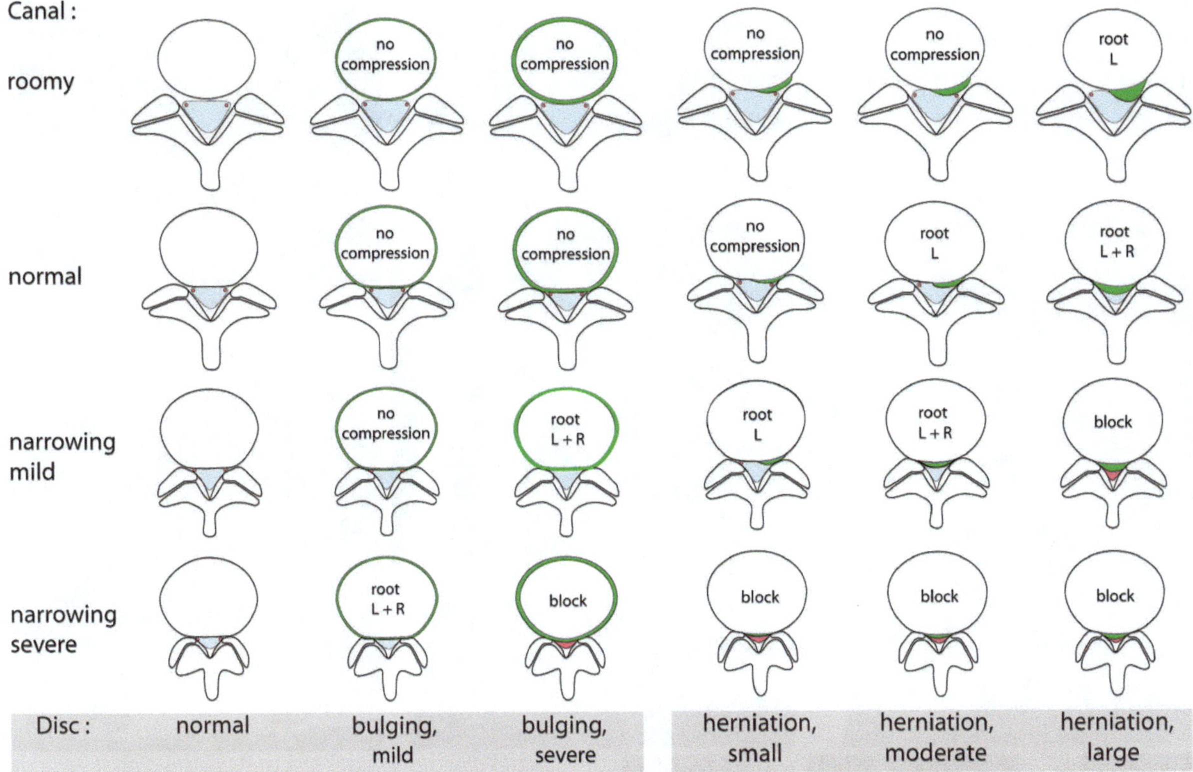

Fig. 4.13 Spectrum of possible combinations of disc pathology and canal narrowing. Canal dimensions in vertical columns ranging from roomy canal to severe narrowing. Disc pathology in horizontal rows ranging from normal via bulging to large herniation. Disc displacements shown in *green*, dural sac in *blue*, traversing nerve roots in *red*. Obliteration of nerve roots indicates root compression. *Red dural sac* indicates CSF block. In roomy canal nerve root compression occurs only in case of large herniation, and CSF block is very unlikely to occur. In severely narrowed canal root compression occurs very easily, even with normal postural disc bulging in extension. Diagram illustrates wide range of combinations causing, or failing to cause, compression of single nerve root or entire cauda equina

4.2.1 Why Is Narrowing of the Spinal Canal Seen So Rarely at L5-S1?

In a myelographic study (Sortland et al. 1977) the distribution of the levels of complete or incomplete myelographic block were as follows: L1–2 7%; L2–3 16%; L3–4 38%; L4–5 34%; L5-S1 5%. Many of these cases featured narrowing at multiple levels: narrowing of the spinal canal limited to L5-S1 is exceedingly rare. There are two reasons for this:

- The bony AP diameter of the spinal canal at S1 is about the same as at the higher levels, but the transverse interfacet and interflaval diameters are greater here than at any other level.
- At the same time the dural sac is tapering towards its termination or cul-de-sac (see Fig. 3.8).

For these reasons lateral encroachment by the articular masses which often contributes to spinal canal narrowing in the lower lumbar region, although it is frequently present at the lumbosacral transition, has relatively less effect upon the available intraspinal space, so that compression of the dural end-sac and the cauda equina by narrowing of the central spinal canal at this level is rare.

Hypertrophy of the S1 facets can however cause marked narrowing of the lateral recesses at the entrance to the sacral canal, and involve the traversing S1 roots (Schlesinger 1955; see also Sect. 4.3).

4.2.2 Factors Further Contributing to Reduction of Space in the Spinal Canal

Degenerative anterolisthesis: Spondylolisthesis is the condition in which a vertebral body moves forward (anterolisthesis) or backward (retrolisthesis) relative to

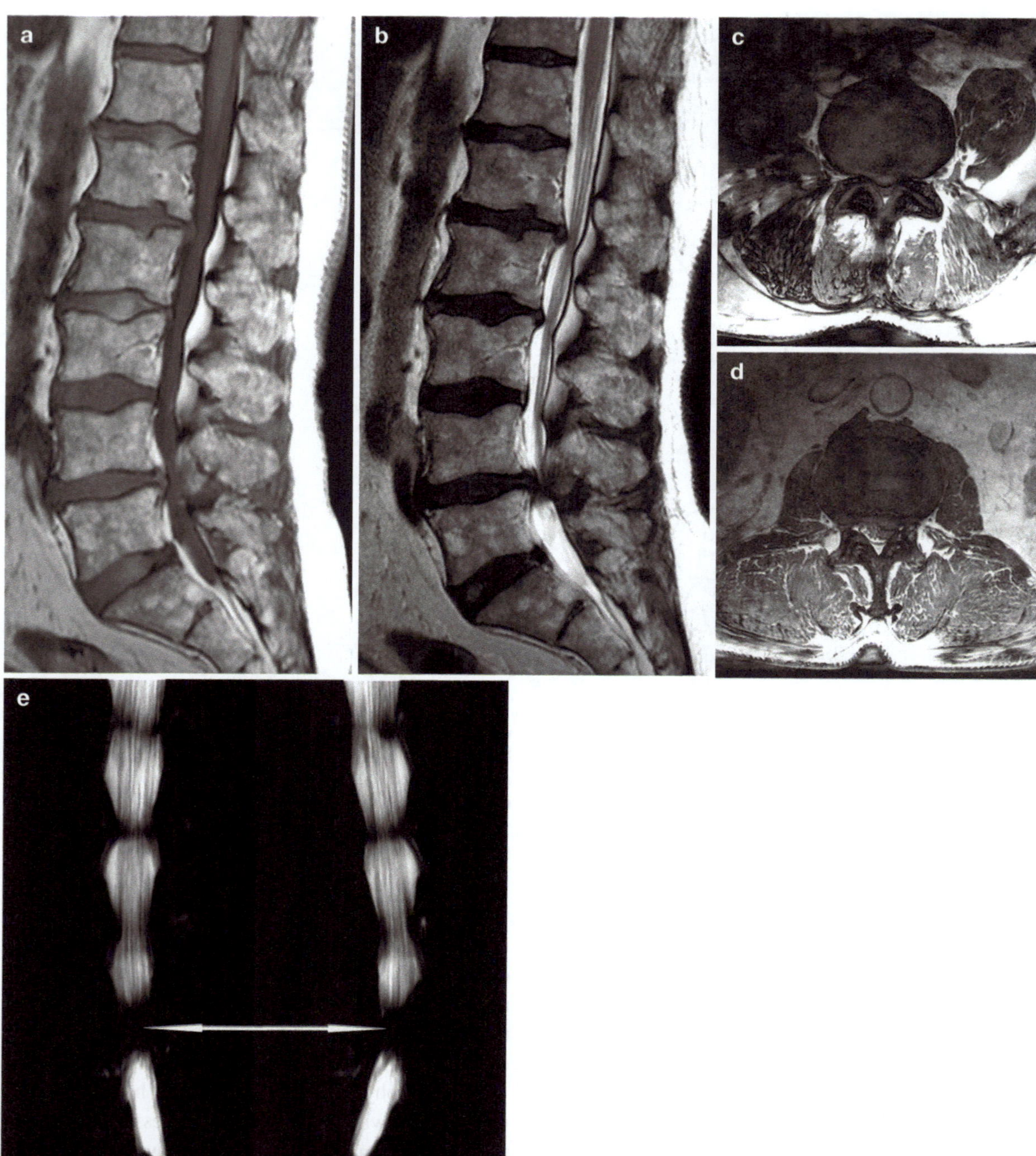

Fig. 4.14 Combination of relative stenosis and disc protrusion. *Presentation*: patient, male, 75 years, had long-standing backache irradiating to lateral side of right leg on walking, relieved by lumbar flexion. No pain when sitting or cycling. SLR somewhat limited at right, no neurologic deficit. No radicular pain at left. *MRI*: sagittal T1- (**a**) and T2-weighted images (**b**) show relative spinal stenosis: bony AP diameter of canal 12 mm. at L3; 13 mm. at L4 and L5. In addition there is disc protrusion with CSF block at L4–5, smaller protrusions at L1–2 and L2–3. Axial T2-weighted image at L4–5 (**c**) confirms protrusion, slightly more pronounced at right, with compression of dural sac. Axial image at L1–2 (**d**) shows left protrusion with flattening of ventrolateral corner of dural sac but apparently not causing symptoms (see presentation). MR myelogram (**e**) confirms CSF block at L4–5 (*arrow*) , shows some dural impressions at L1–2 and L2–3, no clear nerve root compression

the vertebra below. Anterolisthesis is by far the most common, and there are two main circumstances which may cause it: spondylolysis and degenerative facet destruction. Spondylolysis will be discussed in more detail below.

Degenerative changes of the spine can lead to bony hypertrophy of the facets and other structures, but also to erosion of the facet surfaces. The facets guide and limit spinal mobility, and by the overlap of the inferior articular process of the upper vertebra over the superior articular process of the lower vertebra, anterior slipping of the upper vertebra is prevented. The shape of the facet joint surfaces in the axial plane shows considerable individual variation, and when the facets are oriented mainly in the sagittal plane rather than the coronal plane, and additional facet erosion takes place, this facilitates forward slipping of the upper vertebra with respect to its lower neighbour (Fujiwara et al. 2001). This leads to narrowing of the spinal canal, with a pincers-like mechanism of compression upon the dural sac and the nerve roots within it, with the jaws formed by the lower border of the lamina, interlaminar ligaments and fat pad from above and behind, and the posterior border of the vertebral body and the disc from the front and below (Fig. 4.15).

Degenerative anterolisthesis occurs most frequently at the L4–5 level, occasionally at L3–4 or higher, and least frequently at L5-S1.

The nerve roots within the dural sac or the root sleeves may be compressed in the lateral region of the canal by the forward movement of the inferior articular processes of the upper vertebra, leading to radicular pain which is often bilateral. In more severe narrowing the entire dural sac may be compressed by the forward movement of the lamina and its investing ligaments, leading to neurogenic claudication (Fig. 4.15).

The emerging roots in the intervertebral foramina are also at risk of compression by disrupted disc material in anterolisthesis (see below).

Spinal epidural lipomatosis: Abnormal accumulation of epidural fat occurs most frequently in the mid-thoracic region and in the lumbosacral transition. The most common cause is long-term steroid administration or increased endogenous steroid production (Cushing's disease), but the condition may also be associated with morbid obesity, or may be idiopathic in nature (Robertson 1997; Lisai et al. 2001; Fogel et al. 2005).

In the lower lumbar region epidural fat is normally seen dorsal to the dural sac, as a fat pad filling in the interlaminar space and decreasing in size toward L5-S1, as the dural end-sac moves backward at this level (see Fig. 3.8). At the same level and for the same reason the epidural space ventral to the dural sac widens, and in normal individuals fat can be seen from about the L5-S1 level downward, gradually filling in the sacral canal as the dural end-sac tapers to its termination. There are individual variations, but as a rule no epidural fat is visible in the anterior epidural space higher than about halfway the L5 vertebral body. Dorsal epidural fat is seen only in the interlaminar space, and no fat is normally visible between the posterior border of the dural sac and the vertebral lamina.

Like other factors involving intraspinal dimensions, epidural lipomatosis can be present in varying degrees. In the most severe forms, the dural end-sac is concentrically compressed and collapsed by the mass of epidural fat, being seen only as a thin linear structure in the sagittal MR image and a triangular or Y-shaped remnant on the axial image (Fig. 4.16, see also Fig. 4.1c). In these severe cases which are quite rare, epidural lipomatosis can lead to symptoms of neurogenic claudication.

In less severe cases increase in epidural fat is seen only in the lumbar interlaminar spaces, creating dorsal impressions in the dural surface, especially in lumbar extension or lordosis. These impressions are in themselves usually not sufficient to collapse the dural sac and compress the cauda equina, but may play a contributory role when other factors mentioned above are also in play narrowing the bony and ligamentous dimensions of the spinal canal (see Fig. 4.12).

4.3 Regional Spinal Narrowing

Narrowing of the lateral recess: As described in Chap. 3, the lateral recess actually comprises two levels of the spinal canal (Fig. 4.17a).

The bony lateral recess is well known from standard texts, and is found at the pedicular vertebral level and is described in Chap. 3. Incarceration of the nerve root in the bony lateral recess was described by Schlesinger (1955) and later Epstein et al. (1972) and Ciric et al. (1980, 1985). Isolated narrowing of the bony lateral recess is quite rare however, and most reports dealing with the "lateral recess syndrome" mention concomitant narrowing of the spinal canal proper (Penning 1992).

A little more cranially, at the intervertebral disc level, there is what could be called a "ligamentous lateral

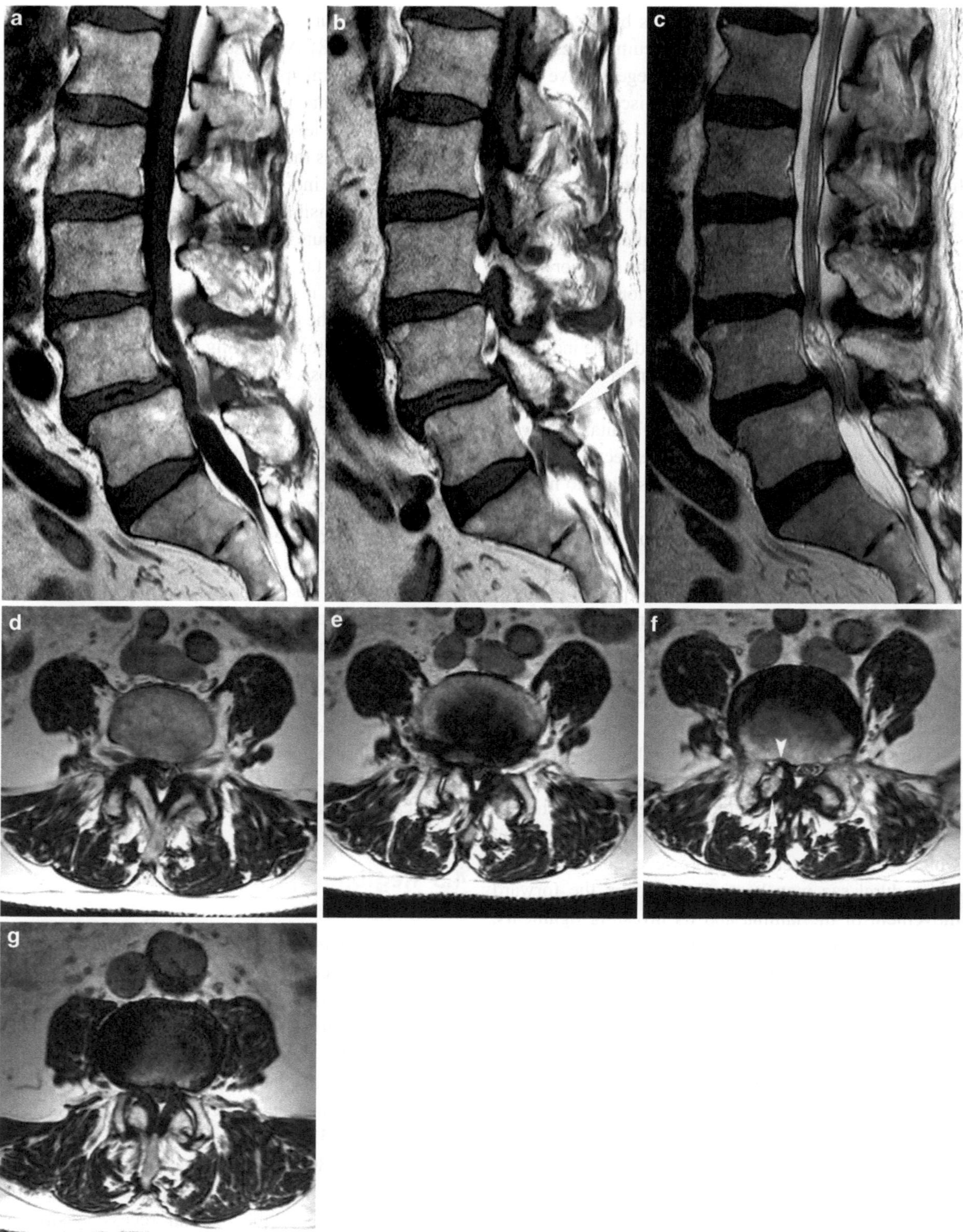

Fig. 4.15 (continued)

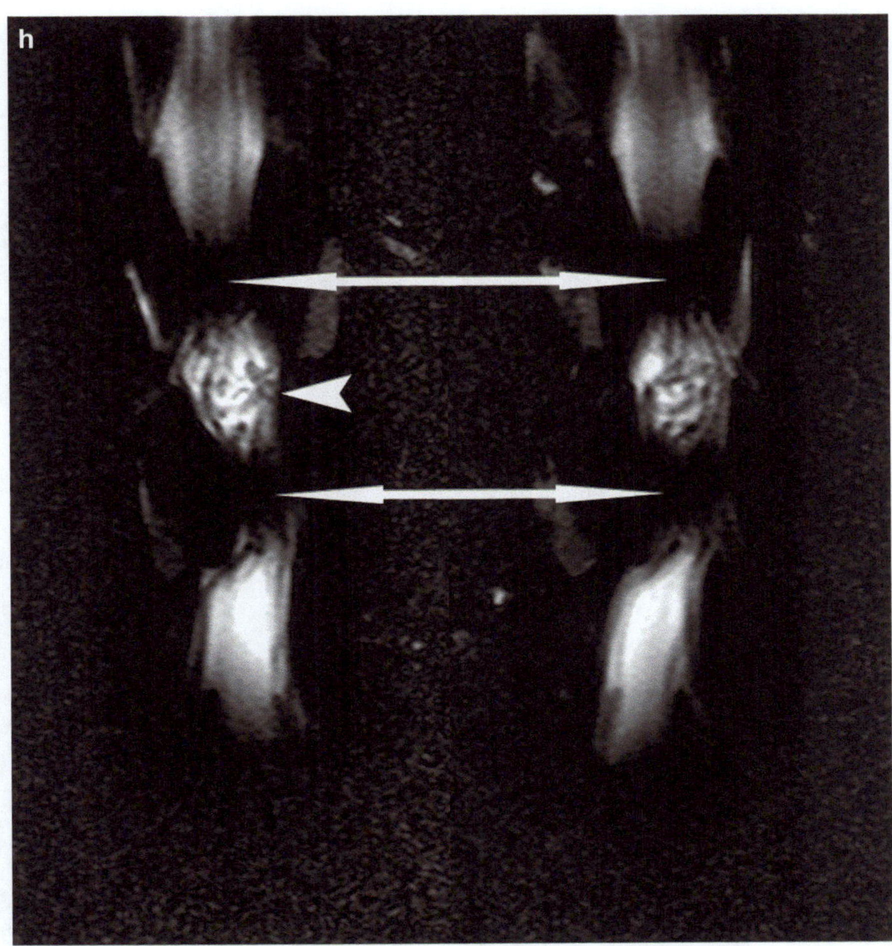

Fig. 4.15 Degenerative anterolisthesis. *Presentation*: patient, male, 79 years, reported weakness of both legs after walking 300 m, relieved by sitting with flexed spine. No radicular symptoms, no neurologic deficit. Decompression proposed but declined. *MRI*: sagittal T1- (**a, b**) and T2-weighted images (**c**) show grade 1 anterolisthesis at L4–5, with CSF block and no widening of L4 bony spinal canal, both unusual for spondylolysis. Right parasagittal cut (**b**) shows severe erosion of right L5 superior articular process (*arrow*). Axial T2-weighted images at lower L4 level (**d**); L4–5 disc level (**e**) and upper L5 level (**f**) show sagittal orientation of facet especially at right, marked anteroposition of L4 inferior articular process (*arrow*) abutting against L5 vertebral body and obliterating right half of spinal canal (*arrowhead*). Axial section at L3–4 (**g**) shows narrowing of spinal canal mainly due to hypertrophy of flaval ligaments. MR myelogram (**h**) confirms two-level CSF block (*arrows*), with dural impressions especially marked at L4–5 right. Note serpentine, so-called redundant roots at L4 level (*arrowhead*)

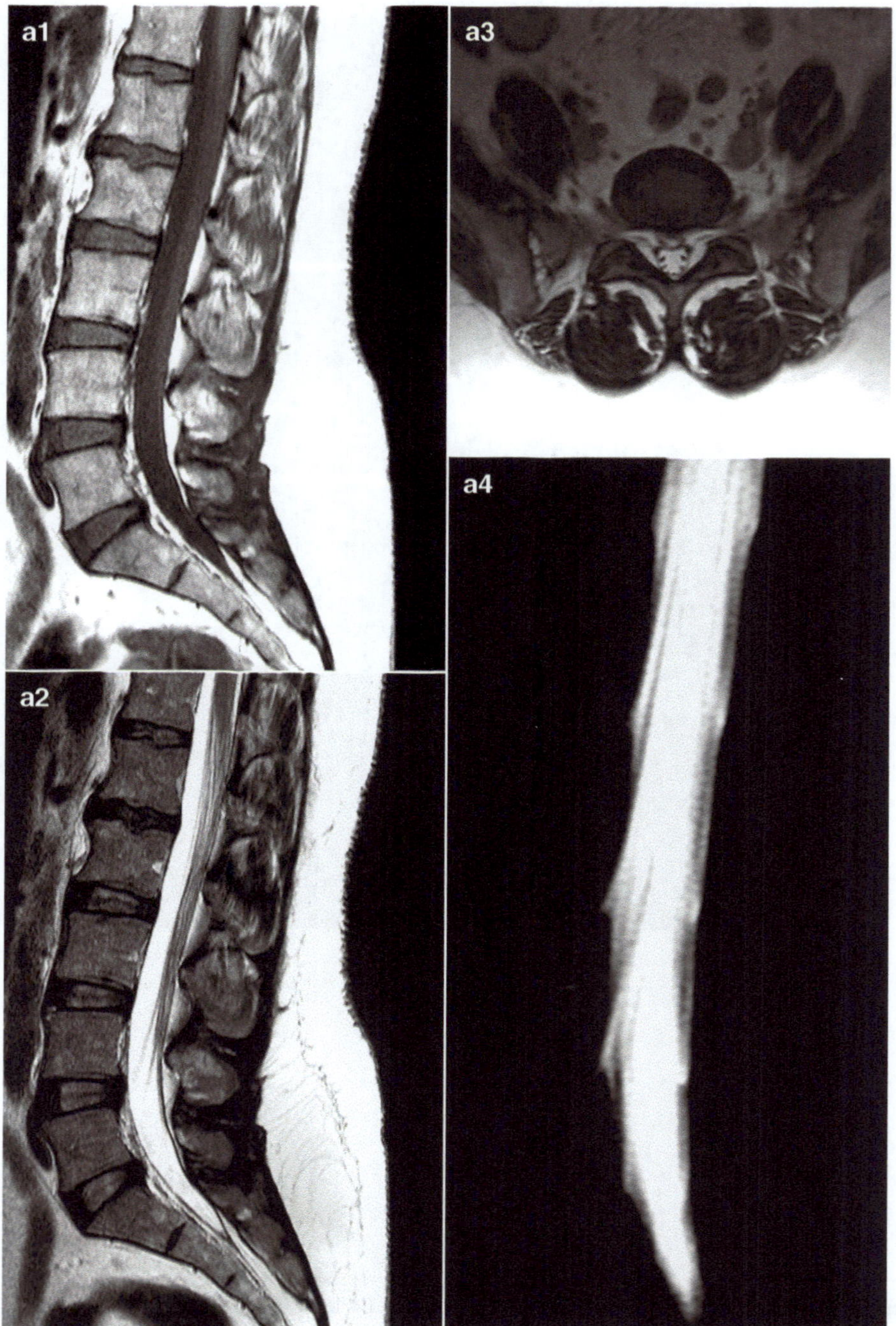

Fig. 4.16 Development of epidural lipomatosis in adipose female. *First presentation*: female, 29 years, MRI performed after fall from stairs, with persistent lumbago with irradiation to left leg, no radicular signs, no neurologic deficit. *First MRI*: sagittal T1- (**a1**) and T2-weighted images (**a2**) as well as T2-weighted axial images at L5-S1 level (**a3**), and MR myelograms (**a4**) show normal dural sac and distribution of epidural fat, no signs of nerve root compression.

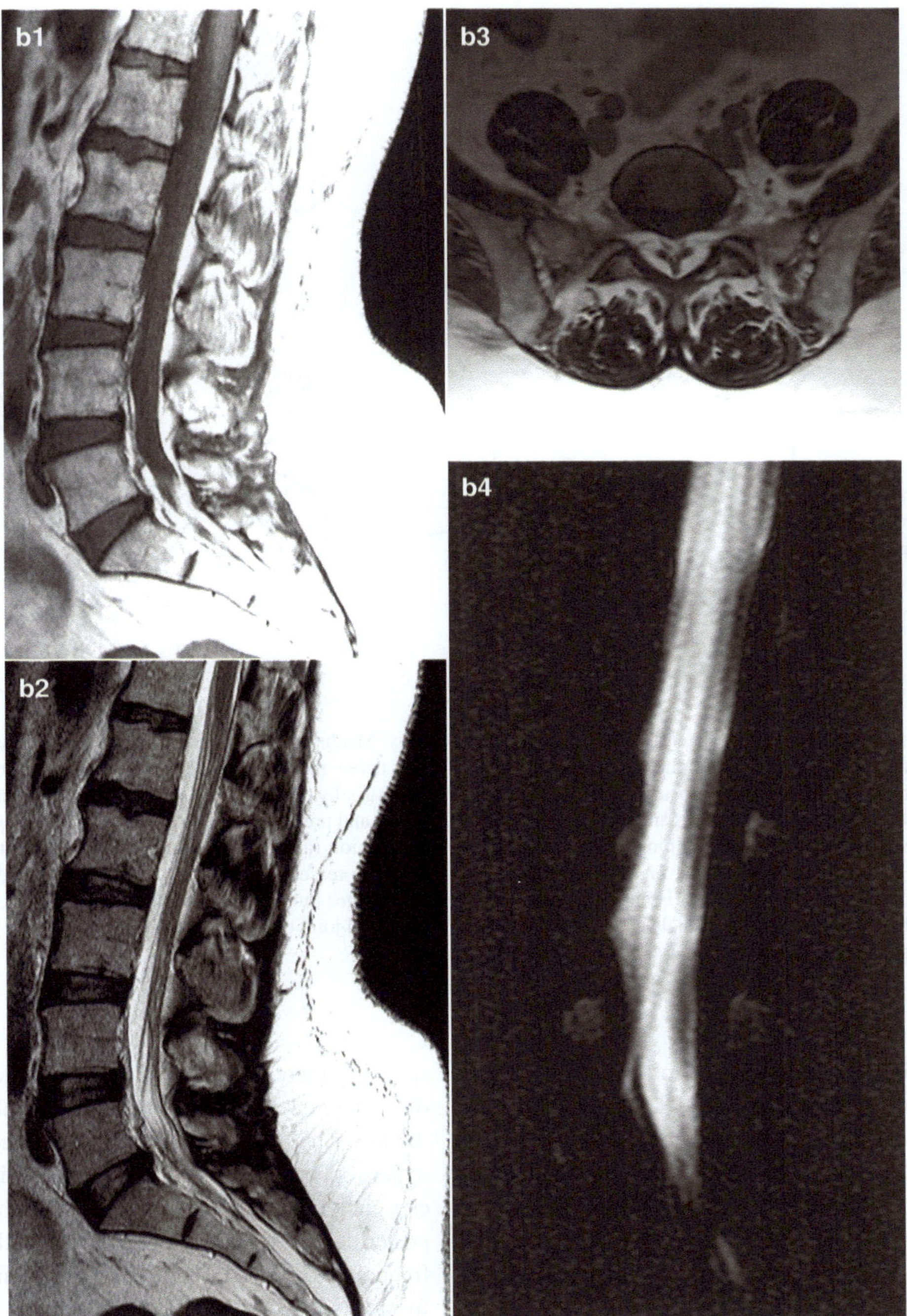

Fig. 4.16 (continued) *Second presentation 2 years later*: patient now reporting a new complaint of back pain irradiating to the buttocks and posterior thighs, provoked by standing and walking, relieved by sitting down. No radicular signs, some loss of strength in left leg, with sensory loss in left S1 dermatome, but normal tendon reflexes. *Second MRI*: sagittal T1-(**b1**) and T2-weighted images (**b2**) show marked increase of epidural fat in lower lumbar and lumbosacral transitional regions (compare with (**a**) and (**b**)). Note also increase in depth of subcutaneous fat. Axial T2-weighted image at L5-S1 (**b3**) shows dural sac now almost collapsed. MR myelogram (**b4**) also shows compression of lumbosacral dural sac progressive caudally

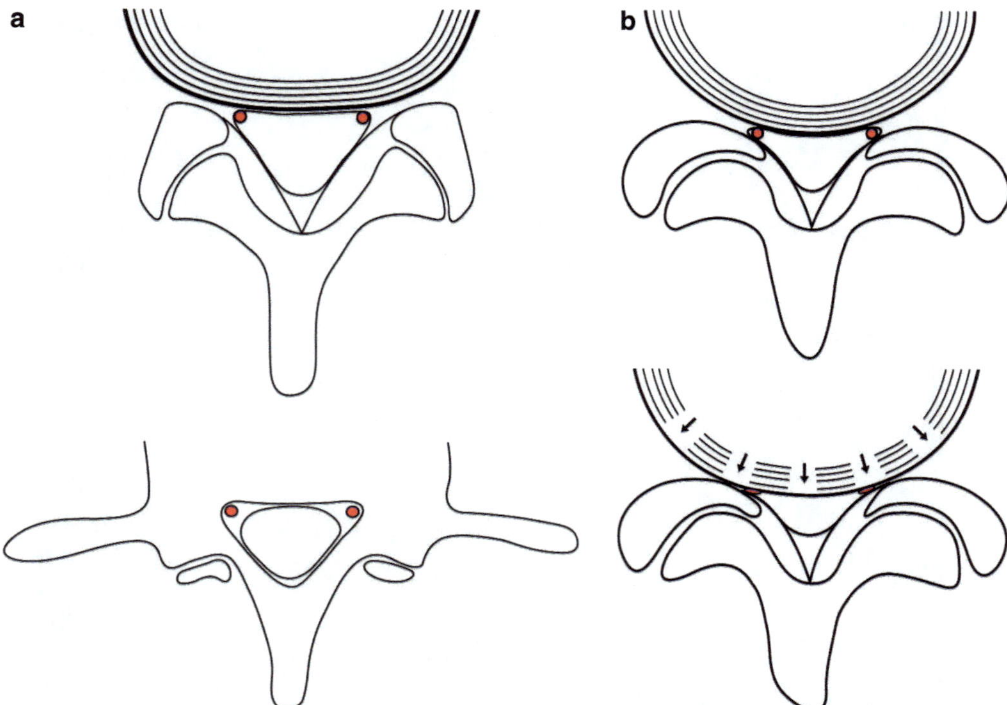

Fig. 4.17 Bony and ligamentous lateral recess. (a) Sectional anatomy. At disc level (*upper image*) the lateral spinal canal is bordered ventrally by the annulus fibrosus and dorsolaterally by the facet joint capsule and the flaval ligament. These structures form a ligamentous lateral recess containing the traversing nerve root (*red*) At the pedicular level (*lower image*) the bony lateral recess containing the root sleeve (*red*) is bordered ventrally by the vertebral body, laterally by the pedicle and dorsolaterally by the base of the superior articular process. (b) Functional anat-omy. Mechanism of posture-dependent compression of travers-ing nerve root (*red*) in the ligamentous lateral recess. Note hypertrophy of facets reducing interflaval diameter (see also Fig. 4.18), and preventing posterior movement of nerve root. In lum-bar flexion (anteflexion, upper image) traversing nerve root is not compressed. In lumbar extension (retroflexion, lower image) disc bulges into spinal canal and compresses nerve root against facet and joint capsule.

recess" which is bordered anteriorly by the annulus fibrosus of the intervertebral disc, dorsolaterally by the facet joint capsule and the flaval ligament (see also Chap. 3). These ligaments attach to the bony structures of the adjacent vertebrae: the annulus fibrosus to the vertebral bodies, and the facet joint capsule and flaval ligament to the articular processes and laminae, respec-tively. The ligamentous lateral recess thus gradually blends into the bony lateral recess which now has a bony lateral border formed by the inner surface of the pedicle (Fig. 4.17a; see also Figs. 3.10 and 3.11). Strictly speaking there is no lateral border to the canal at the disc level, but only fat as the spinal canal opens out in the lower half of the intervertebral foramen. In case of hypertrophy of the facets and their covering ligaments, especially when this is combined with bulging of the posterior disc surface, the lower half of the foramen is frequently occluded so that a true ligamentous recess is formed (see Fig. 4.17e3, e4).

The anatomical distinction between two levels of the lateral recess is of clinical relevance. The bony lat-eral recess on which most attention is usually focused

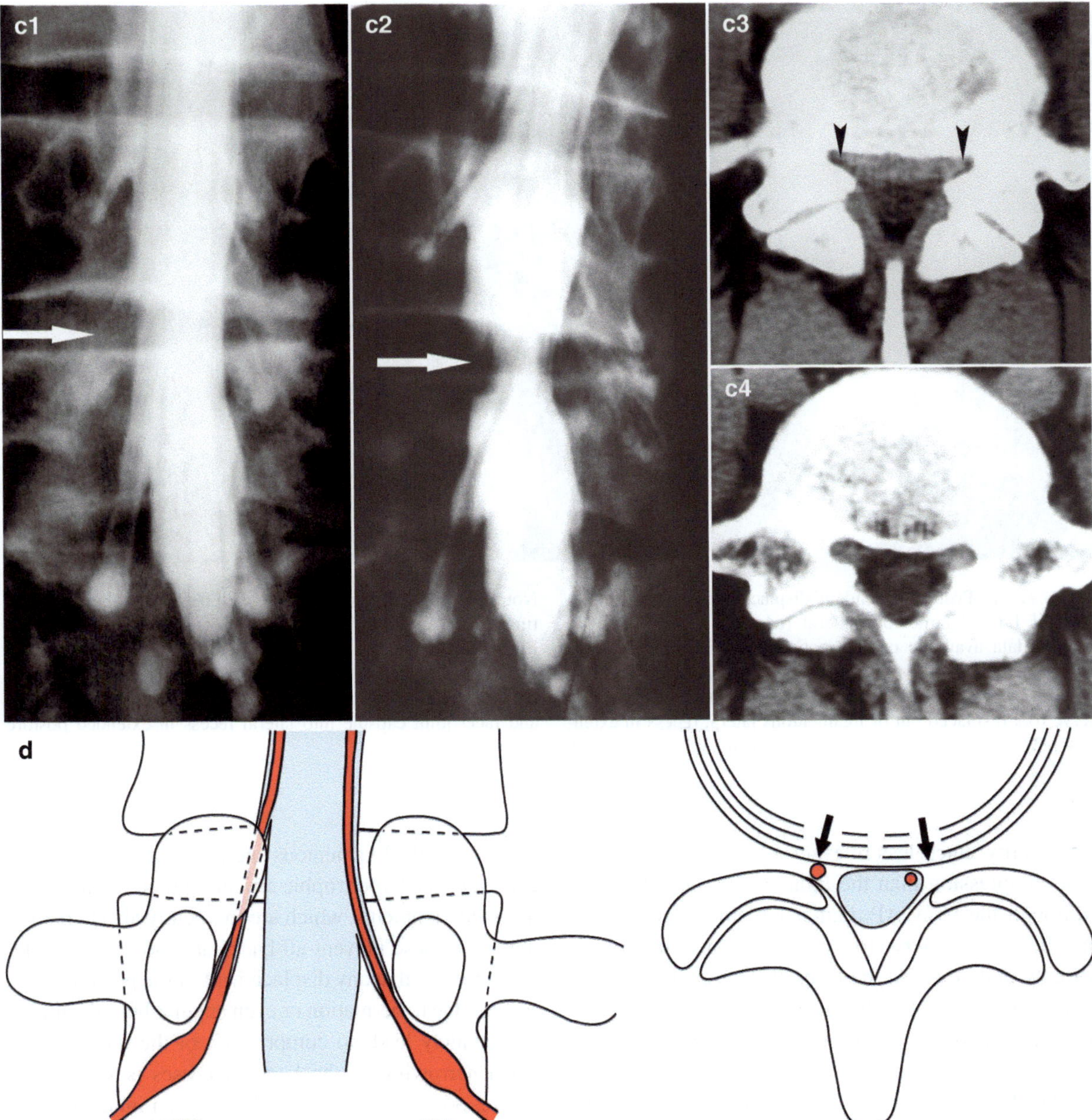

Fig. 4.17 (**c**) Posture-dependent bilateral L5 nerve root compression in L4–5 lateral recesses. *Presentation*: no clinical data available on this patient. Imaging: conventional lumbar myelographic projections show right L5 root sleeve faintly imaged (*arrow*) but not compressed in sitting lumbar flexion (**c1**); compression of same root sleeve and dural sac in extension (*arrow*, **c2**). Identical images on other side, not shown. Note that site of compression is at lower disc level, in ligamentous lateral recess. Axilla of root sleeve located at lower disc level in extension, drawn somewhat cranially in flexion. Consecutive non-contrast CT sections at L4–5 in same patient, at level of lower disc/ entrance to bony lateral recess showing site of root compression by at entrance to lateral recesses by bulging disc (**c3**, *arrowheads*), with lower cut at showing normal L5 roots within bony lateral recess (**c4**). CT was performed with patient supine in extended spinal posture. No flexion views performed. (**d**) Variable positions of traversing nerve roots (red) in lateral recess. Axilla of root sleeve at *left* in coronal diagram is located above disc level, and root crosses disc space within lateral recess, as shown also in axial diagram. Root is vulnerable to compression. Axilla of root sleeve at right in diagrams is located below disc level and traversing nerve root crosses disc space within dural sac, medial to lateral recess. This root is not likely to be compressed by mechanism shown in Fig. 4.17.b.

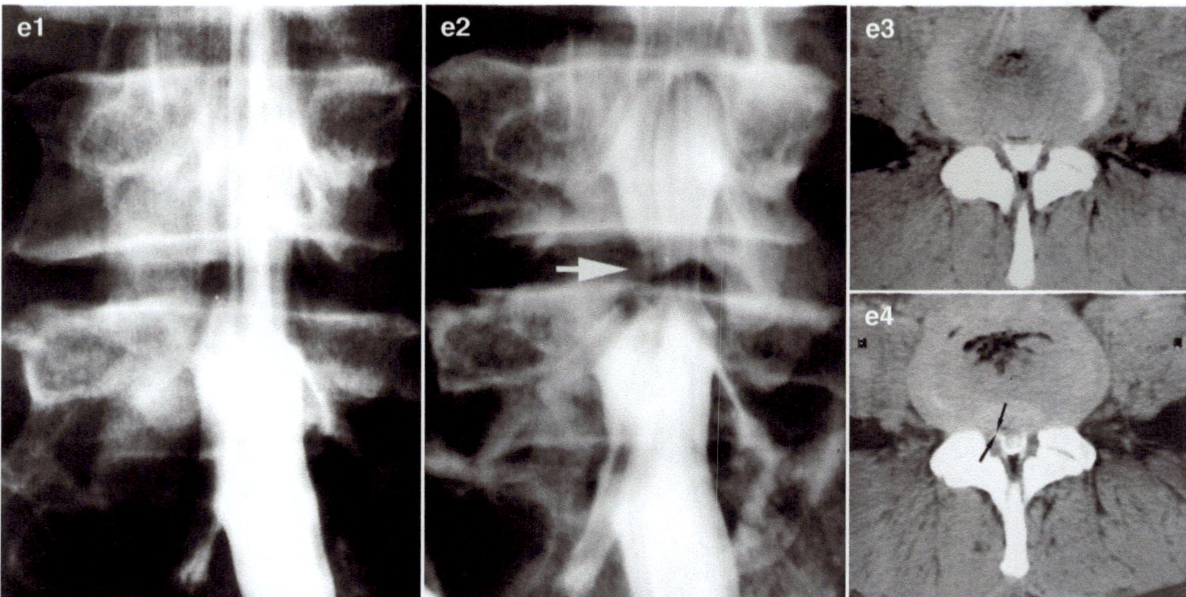

Fig. 4.17 (**e**) Posture-dependent displacement of L5 roots at level of L4–5 ligamentous lateral recesses. *Presentation*: no clinical data available on this patient. *Imaging*: conventional lumbar myelographic projections show normal position of right L5 root sleeve in sitting lumbar flexion (**e1**), with traversing nerve root displaced out of ligamentous lateral recess in extension (**e2**) being somewhat kinked rather than being compressed. Note location of root sleeve axilla well below disc level, permitting greater mobility of intradural root at disc level: compare Fig. 4.17**c1, 2** with 4.17**e1, 2**. CT myelographic sections through ligamentous lateral recess in lumbar flexion (**e3**) and extension (**e4**) illustrate lateral pincers mechanism due to bulging of disc and facet joint capsule into lateral recess in extended posture (*arrows*)

is in reality much less relevant as a location of nerve root compression than the ligamentous lateral recess. Although the bony AP diameter of the lateral recess may be reduced, nerve root compression at this level is actually quite rare. At the level of the ligamentous lateral recess on the other hand, soft tissue changes, often posture-related, can compress the traversing nerve root or root sleeve more easily.

The shape of the bony lateral recess determines the shape of the ligamentous lateral recess. If the superior articular processes are hypertrophic and jut inward into the spinal canal, so will the facet joint capsules and flaval ligaments.

In the lower lumbar region the presence of the lateral recess limits the leeway for the nerve root to move posteriorly. Posterior displacement of the disc surface will quite easily compress the traversing nerve root in this region (Fig. 4.17b; see Sect. 4.1.1).

When the superior articular processes are hypertrophic the bony lateral recesses are narrowed, but also buttresses are formed behind the nerve roots traversing the

disc level in the ligamentous lateral recess. These masses consist of the hypertrophic articular processes and their investing ligaments, which are frequently also hypertrophic, and these prevent all backward movement of the nerve root so that any displacement of the posterior disc surface due to herniation or even annular bulging almost immediately leads to compression of the root. In fact, when narrowing of the lateral recesses is sufficiently severe, posture-dependent bulging of an intact annulus fibrosus can be sufficient to produce nerve root compression in the lateral recess in the upright lordotic posture: standing, walking (Fig. 4.17b, c).

Another anatomic point is of diagnostic relevance here. Nerve root compression in the lateral recess can only occur if the traversing nerve root is actually within the lateral recess. This is by no means always the case, as Figs. 4.17d and e show.

Nerve root compression in lateral recess narrowing is often difficult to assess in axial CT and especially MRI sections, and myelography has been reported to be helpful (Bartynski and Lin 2003). Comparison of

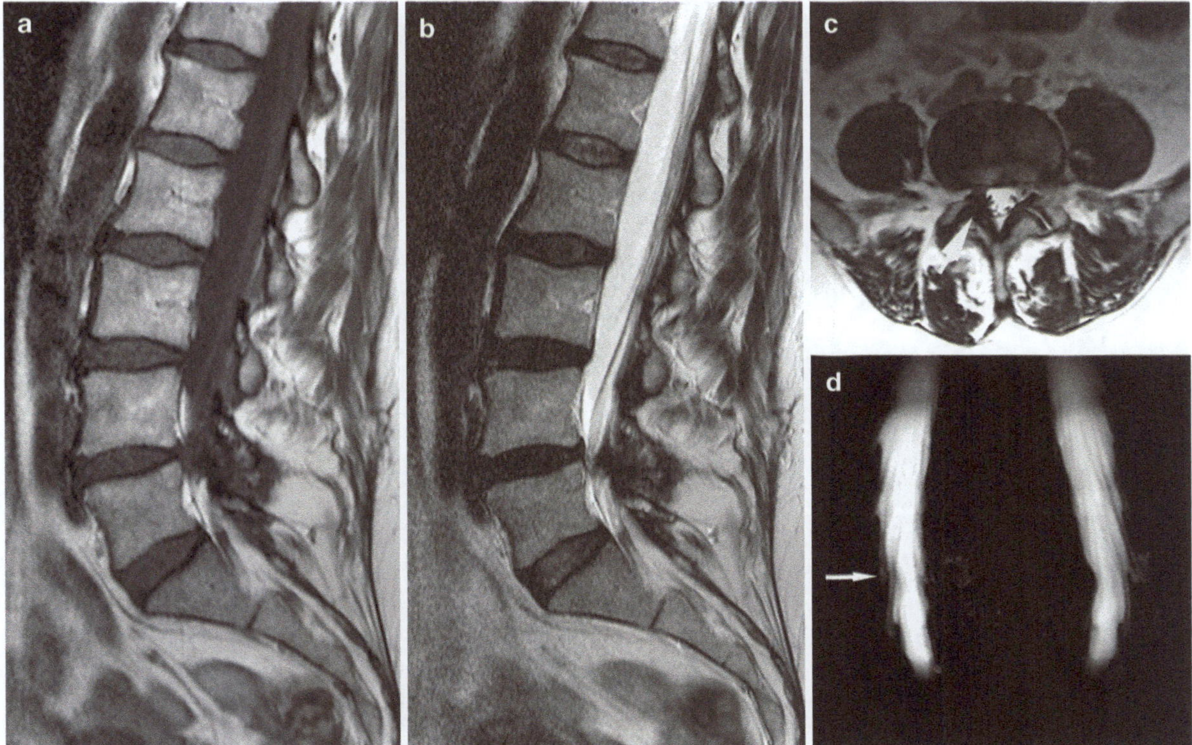

Fig. 4.18 *MRI,* CT and conventional myelographic images in a patient with bony spurring at entrance to right L5 lateral recess. *Presentation*: patient, female, 55 years, reported backache irradiating to right leg in L5 dermatome with paresthesia and tingling of foot. No posture-dependency of complaints, no neurological deficit, no limitation of straight-leg-raising. *MRI*: T1- (**a**) and T2-weighted right para-sagittal MR images (**b**) show dorsal impression upon dural sac at L4–5, effect on nerve root not clear. Axial T2-weighted image (**c**) appears to show flaval hypertrophy at right (*arrow*). MR myelographic images (**d**) show interrupted right L5 root sleeve filling on oblique view (*arrow*) presented at left; also dorsal dural impression on oblique view presented at right.

myelography, CT and MR myelography in such a case is presented in Fig. 4.18.

Foraminal narrowing: Within the intervertebral foramen the emerging nerve root may be compressed by migrated material from a herniated disc as described in Sect. 4.1, but the confines of the foramen itself may also be distorted or narrowed. The foramen is bordered by bony elements belonging to two adjacent vertebrae: the posterior vertebral body, lower pedicular border and inferior articular process of the upper vertebra; and the upper pedicular border and superior articular process of the lower vertebra. In addition, the posterior surface of the intervertebral disc, flaval ligaments and facet joint capsules border the lower half of the foramen (see Fig. 3.10).

As Fig. 4.19 shows, there can be considerable individual variation in the A-P diameter of the normal foramen. Narrowing of the foramen can occur due to bony spurring: degenerative osteophyte formation from the articular processes or the vertebral body. The lumbar foramina are normally quite roomy however, and the reduction in space in these cases is seldom sufficient by itself to compromise the nerve root.

In spondylolisthesis there is anterior slippage (anterolisthesis, Table 4.1) or posterior slippage (retrolisthesis) of the upper vertebral body with respect to the lower vertebra. The alignment of the vertebral bodies changes, and this can result in significant deformation and narrowing of the foramen, especially when the disc is disrupted.

Anterolisthesis: This is the most common direction of olisthesis or slipping, and can be caused by degenerative facet destruction, as described above, or by spondylolysis. In the latter condition a fracture, considered

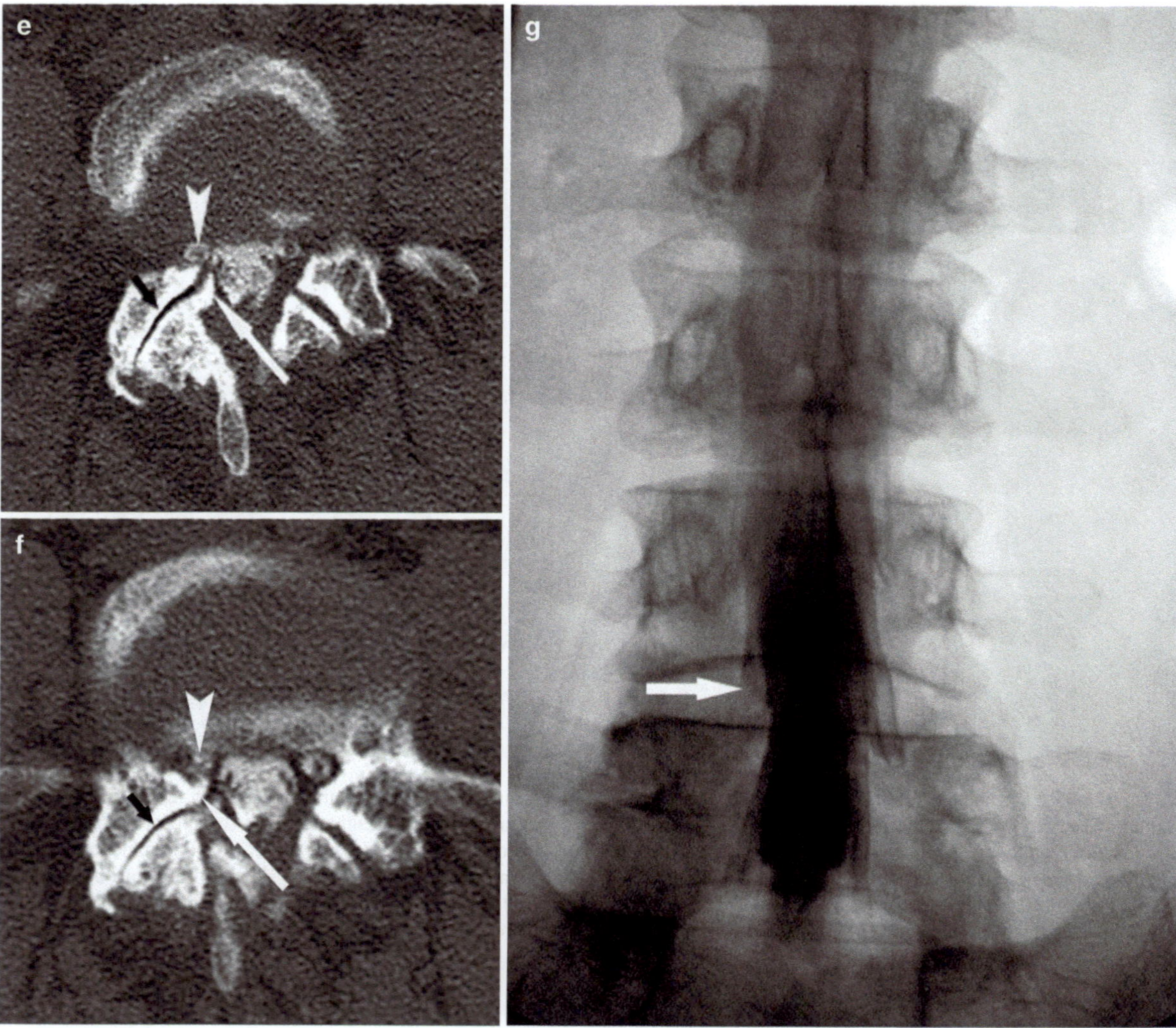

Fig. 4.18 Post-contrast thin-section CT cuts (**e, f**) reveal the cause to be an osteophyte (*arrow*) impossible to identify on the MR images. Right L5 root (*arrowhead*) still uncompressed at lower disc level in (**e**), barely visible at entrance to bony lateral recess in (**f**). Note normal root at left. Gas in right L4–5 facet joint space indicated by *black arrows*. Conventional myelographic image (**g**) confirms right L5 nerve root compression (*arrow*).

by many to be stress-related and usually bilateral, occurs in the pars interarticularis or isthmus connecting the superior and inferior articular processes, almost invariably involving the L5 vertebra, seen infrequently at L4. This pars defect permits the upper vertebral body to slip forward as it does in degenerative anterolisthesis, but there is an important difference.

In degenerative anterolisthesis as described previously, the spinal canal is narrowed by the forward movement of the lamina of the upper vertebral body

Fig. 4.19 Variability in lower foraminal dimensions. *Left column* (a, c, e) roomy lower foramen, open laterally (*upper left, arrows*), roomy lateral recess (*middle*), backward tilted superior articular process (*scout view left, arrows*). *Right column* (b, d, f) almost complete closure of lower foramen (*upper right, black arrows*), with formation of a lateral recess, without involvement of L5 root in dural sac (*open arrow*) or L4 root outside foramen (*white arrow*), normal bony lateral recess, middle right, note more vertically oriented articular processes (*scout view right, arrows*).

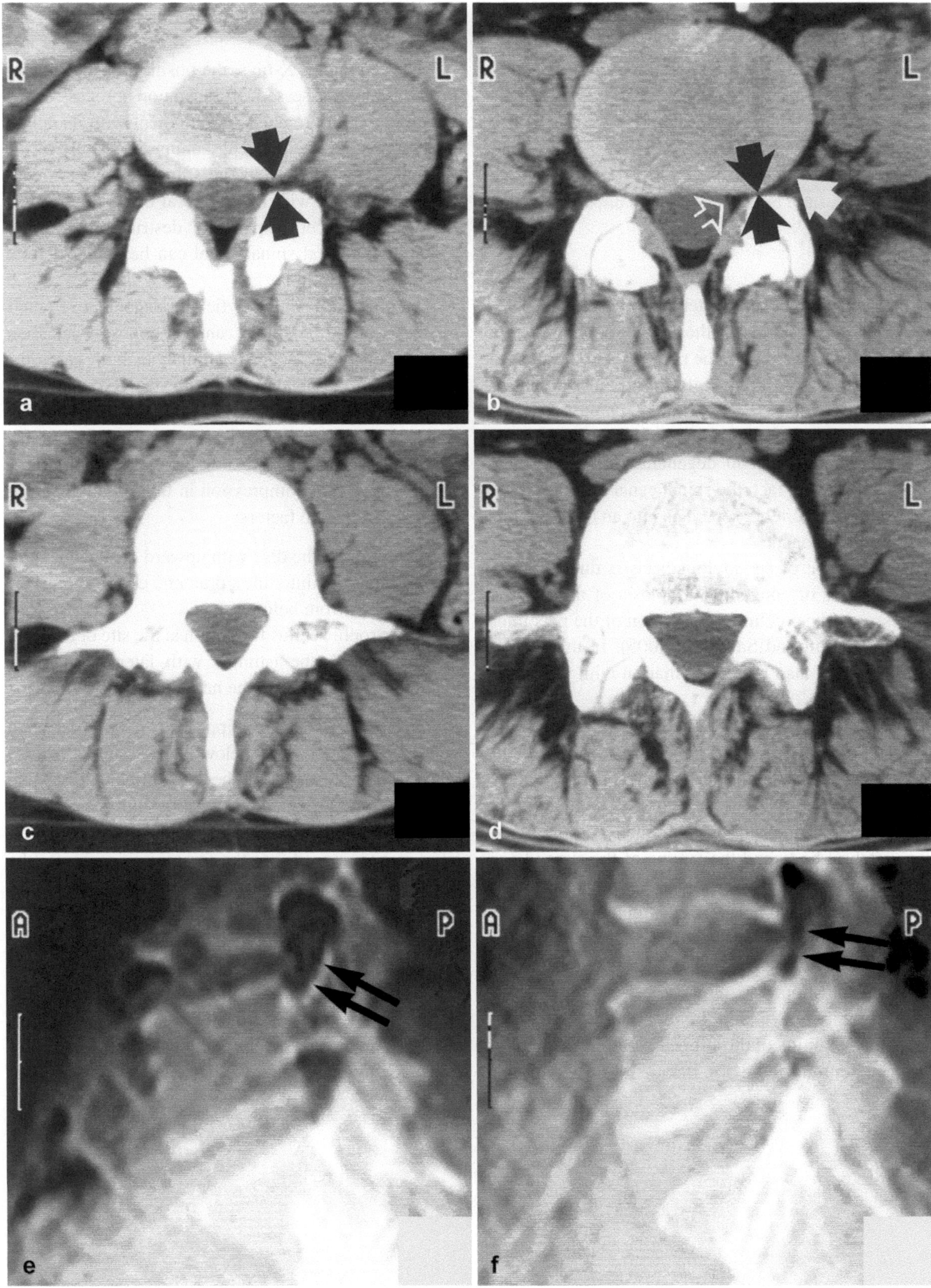

Table 4.1 The commonly used Meyerding grading scale (Wiltse and Winter 1983) divides the A-P diameter of the upper endplate of the lower vertebra into four segments

Grade	Displacement of upper vertebral body
Grade I	<25%
Grade II	25–50%
Grade III	50–75%
Grade IV	75–100%

Grades are classified based on the forward displacement of the upper vertebral body

with respect to the lower vertebral body (see Fig. 4.15). In spondylolytic anterolisthesis the upper vertebral body moves forward with the pedicles and the superior articular processes, but the inferior articular processes, lamina and spinous processes are separated from the remainder of the vertebra and remain behind. The scissors mechanism seen in degenerative anterolisthesis does not occur; in fact, the spinal canal becomes wider as the slipping vertebra separates into an anterior and a posterior component.

A third type of spondylolisthesis is due to one of several forms of congenital dysplasia of the articular processes with sometimes elongation of the pars interarticularis (Butt and Saifuddin 2005). In this type of slip there may also be a combination with an isthmic defect.

Spondylolysis is often difficult to see on axial and even on sagittal MR images. The easiest way to distinguish between spondylolytic and degenerative anterolisthesis is usually to measure the AP diameter of the bony spinal canal: if the distance between the posterior vertebral body and the lamina of the slipped vertebral body is increased when compared to the vertebrae above and below, we are dealing with spondylolysis, or – rarely – isthmic lengthening. If the distance between the posterior vertebral body and the lamina of the slipped vertebra is normal (compared to the vertebrae above and below) and the distance between the lamina of the slipped vertebra and and the posterior contour of the disc below is reduced, the slip

is most likely due to destruction or dysplasia of the facets (Fig. 4.20).

On plain lateral X-rays, the position of the spinous process can be assessed. If the spinous process of the slipping vertebra remains in alignment with its neighbours above and below, lengthening or fracture of the isthmus is most likely. If the spinous process moves forward together with the vertebral body, this is most likely due to facet dysplasia or destruction, and narrowing the central spinal canal can be deduced from this on the plain films.

The effect of spondylolytic and degenerative anterolisthesis upon the spinal canal is opposite, but their effect upon the foramen is similar. In both cases the exiting nerve or dorsal root ganglion can be compressed between the anterior surface of the inferior articular process of the vertebra which moves forward, and the posterior disc surface (Fig. 4.20b4; Jinkins and Rauch, 1994). Nerve root compression in this situation can be exacerbated by two factors:

- Disruption of the disc with upward displacement of disc material into the foramen, compressing the nerve root from below.
- Hypertrophic callus formation at the site of the fracture through the isthmus with later ossification, which may compress the nerve dorsally.

Retrolisthesis: Backward slippage of a vertebral body with respect to the body below is generally associated with decreased height of the intervertebral disc, and results from the overlapping relationship of the facets. The tip of the superior articular process of the lower vertebra moves upward into the foramen to compress the dorsal root ganglion against the lower border of the pedicle above, and the likelihood of this is increased in case of degenerative hypertrophy of the articular process.

Alternatively the distance of slippage can be expressed as a percentage of the A-P diameter of the end-plate.

The most severe grade of slip is called spondyloptosis, in which the upper vertebral body is displaced anterior to the lower vertebra.

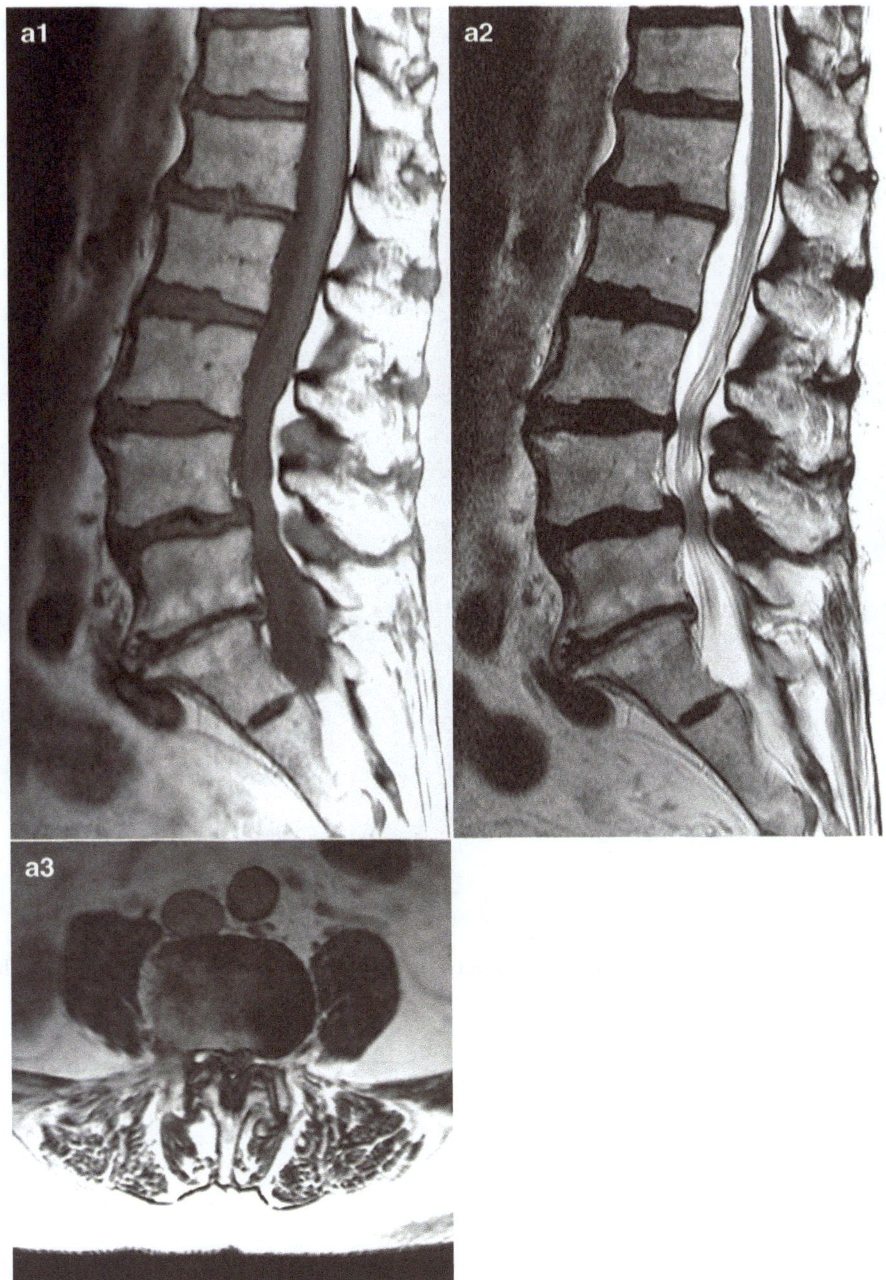

Fig. 4.20 Degenerative and spondylolytic anterolisthesis. (**a**) Degenerative anterolisthesis. *Presentation*: patient, female, 75 years, suffered from long-standing low back pain with irradiation to both legs, sometimes feet. No radicular signs, no neurologic deficits. *MRI*: sagittal T1- (**a1**) and T2-weighted images (**a2**) show grade 1 anterolisthesis at L4–5. Mid-sagittal bony AP diameter at L3 14 mm, at L4 15 mm and at L5 17 mm: therefore no spondylolysis. Disrupted L4–5 disc, bulging L3–4 disc, dorsal impression upon dural sac due to flaval hypertrophy (axial image **a3**).

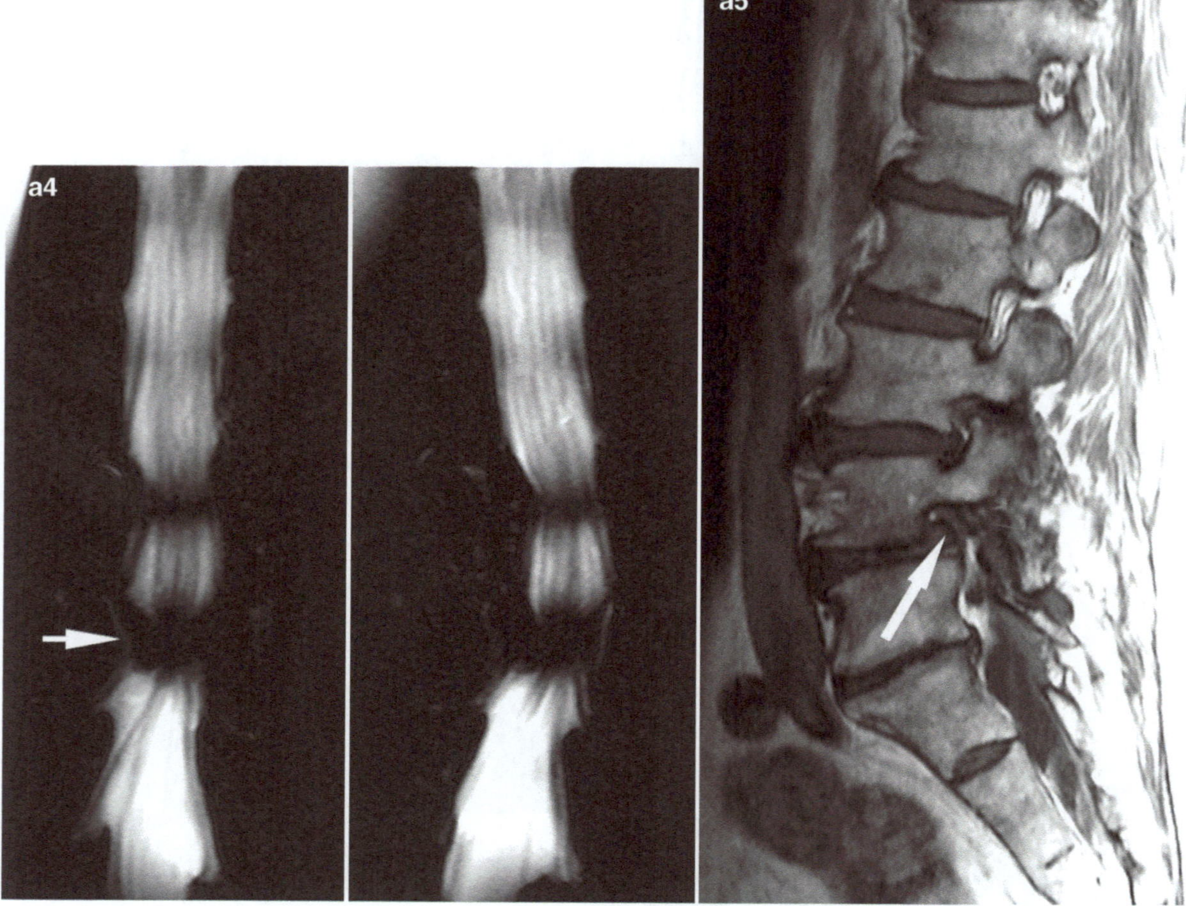

Fig. 4.20 Compression of dural sac with myelographic block at L4–5 (**a4** *arrow*), partial at L3–4. Disrupted L4–5 disc compressing L4 nerve root in foramen (**a5,** *arrow*).

Fig. 4.20 (**b**) Spondylolytic anterolisthesis. *Presentation*: patient, female, 37 years, reported long-standing low back pain with recent irradiation to left leg with sensory loss in left L5 dermatome. No limitation of SLR. *MRI*: sagittal T1- (**b1**) and T2-weighted images (**b2**) show grade 2 anterolisthesis at L5-S1. Mid-sagittal bony AP diameter at L4 is 18 mm, increasing to 30 mm at L5: therefore, spondylolysis or isthmic lengthening. Note disruption of L5-S1 disc, no dural compression. Widening of spinal canal also well seen on axial image at level of L5 spondylolysis (**b3**). Disrupted L5-S1 disc compressing left L5 dorsal root ganglion in foramen (**b4**, *arrow*)

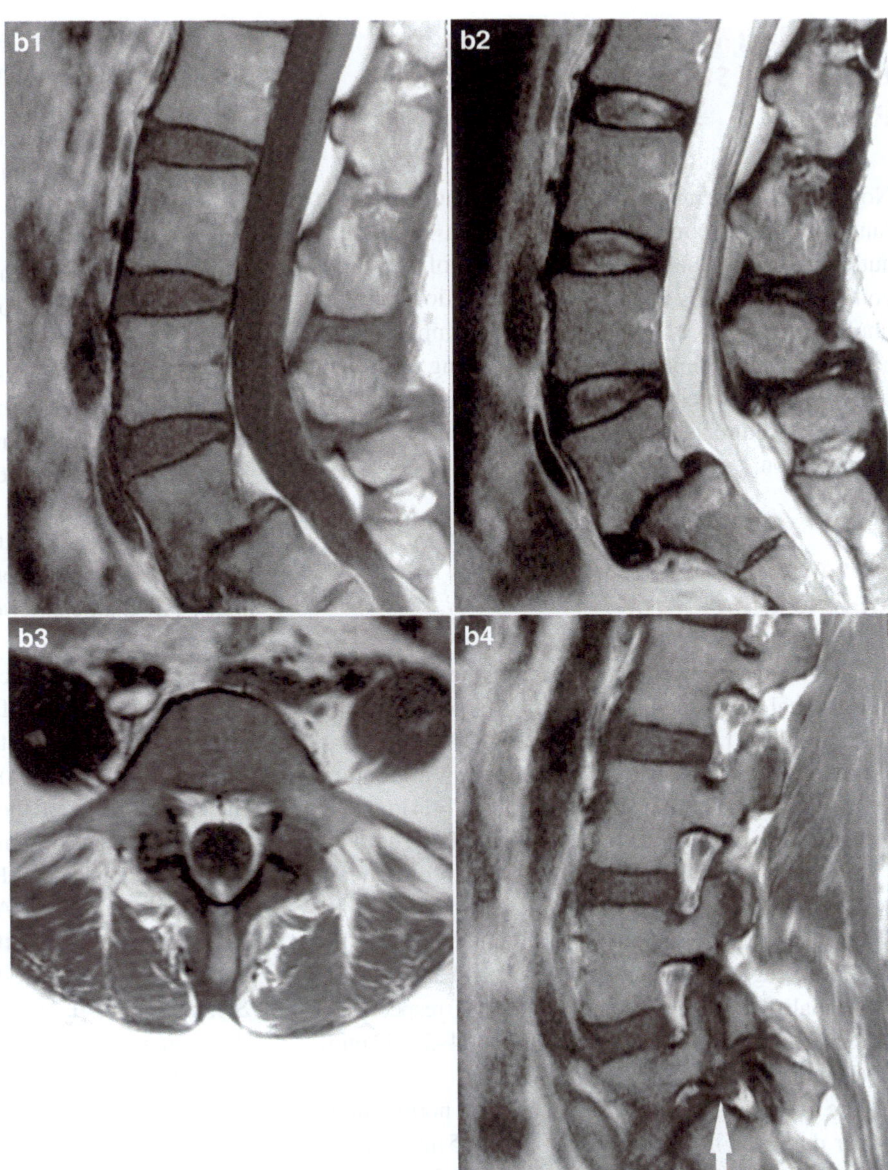

Appendix : Morphometrics of Lumbar Intraspinal Structures, A Literature Review

Note: Measurements can be misleading; note the wide range of normal limits frequently given by various authors. In individual cases the likelihood of nerve root compression usually depends on combinations of morphologic changes, which are difficult or impossible to capture in measurements. Instead of relying overmuch on simple measurements it is better to focus on key anatomic features such as nerve root or cauda equina compression.

Measurements in Normals and Patients, Static

- The average bony A-P diameter of the lumbar spinal canal measured in Caucasian skeletons is 17 mm (range 11–21 mm) (Eisenstein 1977).
- The average bony AP canal diameter in a group of individuals without back complaints is 14.4 mm (SD 1.4 mm) at L4 and 14.5 mm (SD 1.9) at L5. The average bony AP canal diameter in a group of patients with back complaints is 14.5 mm (SD 1.4 mm) at L4 and 15.7 mm (SD 2.8) at L5 (Wilmink et al. 1988).
- The average A-P dural diameter at L3–4 and L4–5 in normals is 13.9 mm and 14.6 mm, respectively (Schönstrom). In lordosis this value at L4–5 is 12 mm. (Penning and Wilmink 1987).
- The average cross-sectional area of the normal lumbar dural sac in lordosis at L4–5 is 145 mm² (range 86–230 mm²) (Penning and Wilmink 1987).
- The average cross-sectional area of the normal lumbar dural sac, measured at the level of the facets, is 178 mm² (Schönstrom et al. 1985).
- The average cross-sectional area of the retrodural fat pad at L4–5 is 33 mm² (range 18–58 mm²) (Penning and Wilmink 1987).
- The interflaval diameter is the distance between the inner borders of the flaval ligaments, measured on a line connecting the inner borders of the left and right facet joint space. The average interflaval diameter at L4–5 in normals is 14 mm (range 12–19 mm) (Penning and Wilmink 1987).
- The average interflaval diameter at L4–5 in normals is 14.6 mm (SD 3.8). In patients with sciatica the same average value is 11.2 mm. The borderline value is 11 mm (Wilmink et al. 1988).
- A lateral recess height (AP diameter) of 5 mm or more is normal. A height of 3–4 mm suggests lateral recess stenosis and a height of 2 mm or less is pathologic (Ciric et al. 1980).
- The normal foraminal height varies from 20 to 23 mm, and the A-P diameter of the upper foramen at the level of the dorsal root ganglion varies from 8 to 10 mm (Hasegawa et al. 1993).
- Absolute stenosis exists when the minimum bony AP diameter of the lumbar spinal canal, measured at the pedicular level, is smaller than 10 mm. Relative stenosis exists when the same diameter is between 10 and 12 mm (Verbiest 1976b).
- Bony AP diameters of the spinal canal of 12 mm or less were measured in only 4.7% of vertebral specimens. AP diameters were never less than 11 mm (Eisenstein 1977).
- In 24 patients with clinical signs of stenosis the average bony AP diameter of the lumbar spinal canal was 14 mm. In only two was the diameter less than 12 mm (Schönstrom et al. 1985).
- The AP diameter of the dural sac correlates better with clinical signs of stenosis than the bony AP diameter of the spinal canal (Penning 1992).
- The average minimal AP dural diameter at L3–4 and L4–5 in patients with stenosis is 9.1 mm. In normals these values are 13.9 and 14.6 mm, respectively (Schönstrom et al. 1985).
- The average cross-sectional area of the lumbar dural sac in patients with symptoms of spinal stenosis is 90 mm² (Schönstrom et al. 1985).
- Myelographic block occurs when the cross-sectional area of the dural sac at L4–5 is reduced below 40 mm² (Wilmink 1989).
- Intradural fluid transmission in a cadaver experiment was blocked when average cross-sectional area of the dural sac at L4 was reduced below 45.8 mm² (Schönstrom et al. 1984).

Measurements in Normals and Patients, Dynamic

- The increase in backward bulge of the normal L4–5 disc in extension in normals is about 1 mm (Penning and Wilmink 1981).

- The average inward bulge at L4–5 of the retrodural structures into the canal in extension compared to flexion in normals is about 2 mm (Penning and Wilmink 1981).
- The average craniocaudal movement of the dural end-sac in flexion–extension movements is 7.9 mm, maximum 25 mm (Penning and Wilmink 1981).
- The average decrease in length of the lumbar spinal canal when moving from flexion to extension in normal individuals is 16.6 mm (Penning and Wilmink 1981).
- The average reduction in cross-sectional area of the lumbar dural sac at L3–4 when moving from lumbar flexion to extension is 40 mm^2. The average reduction of the same area when going from unloaded to loaded spine is 50 mm^2 (Schönstrom 1988).
- The average reduction in A-P diameter of the dural sac in lumbar extension at L4–5 in a group of patients with sciatica is 3.6 mm: from 18.5 to 14.9 mm (Penning and Wilmink 1981).
- In normal individuals, the reduction of AP dural diameter when going from flexion to extension is about 9%. In severe stenosis it is about 67% (Sortland et al. 1977).
- In normal individuals, the AP dural diameter at L4–5, which is 12.6 mm on average, is reduced by 2.2 mm on average (17%) when going from flexion to extension. In individuals with stenosis the average AP dural diameter is 10.7 mm in flexion, reduced by 4.2 mm (39%) in extension (Wilmink et al. 1984).
- In a group of patients with clinical and myelographic signs of stenosis: the average AP diameter of the dural sac decreased from 10 mm (8–13) in flexion to 7 mm (5–11 mm) in extension (reduction by 30%). The retrodural fat pad bulged forward by about 2 mm in extension; the disc and the flaval ligaments bulged inward by about 1 mm.
- The interflaval diameter (the distance between the inner borders of the flaval ligaments, measured on a line connecting the inner borders of the left and right facet joint space) was reduced from 11 to 9 mm. The cross-sectional area of the dural sac at L4–5 was reduced from 105 to 66 mm^2 (37%) (Penning and Wilmink 1987).
- The mean reduction in A-P diameter of the dural sac in lumbar extension at L4–5 in a group of patients with sciatica is 3.6 mm; from 18.5 to 14.9 mm. In a subgroup of patients with normal myelograms the degree of reduction was about 3 mm (Penning and Wilmink 1981).

- A myelographic block in lumbar extension can be reduced by flexion of the lumbar spine (Teng and Papatheodorou 1963; Yamada et al. 1972).

Imaging Features of Compression of Individual Nerve Roots and Cauda Equina

Compression of an intradural nerve root is indicated by one or more of the following:

- Sectional images in axial plane:
  - Flattening of ventrolateral dural angle
  - Obliteration of fat adjacent to dural sac and around root sleeve
  - Nerve root enhancement
- Myelographic images:
  - Nerve root swelling
  - Cut-off of root sleeve filling
  - Dural impression
  - (Wilmink 1989)

Cauda equina compression is indicated by:

- Obliteration of CSF at site of compression: myelographic block
- Presence of coiled and elongated "redundant" roots adjacent to level of compression
- Reduction of transverse dural area <40 mm^2 (Wilmink 1989)

References

Asquier C, Troussier B, Chirossel JP et al (1996) Femoral neuralgia due to degenerative spinal disease. A retrospective clinical and radio-anatomical study of one hundred cases. Rev Rhum Engl Ed 63(4):278

Baddeley H (1976) Radiology of lumbar spinal stenosis. Sector, London

Bartynski WS, Lin L (2003) Lumbar root compression in the lateral recess: MR imaging, conventional myelography, and CT myelography comparison with surgical confirmation. AJNR Am J Neuroradiol 24(3):348

Boden SD, Davis DO, Dina TS et al (1990) Abnormal magnetic-resonance scans of the lumbar spine in asymptomatic subjects. A prospective investigation. J Bone Joint Surg Am 72(3):403

Boos N, Rieder R, Schade V et al (1995) 1995 Volvo Award in clinical sciences. The diagnostic accuracy of magnetic resonance imaging, work perception, and psychosocial factors in identifying symptomatic disc herniations. Spine 20(24):2613

Butt S, Saifuddin A (2005) The imaging of lumbar spondylolisthesis. Clin Radiol 60(5):533

Ciric I, Mikhael MA (1985) Lumbar spinal-lateral recess stenosis. Neurol Clin 3(2):417

Ciric I, Mikhael MA, Tarkington JA et al (1980) The lateral recess syndrome. A variant of spinal stenosis. J Neurosurg 53(4):433

Eisenstein S (1977) The morphometry and pathological anatomy of the lumbar spine in South African negroes and caucasoids with specific reference to spinal stenosis. J Bone Joint Surg Br 59(2):173

Eisenstein S (1980) The trefoil configuration of the lumbar vertebral canal. A study of South African skeletal material. J Bone Joint Surg Br 62-B(1):73

Epstein JA, Epstein BS, Rosenthal AD et al (1972) Sciatica caused by nerve root entrapment in the lateral recess: the superior facet syndrome. J Neurosurg 36(5):584

Fardon DF, Milette PC (2001) Nomenclature and classification of lumbar disc pathology. Recommendations of the Combined task Forces of the North American Spine Society, American Society of Spine Radiology, and American Society of Neuroradiology. Spine 26(5):E93

Fogel GR, Cunningham PY 3rd, Esses SI (2005) Spinal epidural lipomatosis: case reports, literature review and meta-analysis. Spine J 5(2):202

Fries JW, Abodeely DA, Vijungco JG et al (1982) Computed tomography of herniated and extruded nucleus pulposus. J Comput Assist Tomogr 6(5):874

Fujiwara A, Tamai K, An HS et al (2001) Orientation and osteoarthritis of the lumbar facet joint. Clin Orthop Relat Res 385:88

Hasegawa T, An HS, Haughton VM (1993) Imaging anatomy of the lateral lumbar spinal canal. Semin Ultrasound CT MR 14(6):404

Herzog RJ (1996) The radiologic assessment for a lumbar disc herniation. Spine 21(24 Suppl):19S

Jensen MC, Brant-Zawadzki MN, Obuchowski N et al (1994) Magnetic resonance imaging of the lumbar spine in people without back pain. N Engl J Med 331(2):69

Jinkins JR, Rauch A (1994) Magnetic resonance imaging of entrapment of lumbar nerve roots in spondylolytic spondylolisthesis. J Bone Joint Surg Am 76(11):1643

Lisai P, Doria C, Crissantu L et al (2001) Cauda equina syndrome secondary to idiopathic spinal epidural lipomatosis. Spine 26(3):307

Mixter WJ, Barr JS (1934) Rupture of the intervertebral disc with involvement of the spinal canal. New Engl J Med 211(5):210

Modic MT, Obuchowski NA, Ross JS et al (2005) Acute low back pain and radiculopathy: MR imaging findings and their prognostic role and effect on outcome. Radiology 237(2):597

Modic MT, Ross JS, Obuchowski NA et al (1995) Contrast-enhanced MR imaging in acute lumbar radiculopathy: a pilot study of the natural history. Radiology 195(2):429

Paine KW, Haung PW (1972) Lumbar disc syndrome. J Neurosurg 37(1):75

Papp T, Porter RW, Aspden RM (1995) Trefoil configuration and developmental stenosis of the lumbar vertebral canal. J Bone Joint Surg Br 77(3):469

Penning L (1992) Functional pathology of lumbar spinal stenosis. Clin Biomech 7:3

Penning L, Wilmink JT (1981) Biomechanics of lumbosacral dural sac. A study of flexion-extension myelography. Spine 6(4):398

Penning L, Wilmink JT (1987) Posture-dependent bilateral compression of L4 or L5 nerve roots in facet hypertrophy. A dynamic CT-myelographic study. Spine 12(5):488

Ramani P (1976) Variations in size of bony lumbar canal in patients with prolapse of lumbar intervertebral; discs. ClinRadiol 27(3):301

Robertson SC, Traynelis VC, Follett KA et al (1997) Idiopathic spinal epidural lipomatosis. Neurosurgery 41(1):68

Sanderson SP, Houten J, Errico T et al (2004) The unique characteristics of "upper" lumbar disc herniations. Neurosurgery 55(2):385

Schlesinger PT (1955) Incarceration of the first sacral nerve in a lateral bony recess of the spinal canal as a cause of sciatica. J Bone Joint Surg Am 37-A(1):115

Schönstrom N, Bolender N-F, Spengler D et al (1984) Pressure changes within the cauda equina following constriction of the dural sac. Spine 9:604

Schönstrom N. et al (1988). Dynamix changes in the dimensions of the lumber spinal canal. In: The narrow lumber spinal canal and the size of the cauda equina in man. Gothenburg University Press, Göteborg

Schönstrom NS, Bolender NF, Spengler DM (1985) The pathomorphology of spinal stenosis as seen on CT scans of the lumbar spine. Spine 10(9):806

Singh K, Samartzis D, Vaccaro AR et al (2005) Congenital lumbar spinal stenosis: a prospective, control-matched, cohort radiographic analysis. Spine J 5(6):615

Sortland O, Magnaes B, Hauge T (1977) Functional myelography with metrizamide in the diagnosis of lumbar spinal stenosis. Acta Radiol Suppl 355:42

Spangfort EV (1972) The lumbar disc herniation. A computer-aided analysis of 2,504 operations. Acta Orthop Scand Suppl 142:1

Teng P, Papatheodorou C (1963) Myelographic findings in spondylosis of the lumbar spine. Br J Radiol 36:122

van den Hauwe L (2007) Pathology of the posterior elements. In: Van Goethem J, van den Hauwe L, Parizel P (eds) Spinal imaging. Springer, Berlin

Van Gelderen C (1948) Ein orthotisches (lordotisches) kaudasyndrom. Acta Psychiat 23:57

Verbiest H (1949) Sur certaines formes rares de compression de la queue de cheval. 1. Les sténoses ossueuses du canal vertébral. Malone, Paris

Verbiest H (1954) A radicular syndrome from developmental narrowing of the lumbar vertebral canal. J Bone Joint Surg 36 B (2):230

Verbiest H (1976a) Neurogenic intermittent claudication. With special reference to stenosis of the lumbar spinal canal. Elsevier, Amsterdam

Verbiest H (1976b) Fallacies of the present definition, nomenclature and classification of the stenoses of the lumbar vertebral canal. Spine 1(4):217

Wilmink JT (1989) CT morphology of intrathecal lumbosacral nerve-root compression. AJNR Am J Neuroradiol 10(2):233

Wilmink JT, Korte JH, Penning L (1988) Dimensions of the spinal canal in individuals symptomatic and non-symptomatic for sciatica: a CT study. Neuroradiology 30(6):547

Wilmink JT, Penning L, van den Burg W (1984) Role of stenosis of spinal canal in L4-L5 nerve root compression assessed by flexion-extension myelography. Neuroradiology 26 (3):173

Wiltse LL, Winter RB (1983) Terminology and measurement of spondylolisthesis. J Bone Joint Surg Am 65(6): 768

Yamada O et al (1972) Intermittent cauda equina compression due to narrow spinal canal. J Neurosurg 37:83

5.1 Introduction

Lumbar disc herniation with protrusion or extrusion of the nucleus pulposus is often classified under degenerative spinal conditions but has a different epidemiological profile. Herniations occur with higher frequency in the middle-age group and even in adolescents, and sometimes without other degenerative spinal features such as spondylosis and spondylarthrosis, whereas the incidence of the latter manifestations appears to have a more linear relationship with increasing age (Boden et al. 1990).

Not all degenerative lumbar spinal conditions are amenable to operative therapy. Surgical interventions in patients with sciatica and related complaints, with the exception of those performed for the purpose of spinal stabilisation, are usually aimed at relieving compression of a nerve root or of multiple roots. As discussed in Chap. 4, such compression can be due to one of many possible combinations of degenerative lumbar spinal changes. These form a morphologic spectrum ranging from a case of a large disc herniation causing nerve root compression in an otherwise normal spinal canal, to a case with a severely narrowed spinal canal, in which mild degenerative annular bulging or even the slight posterior displacement of the normal annulus fibrosus in spinal extension, is sufficient to produce cauda equina compression. Between these two extremes, many intermediate conditions and combinations are possible (see Fig. 4.13). In the first case of a herniated disc in a normal canal, surgical removal of the herniation or reduction of its volume by one of various percutaneous techniques is sufficient to relieve symptoms. In the last case, when narrowing of the spinal canal by bony or ligamentous pathology plays a substantial or predominant role, more extensive decompressive procedures such as flavectomy and facetectomy or more extensive laminectomy may be necessary.

5.2 Pre-Operative Imaging

When diagnostic imaging performed in a patient with sciatica or a related complaint demonstrates an intraspinal lesion (herniated disc, spinal canal narrowing or combination) and surgical therapy is contemplated, the following two questions first need to be addressed:

1. Is the spinal lesion responsible for the presenting symptoms or are we dealing with a chance finding of an incidental disc herniation or insignificant spinal narrowing?
2. Is the condition likely to show an early favourable response to conservative therapy, or is conservative management likely to fail in the long run, and is early surgery preferable?

5.2.1 Is the Lesion Responsible for the Presenting Symptoms?

This question directly determines patient selection for a possible spinal operation. It is important to bear in mind that there is no one-to-one relationship between the presence of radicular pain on the one hand, and that of a lumbar disc herniation on the other. The one can be present without the other, and *vice versa* (see Chap. 4).

There are many potential causes of low back pain irradiating to the leg: the nerve root may be compressed

J. T. Wilmink, *Lumbar Spinal Imaging in Radicular Pain and Related Conditions*
DOI: 10.1007/978-3-540-93830-9_5, © Springer-Verlag Berlin Heidelberg 2010

by a herniated disc, by narrowing of the spinal canal, of the lateral recess or the intervertebral foramen, by scar formation, or a neoplasm. Besides mechanical compression of the root, inflammatory factors are considered to play a role in the pathogenesis of sciatica (see Chap. 1). Non-radicular so-called pseudoradicular pain can originate in structures such as the hip or the sacro-iliac joint or the spinal facets, and can be referred to the lower extremity in a deceptive fashion. A presentation of intermittent claudication in arterial occlusive disease of the lower extremities can mislead the unwary observer into diagnosing neurogenic claudication due to cauda equina compression in spinal stenosis.

Disc abnormalities can be seen with considerable frequency in individuals without any complaints of low back pain or sciatica, who are undergoing spinal imaging for other medical reasons, or taking part in volunteer studies. This applies in similar frequencies to all techniques suitable for imaging such abnormalities.

Hitselberger and Witten (1968) reported lumbar and cervical abnormal myelographic findings in 110 out of 300 patients undergoing intradural contrast administration for diagnosis of acoustic neuroma and without symptoms of nerve root compression. Wiesel et al. (1984) found disc herniations in 35% of CT studies from 52 asymptomatic individuals, and Boden et al. (1990) reported MRI findings of herniated discs or spinal stenosis in one-third of a group of 67 people who had no complaints related to these conditions, with the incidence of stenosis especially increasing with age. In a 7-year follow-up study, Borenstein et al. (2001) concluded that people with such an asymptomatic disc herniation were not at increased risk of developing low back pain.

On the other hand, Modic et al. (1995) documented normal lumbar spinal MRI findings in 5 out of 25 patients with clinical signs and symptoms of an acute lumbar radiculopathy.

Sometimes in a patient with sciatica, a disc herniation can be seen on the side opposite to the clinical symptoms, apparently a chance finding unrelated to the symptoms (Figs. 5.1 and 5.2a). An injudicious decision to operate may result in the removal of an asymptomatic disc herniation while the true cause of the pain, whatever it may be, remains untreated.

A review is now given of imaging features which may be helpful in determining whether or not a given spinal lesion is likely to be associated with occurrence of sciatica and related symptoms.

5.2.1.1 Radiologic Features of a Disc Lesion Related to Clinical Significance: Shape and Size

As set out in Chap. 4, disc displacements can be classified as diffuse bulges or more localised herniations. Herniations can be protrusions which are still contained within the outer annular fibres, or extrusions no longer contained by the annulus fibrosus. Extrusions are usually larger than protrusions (Fries et al. 1982).

In a study by Jensen et al. (1994) featuring 98 asymptomatic volunteers and 27 patients with back pain, the classification revealed the following clinical correlations: disc bulges were seen in 52% of the volunteers and 76% of the patients; disc protrusions in 27% of volunteers and 54% of patients. The difference in prevalence of bulges and protrusions between patients and volunteers appears insufficiently great to be diagnostically useful in individual cases. Disc extrusions, however, were seen in only 1% of volunteers and in 26% of patients. The virtual absence of disc extrusions in the volunteer group in this study suggests that the finding of an extrusion reliably indicates a symptomatic disc lesion. As always there are exceptions to the rule, however: Fig. 5.2b illustrates another case of an extrusion, this time modest-sized and in the roomy central region of the spinal canal, and apparently not causing symptoms (see also Fig. 4.3d,g).

Porchet et al. (2002) studied 394 patients with sciatica and/or back pain, and found a correlation between the severity of leg pain and disability, with the severity of disc abnormality (normal, bulging, protruded, extruded, sequestrated). There was an inverse relationship with the severity of back pain. Beattie et al. (2000) studying 408 patients with low back pain and/or radiculopathy, found a strong correlation only between the presence of disc extrusion causing severe nerve root compression, with distal leg pain.

However, Karppinen et al. (2001), reporting on 160 patients, found no correlation of the degree of disc abnormality on the one hand, with the intensity of back and leg pain and the degree of disability on the other.

Modic et al. (2005) studied 246 patients with low back pain or sciatica, and also found no relationship between the number or extent of herniations and patients' signs and symptoms. In this study the prevalence of disc herniations did not differ significantly between those with only low back pain and those with sciatica: herniations were present in 57% and 62% respectively.

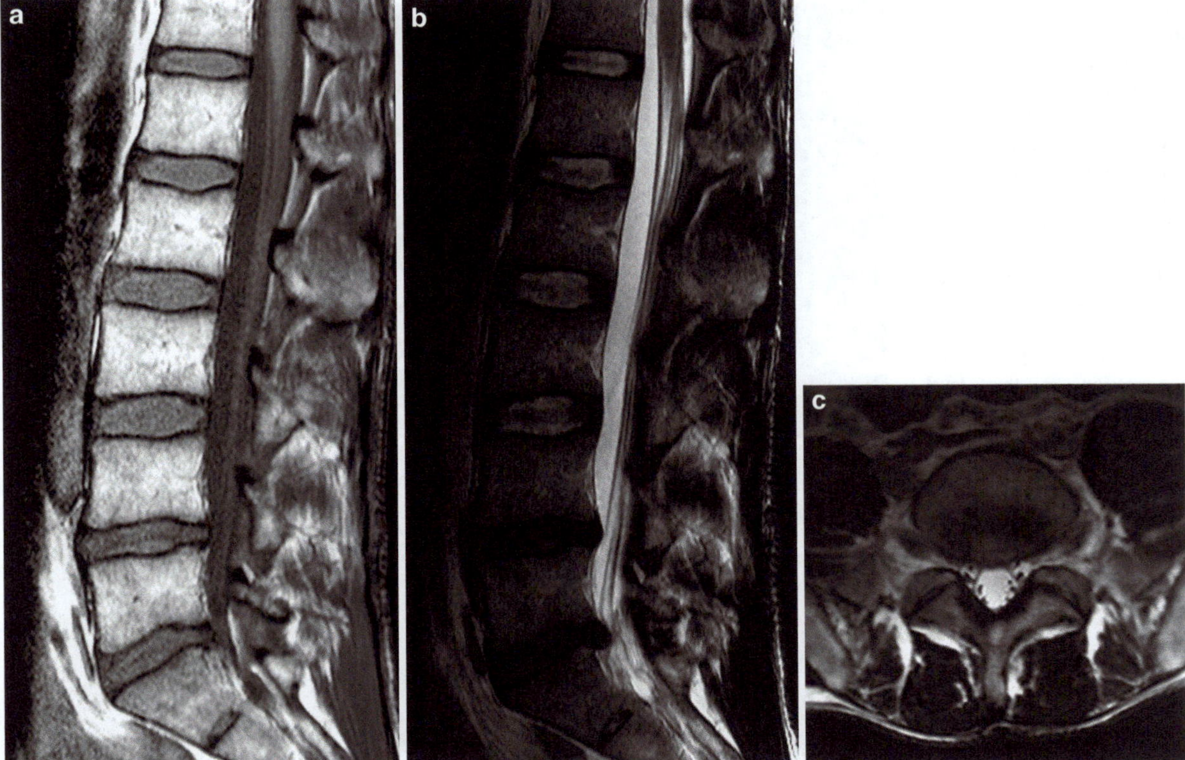

Fig. 5.1 Disc extrusion contralateral to side of symptoms. *Presentation*: patient, male 29 years, described pain in left buttock irradiating to lateral side of thigh, calf and foot. Straight-leg-raising was limited on left side, with crossed SLR sign upon raising of right leg, also some motor and sensory loss in left leg with radicular distribution. No pain on right. *MRI*: small L5-S1 extrusion demonstrated in sagittal T1 (**a**) and T2-weighted images (**b**).

5.2.1.2 Assessment of Relative Size of the Herniation with Respect to Dimensions of the Canal

As the conflicting findings mentioned above indicate, the likelihood of a disc herniation causing symptoms and the severity of symptoms of nerve root compression, appear to depend not only on the volume of the displaced disc material. Variations in roominess of the spinal canal also play a role. The level of the herniation is also of significance: at L4–5 and L5-S1, where most disc herniations occur, the shape of the spinal canal is triangular, so that in the central region there is more room than in the lateral recess (see Fig. 5.2b). A small herniation can easily compress a nerve root within the confined space of the lateral recess (Fig. 5.2c); even a bulging disc can cause compression of a nerve root here (see Chap. 4) (see also Fig 4.3h).

Thelander et al. (1994) compared different methods of relating the size of a disc herniation to the size of the spinal canal in 30 patients (using CT measurements of areas as well as linear measurements in either one or two directions), and found significant correlations of the relative size of the hernia with the degree of sciatica. Linear measurements of the hernia and canal in two perpendicular directions were found to be practical and accurate.

Carlisle et.al. (2005) performed a retrospective study comparing the degree of canal compromise by a disc herniation in 44 patients who had undergone surgery, with 44 other patients from the same pool who had not been operated. The area of the herniation at the level of maximal compromise was calculated as a percentage of the area of the spinal canal at the same level. The overall canal compromise in the operated group was 47%, against 32% compromise in the non-operated group. The trend was thus for surgically treated patients to have larger herniations than those treated non-operatively. This trend was more marked in central herniations at all levels than in laterally located herniations at L4–5, probably because in the lateral

Fig. 5.1 Axial images (**c-e**) show broad-based L5-S1 extrusion somewhat right of midline, some flattening of right S1 root sleeve (*arrows*), with thinning of CSF around right S1 root visible on right oblique myelographic projection (**f**, *arrow*), no root compression or swelling. Patient had previously undergone left L4–5 laminectomy, see post-operative dorsolateral bulging of dural sac (*long arrows* in **f**). No root compression at this level. Asymptomatic right L5-S1 extrusion. No explanation for left-sided symptoms

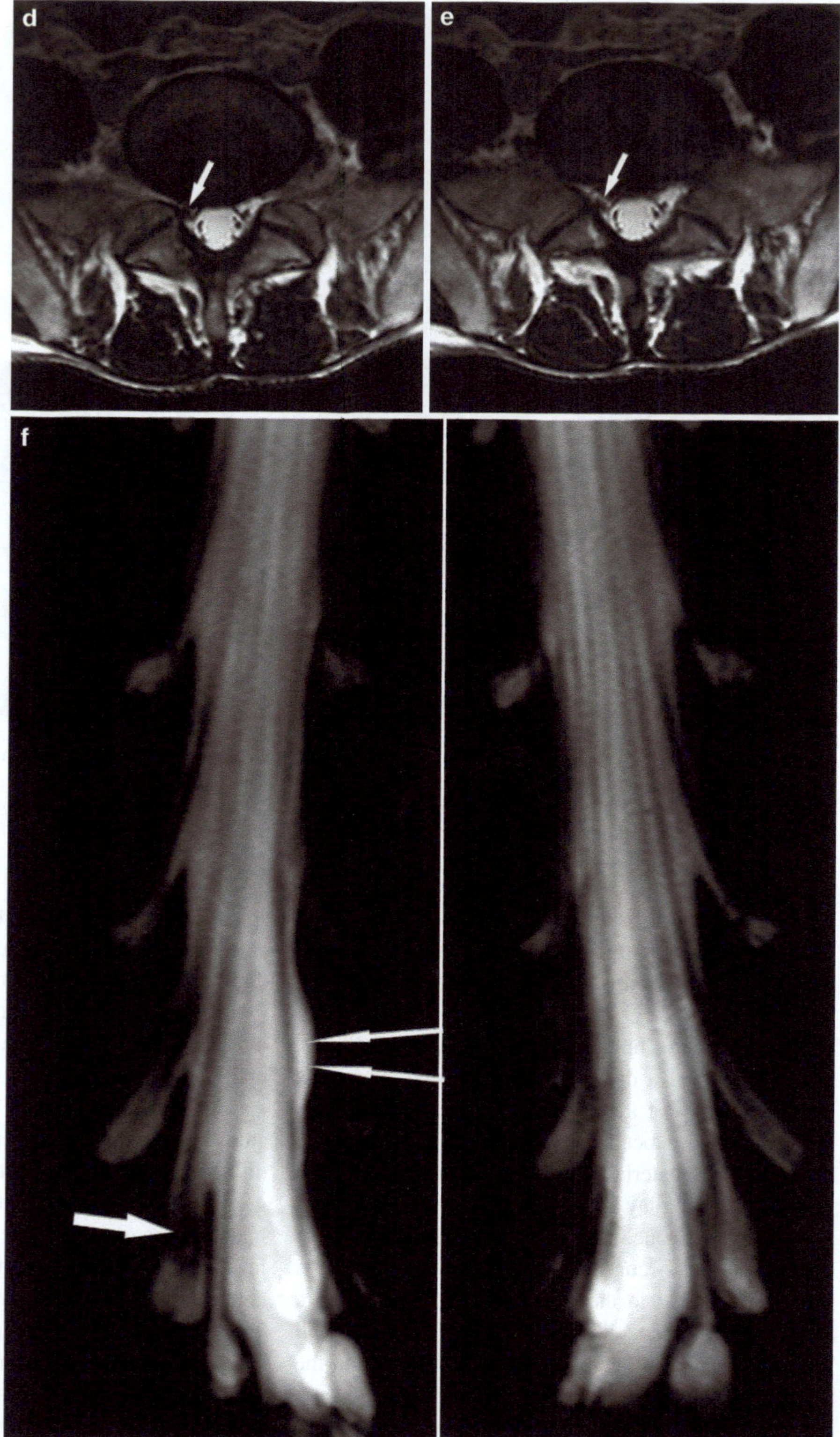

Fig. 5.2 Ratio of size of extruded disc to local spinal dimensions determines risk of root compression: three cases. *Presentation case **a***: patient complained of left sciatica. No other clinical date available. *CT*: CT (**a**) shows L4–5 disc herniation centred in right paracentral zone impressing upon dural sac. Note roomy spinal canal, note ventrolateral angle of dural sac containing traversing nerve root flattened by herniation but not obliterated (estimated location of right L5 intradural root indicated by *arrow*). No effacement of epidural fat adjacent to dural sac. Asymptomatic right L4–5 disc herniation. Cause of left-sided complaints not clear from this study.

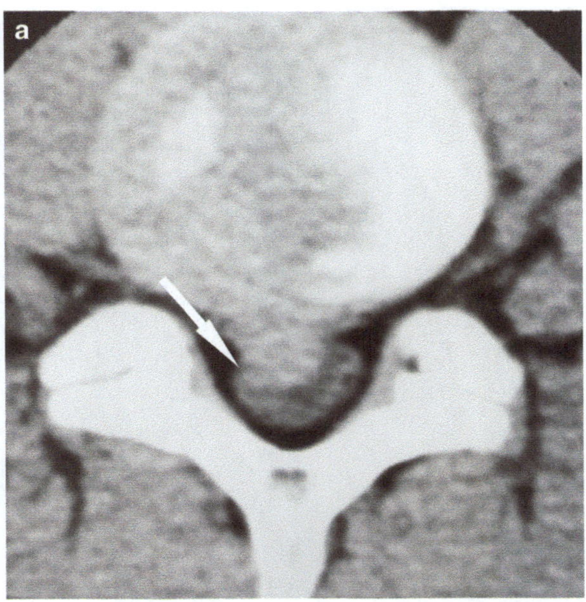

recess which is present at L4–5 the location is more relevant than the size of the herniation alone.

With regard to dimensions of the spinal canal, a plethora of measurements has been suggested (see Appendix Chap. 4). It is unwise, however, to rely overmuch on spinal measurements.

Verbiest, as described in Chap. 4, regarded a midsagittal A-P diameter of the bony spinal canal less than 10 mm to represent 'absolute stenosis'; i.e. sufficient to cause cauda equina compression and neurogenic claudication by itself. In case of 'relative stenosis' with a bony A-P spinal diameter of 10–12 mm, additional pathology such as small disc protrusions or vertebral osteophytes would be necessary to produce symptoms. This definition of 'relative' stenosis can of course be expanded to include larger canal dimensions when combined with larger disc displacements or greater bony spurring.

As also mentioned in Chap. 4, Ciric et al. regarded an A-P diameter of the bony lateral recess of 3–4 mm to be suggestive of lateral recess narrowing, and less than 2 mm to be definitely pathologic. This is again a limited point of view, as it focuses only on bony dimensions and excludes ligamentous hypertrophy or disc bulging, for instance, as a relevant factor in producing nerve root compression within the lateral recess.

5.2.1.3 Imaging of Nerve Root Compression: MR Myelography

We can also see if it is possible to correlate the occurrence of sciatica and related complaints with compression of the dural sac and the traversing nerve root.

Boos et al. (1995) compared various MRI findings and psychosocial features in 46 patients with low back pain and sciatica with the same features in 46 matched asymptomatic controls, finding disc herniations in 96% of patients but also 76% of matched controls! Severe extrusions were found in 35% of patients and 13% of controls. The only significant difference regarding MRI findings between the groups was that of nerve root compromise, which occurred in 96% of the study group and 22% of the control group ($p < 0.0001$).

Weishaupt et al. (1998) studied 60 asymptomatic volunteers, finding bulging discs in 37; protrusions in 40; extrusions in 11, and nerve root compression in only one.

Karppinen et al. (2001) studied 160 patients with sciatica and did not find a relationship of complaints with nerve root compression, however.

In the studies mentioned above, nerve root compression was estimated on standard sectional MR images. Bartynsky et.al. in a study of 26 patients with lateral recess stenosis using CT, MRI and conventional

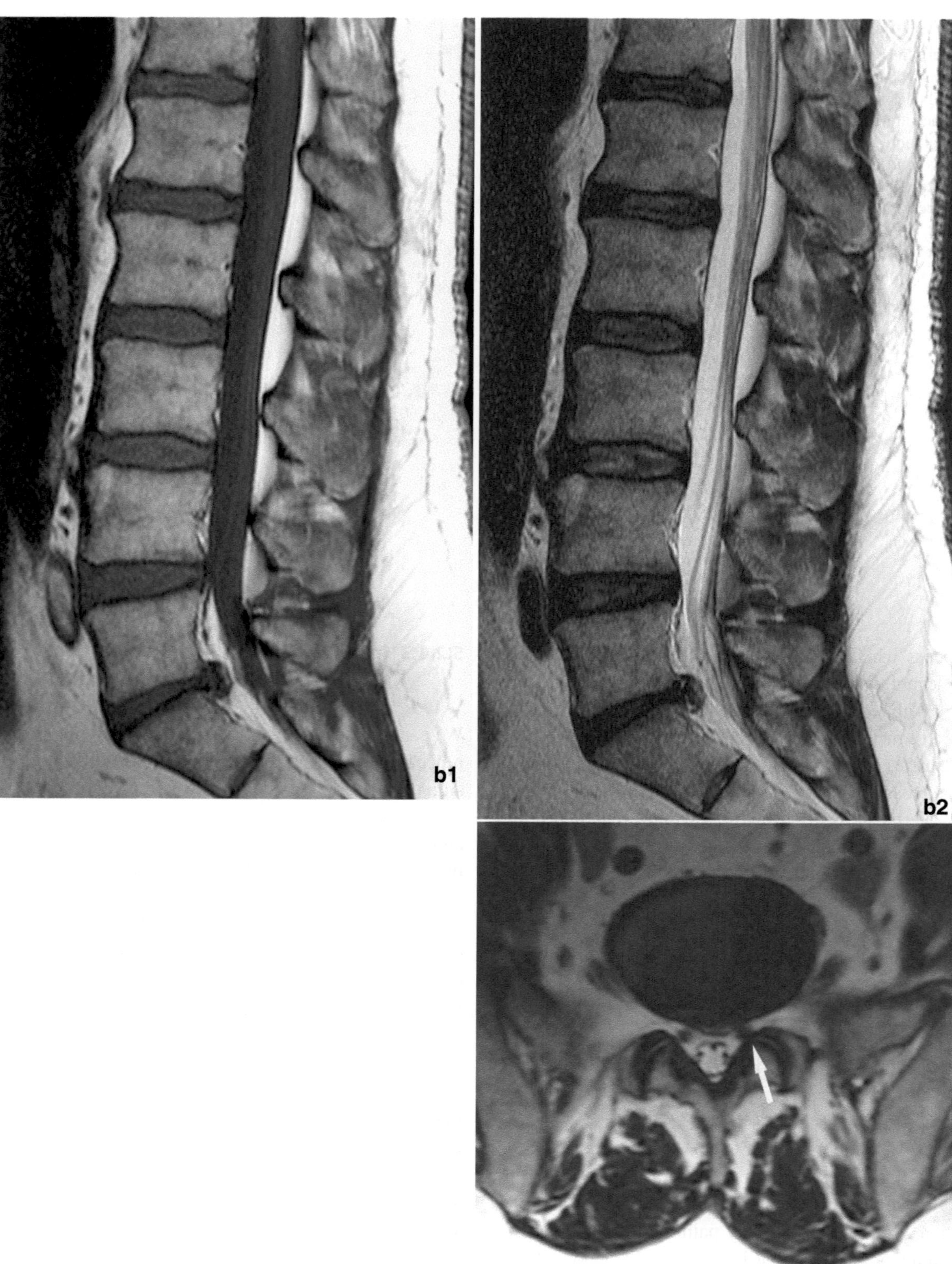

b1
b2
b3

Fig. 5.2 Presentation case (**b**): patient, male 55 years, with long-standing pain radiating from right hip region to anterior right thigh, without signs of L5 or S1 radicular involvement, or neurologic deficit. *MRI*: moderately large L5-S1 central extrusion on sagittal T1 (**b1**) and T2-weighted images (**b2**) normal mid-sagittal bony A-P diameter of 17 mm at level of L5 lamina. Axial T2-weighted image (**b3**) confirms midline herniation and sufficiently roomy central canal, with traversing S1 root sleeves just escaping compression in lateral regions which are somewhat constricted by facet hypertrophy, especially at left (*arrow*). MR myelographic images (**b4**) not helpful because of short S1 root sleeves (*arrows*). Central L5-S1 extrusion in spinal canal just sufficiently roomy to accommodate disc lesion. Cause of irradiating right hip and thigh pain not clear from these images.

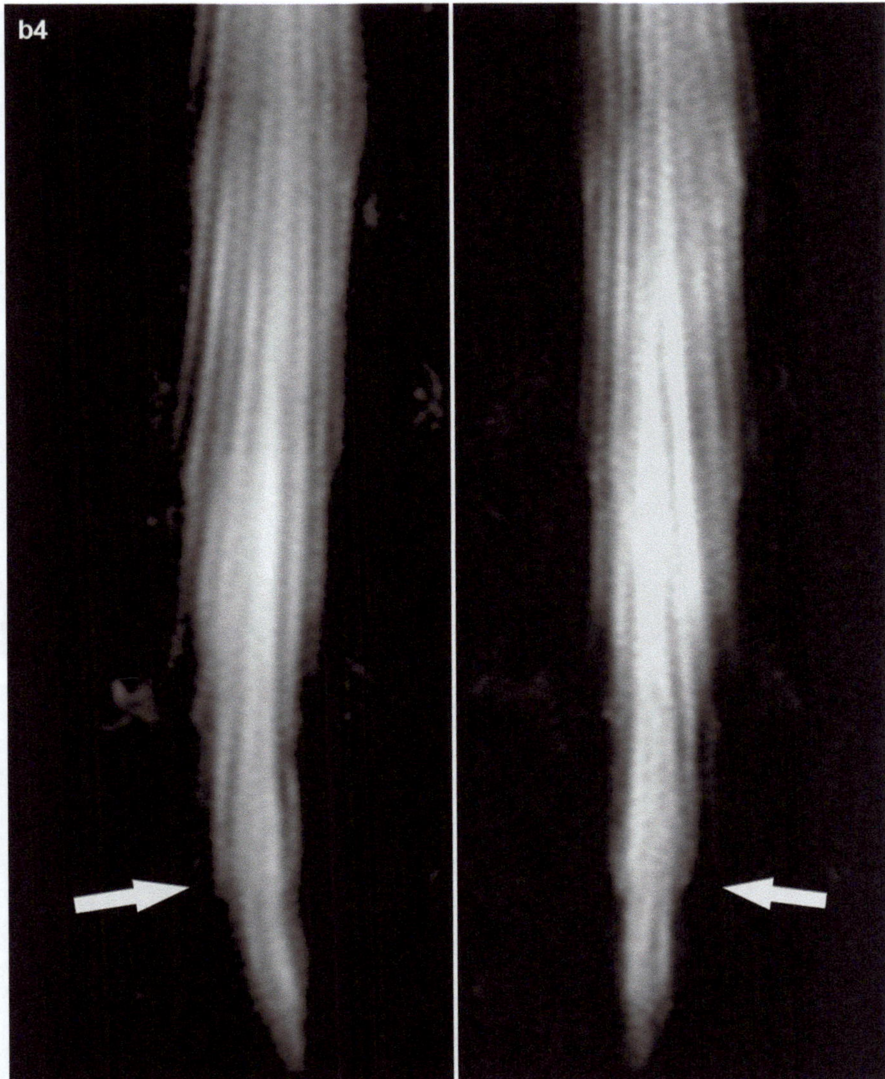

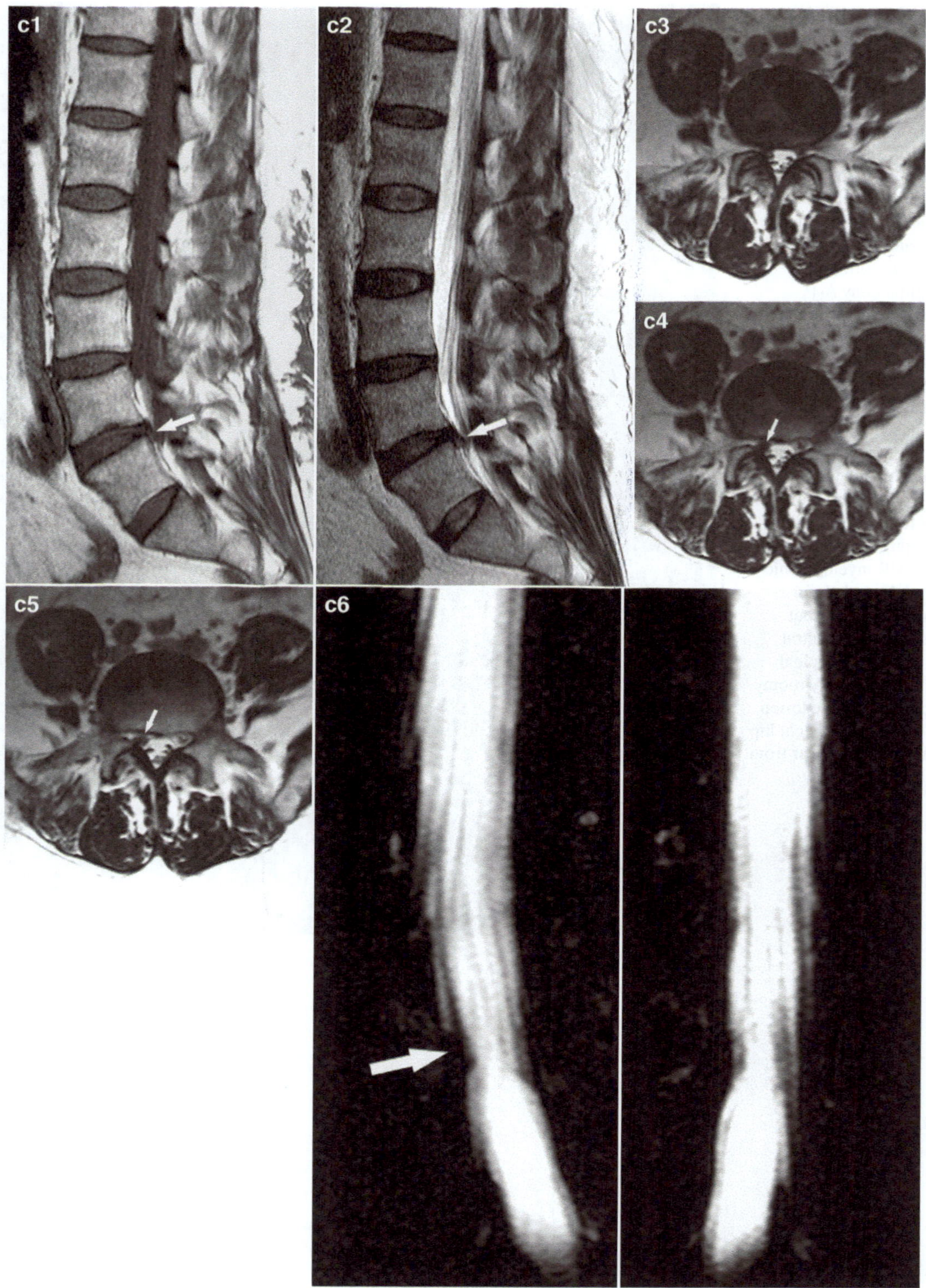

Fig. 5.2 Presentation case (**c**): patient, male 54 years, reported severe pain irradiating from low back to lateral aspect of right thigh and lower leg, and to hallux, with sensory loss in right foot; no limitation of straight-leg-raising. *MRI*: small L4–5 disc extrusion migrated to right L5 lateral recess seen in right parasagittal T1 and T2-weighted images (**c1, 2,** *arrows*) Consecutive axial T2-weighted images show compression of right L5 root in lateral recess by small disc fragment (**c3–5,** *arrows*) and MR myelogram clearly confirms right L5 root compression (**c6,** *arrow*). Small L4-5 extrusion, compressing L5 root due to limited space in lateral recess.

myelography, concluded that myelography provided crucial confirmation of degenerative nerve root impingement in the lateral recess as a cause of radiculopathy.

With the availability of fast spin-echo MRI sequences capable of producing a very bright CSF signal in a rapid acquisition, MR myelography became feasible (Krudy 1992, see also Chap. 2; Figs. 2.14–2.16). This technique provides images of the nerve root sleeves practically equivalent to conventional myelography (Kuroki et al. 1998). MR myelography was evaluated in a study of 43 patients with sciatica, and was reported to improve considerably the confidence of the assessment of nerve root compression in 13 out of 19 (68%) of those cases with questionable nerve root involvement (30% of all 43 cases studied) (Hofman and Wilmink 1996).

Vroomen et al. (2002a) studied 274 patients with sciatica and found nerve root compression demonstrated by MR myelography to be associated with paresis, absence of tendon reflexes, a positive straight-leg-raising test and limitation of spinal flexion.

O'Connell et al. (2003), however, in a study of 207 patients with low back pain and sciatica found routine MR myelography to be of limited value, assisting diagnosis in only 6% of cases.

5.2.1.4 Intravenous Contrast Studies of Nerve Root Enhancement

Enhancement of lumbosacral nerve roots after intravenous injection of gadolinium contrast media in patients with sciatica (Fig. 5.3) has been reported with varying frequency.

Jinkins (1993) saw enhancement of single and multiple nerve roots in seven out of 33 patients with lumbosacral pain syndromes and disc herniations (21%), but also in three patients without herniations.

Toyone et al. (1993) studied 25 patients with sciatica, and observed enhancement of a symptomatic root in 17 (68%), with more diffuse enhancement associated with more severe sciatica. After operation which was performed in 18 patients, enhancement was no longer seen.

Crisi et al. (1993), reporting on 20 patients, described root enhancement from the site of compression up to the conus medullaris in six cases (30%), associated with a larger size of disc herniation but not with greater severity of symptoms. After successful conservative or surgical therapy, follow-up MRI at 1 year showed no

root enhancement.

Taneichi et al. (1994) saw nerve root enhancement positively correlated to severity and short duration of radicular pain in 39% of 115 patients about to undergo spinal surgery. In 6% there was also enhancement of radicular veins. The presence of nerve root enhancement did not predict outcome.

Lane et al. (1996) considered that radicular veins rather than nerve roots were involved in the phenomenon of intradural contrast enhancement.

Vroomen et al. (1998) studied 71 patients with sciatica by post-contrast MRI, and saw segmental or diffuse nerve root enhancement in 25 (35%). Nerve root enhancement proved to be related to neurologic deficit, especially sensory loss, rather than severe pain or limited straight-leg-raising.

Karppinen et al. (2001) found no correlation of root enhancement, which was present in 44% of 160 patients with sciatica on the one hand, with subjective symptoms on the other.

5.2.1.5 Conclusion

There is no single feature which infallibly distinguishes a symptomatic disc herniation on the one hand from a chance finding on the other. The risk of misinterpretation may, however, be minimised by heeding the following guidelines.

Firstly, the anatomic location of the lesion should be matched against the clinical localisation as determined by the dermatome in which pain and/or sensory loss is distributed, and the radicular level of paresis and loss of deep tendon reflexes. Lumbosacral transitional anomalies may confound the issue, and in any case a discrepancy of between the anatomic and the clinical level of a radicular syndrome is not uncommon (Fig. 5.4; Aejmelaeus et al. 1984; see also Chap. 1). The greater the discrepancy, however, the less likely a causal relationship: clearly an S1 radicular syndrome is very unlikely to be the result of an L1–2 disc herniation.

Then the size and localisation of the disc lesion and the dimensions of the spinal canal must be taken into account. A disc extrusion, usually being larger, is much more likely to produce radicular symptoms than a protrusion. An extrusion in a roomy spinal canal, however, especially when located in or near the midline, can easily remain asymptomatic. Close scrutiny of key

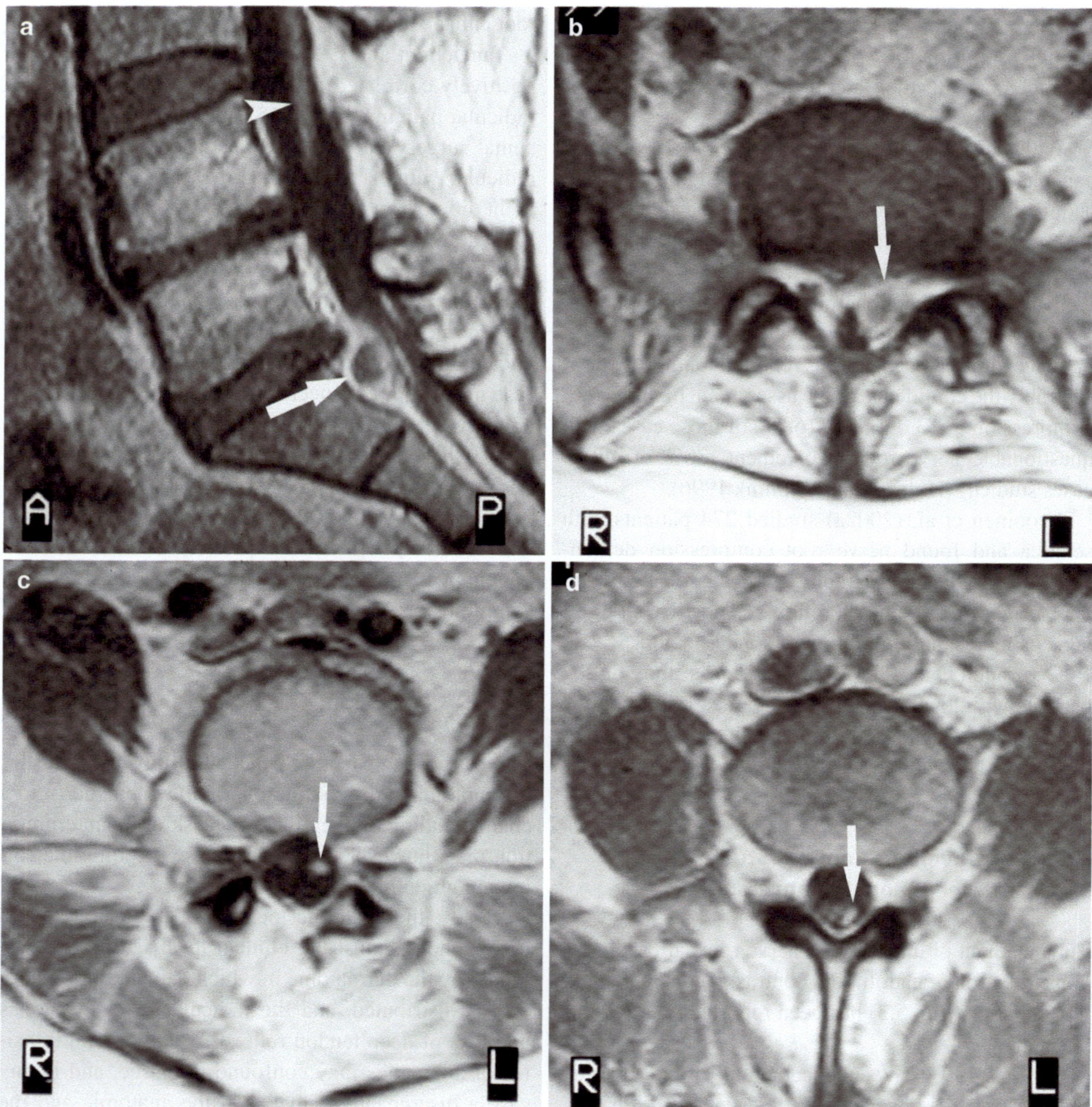

Fig. 5.3 Contrast enhancement of sequestrated disc extrusion and of compressed nerve root. *Presentation*: patient, female 57 years, was referred with left S1 radicular syndrome after two previous surgical procedures at L4–5 level. *MRI*: left sequestrated L5-S1 disc fragment showing rim enhancement on post-gadolinium sagittal (**a**) and axial (**b**) T1-weighted images (*arrows*); compression of left S1 root. Higher axial section (**c**) shows previous L4–5 laminectomy as well as enhancing S1 root (*arrow*), which is also visible at L3 level (**d**). This enhancing root could be followed to conus level and is also partially visualised in a (*arrowhead*)

areas and structures such as the ventrolateral border of the dural sac, the emerging root sleeve and the adjacent epidural fat, looking for evidence of nerve root compression, is more profitable than uncritically performing linear or area measurements.

MR myelography appears to possess value as an ancillary investigation in a subgroup of patients in whom the standard MRI sequences show some disc and/or canal pathology and possible nerve root compression, but where there is insufficient clarity with regard to the state of the nerve root. It is useful to stress that MR myelography provides information only on the state of the intradural root and root sleeve, and can never take the place of the standard MR images which more clearly demonstrate the presence of the offending disc herniation as well as other relevant details of spinal pathology. One could say that the standard MR images show the potential *cause* of root compression, but the MR myelogram better demonstrates the *effect*. The two complement one another.

Another aspect to bear in mind is the influence of postural variations. In a number of cases nerve root compression may take place only when the patient is erect, but is no longer visible when the same patient is lying supine in an MRI or CT scanner. Such posturally induced morphologic changes are usually quite small but may be significant especially in cases of narrowing of the spinal canal or the lateral recess (see Figs. 4.12 and 4.17). Careful questioning of the patient will reveal whether symptoms are markedly posture-dependent, and when indicated, additional imaging can be performed with the patient upright, by conventional contrast myelography or in an open upright MRI system. It is, however, highly unlikely that in a patient with a completely normal aspect of the disc, spinal canal and lateral recesses in the supine position, nerve root compression will be demonstrated in the upright posture.

The phenomenon of contrast enhancement of a (presumably inflamed and irritated) nerve root is of considerable theoretical interest, but the lack of sensitivity and also specificity of this finding make it unsuitable at present as a routine test. The inflammatory changes in and around the compressed nerve root, described in more detail in Chap. 1, are relevant and possibly essential for the production of radicular pain, but apparently only in conjunction with mechanical compression or deformation of the nerve root by a herniated disc or another agent.

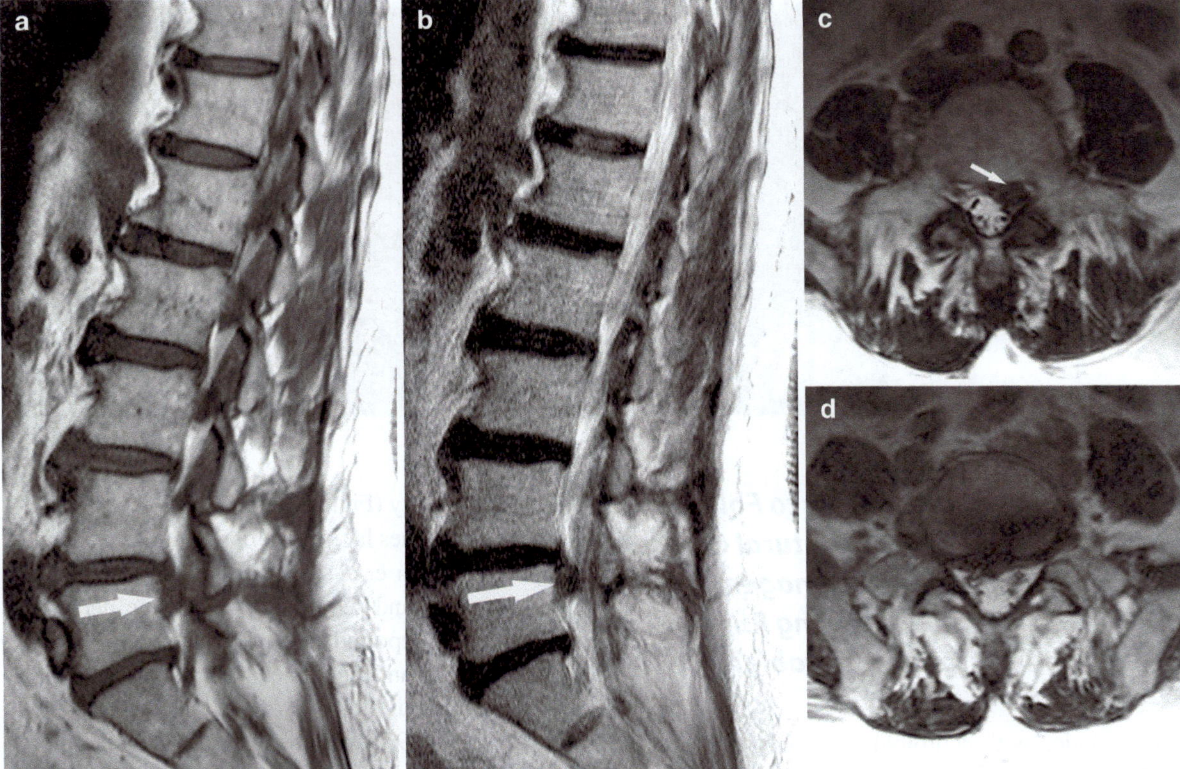

Fig. 5.4 Discrepancy between clinical and radiological levels. *Presentation*: patient, male 63 years, reported pain irradiating from lower back via S1 dermatome to lateral border of the left foot and little toe, with sensory loss in S1 dermatome and absent left ankle jerk, SLR limited on left. *MRI*: left L4–5 extrusion (*arrows*) seen on T1- (**a**) and T2-weighted sagittal images (**b**). Axial T2-weighted image (**c**) shows migration to L5 lateral recess (*arrow*), L5-S1 disc (**d**) shows only insignificant right paracentral protrusion not compressing root. MR myelograms show only L5 root compression, with some swelling of distal intradural root and non-filling root sleeve (**e**, *arrow*). Classic presentation of an S1 radicular syndrome, but in this case due to an L4–5 disc extrusion with L5 root involvement

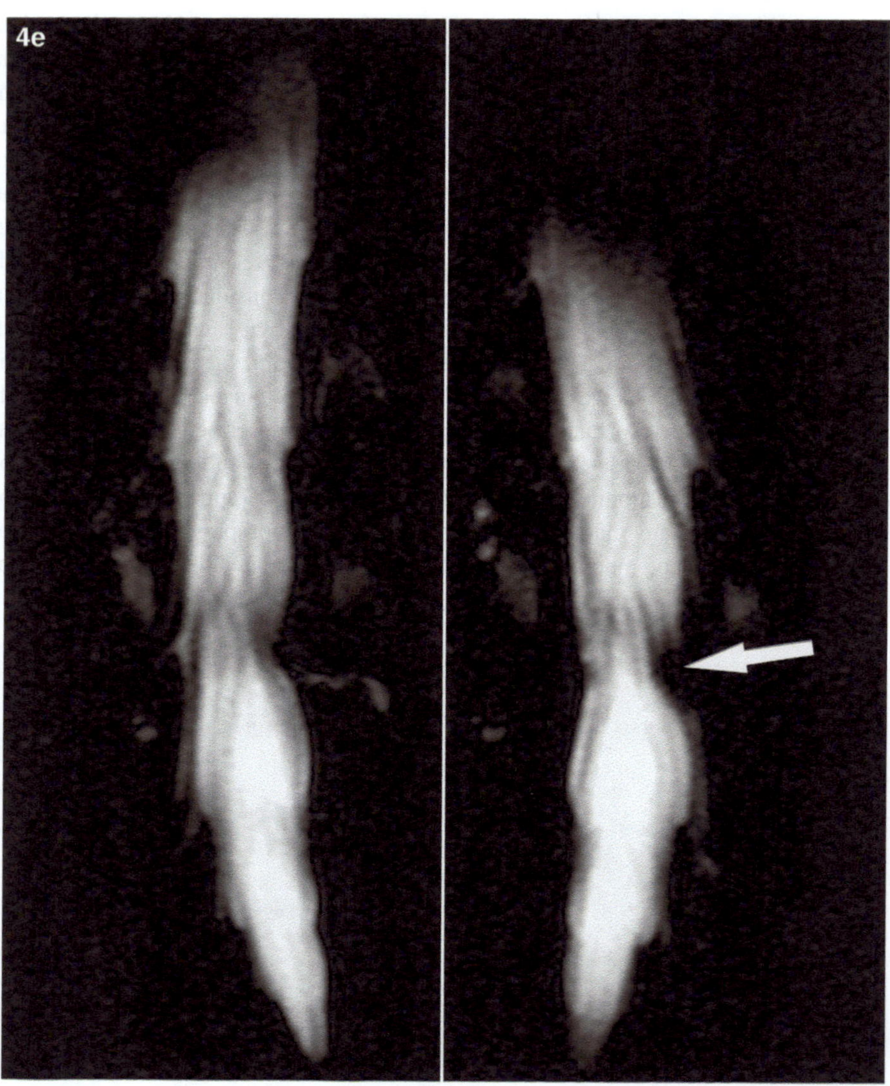

Fig. 5.4 (continued)

5.2.2 Is the Condition Likely to Follow a Favourable Early Natural Course, or Is Conservative Management Likely to Fail in the Long Run, and Is Early Surgery Preferable?

Acute sciatica with neurological symptoms is a transient condition which, with few exceptions, subsides after a relatively short period (Hakelius 1970). Good or excellent outcomes have been reported without surgical therapy in up to 90% of these patients (Saal and Saal 1989; Bush et al. 1992; Bozzao et al. 1992) In follow-up imaging studies the herniation can be seen to diminish in size and eventually disappear entirely or almost completely (Fig. 5.5) with the evolution of MRI findings sometimes lagging behind the improvement of leg pain (Komori et al. 1996). The natural history of disc extrusions and sequestrations causing nerve root compression is reported to be more favourable than that of disc bulges and contained protrusions (Ito et al. 2001; Jensen et al. 2006) especially in young patients (Cowan et al. 1992) and when the extrusion has a high T2 signal (Splendiani et al. 2004). Carragee and Kim (1997) saw the best non-surgical outcomes in younger patients with short duration of symptoms who were not involved in litigation.

With regard to speed of recovery, studies of sciatica patients undergoing conservative treatment revealed that 60% of all patients recovered within 3 months and

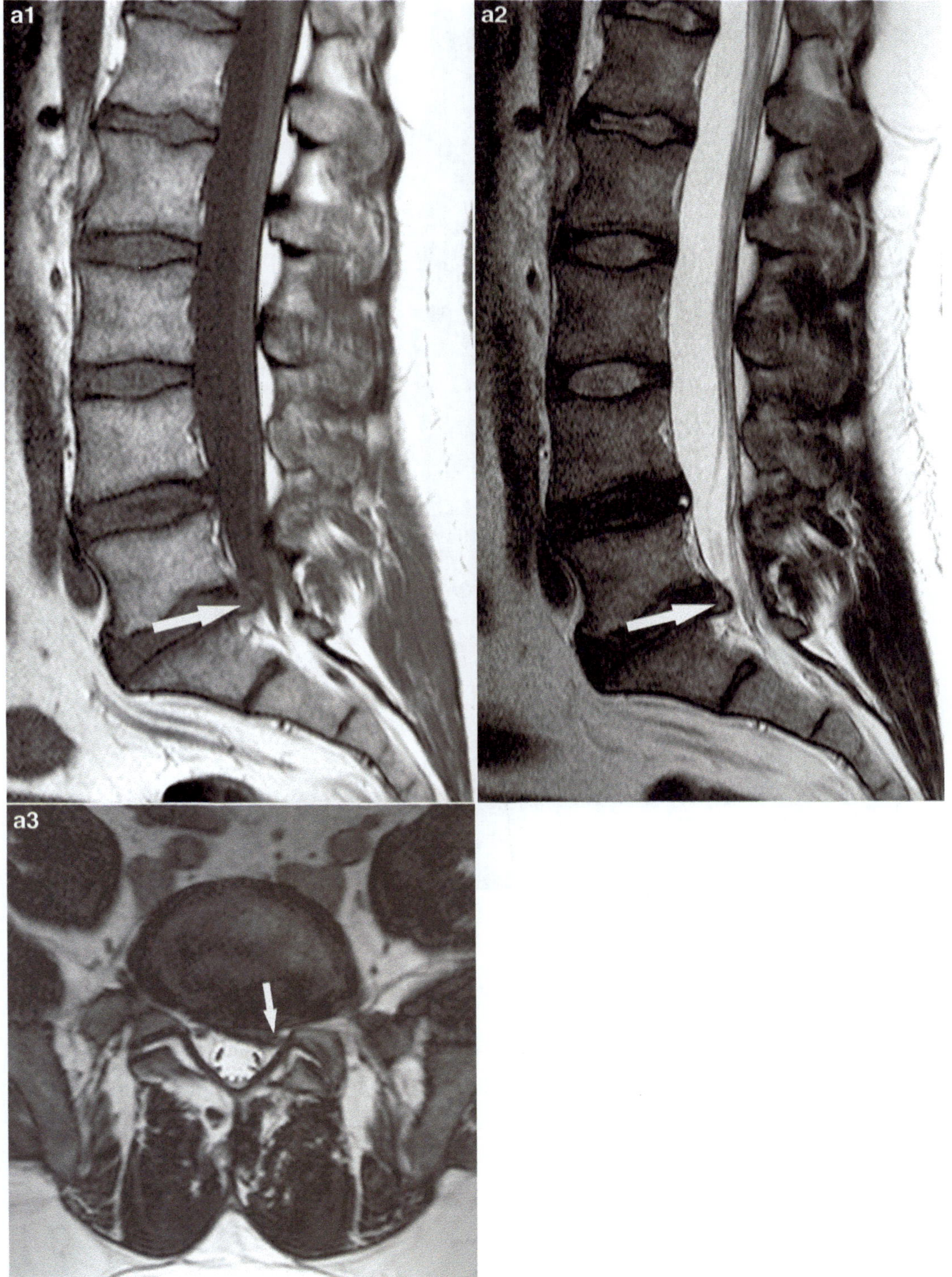

Fig. 5.5 Spontaneous resolution of disc extrusion. *Presentation*: patient, male 37 years, initially reported severe incapacitating left sciatica irradiating to left leg and foot, increasing upon ambulation. Subjective loss of sensation in left lateral thigh, lower leg and foot, especially medial aspect. Weakness was reported of flexion as well as dorsiflexion of left ankle but testing revealed normal muscle strength. No limitation of straight-leg-raising. *MRI*: first MRI study (**a1–4**) shows L5-S1 disc extrusion in sagittal T1 (**a1,** *arrow*) and T2-weighted images (**a2,** *arrow*). Axial T2-weighted image (**a3**) shows traversing left S1 root compressed against L5-S1 facet capsule (*arrow*). MR myelogram (**a4**) shows some swelling of distal intrathecal segment of left S1 root (*arrow*) and cut-off of distal S1 root sleeve filling compared to same root at right *arrow*. Surgery was considered, but the complaints quickly disappeared.

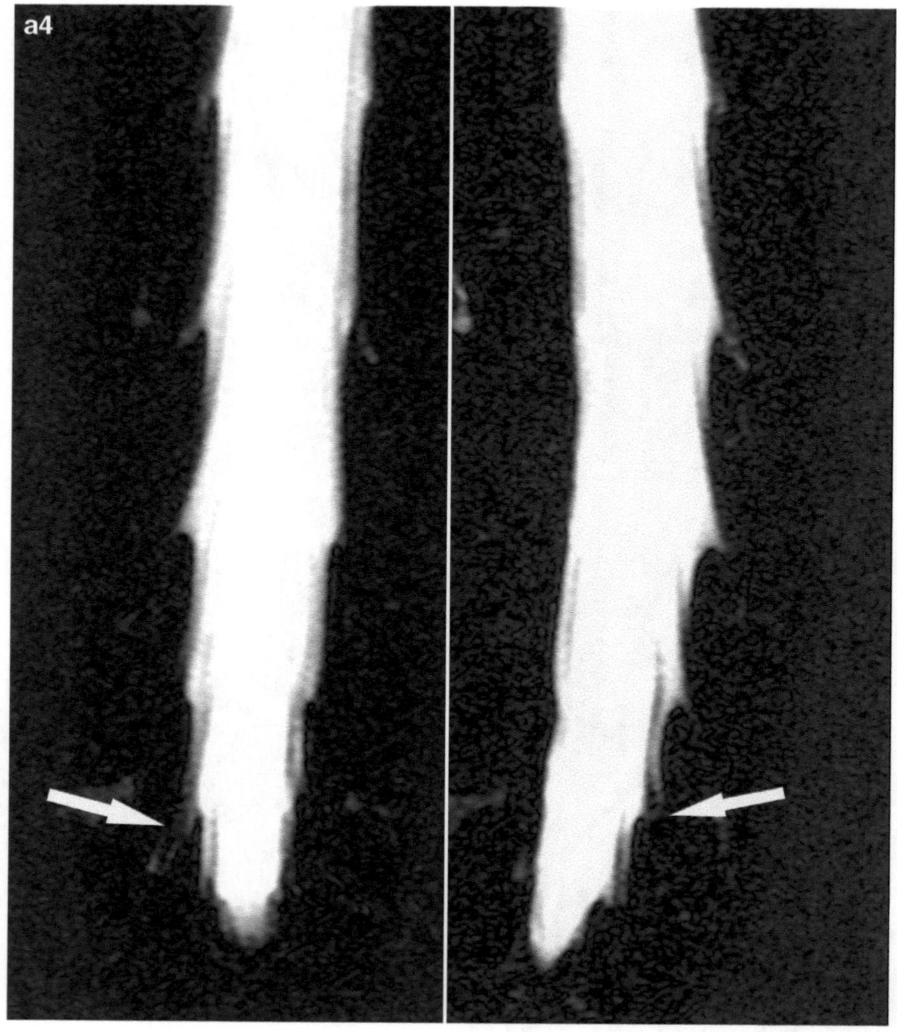

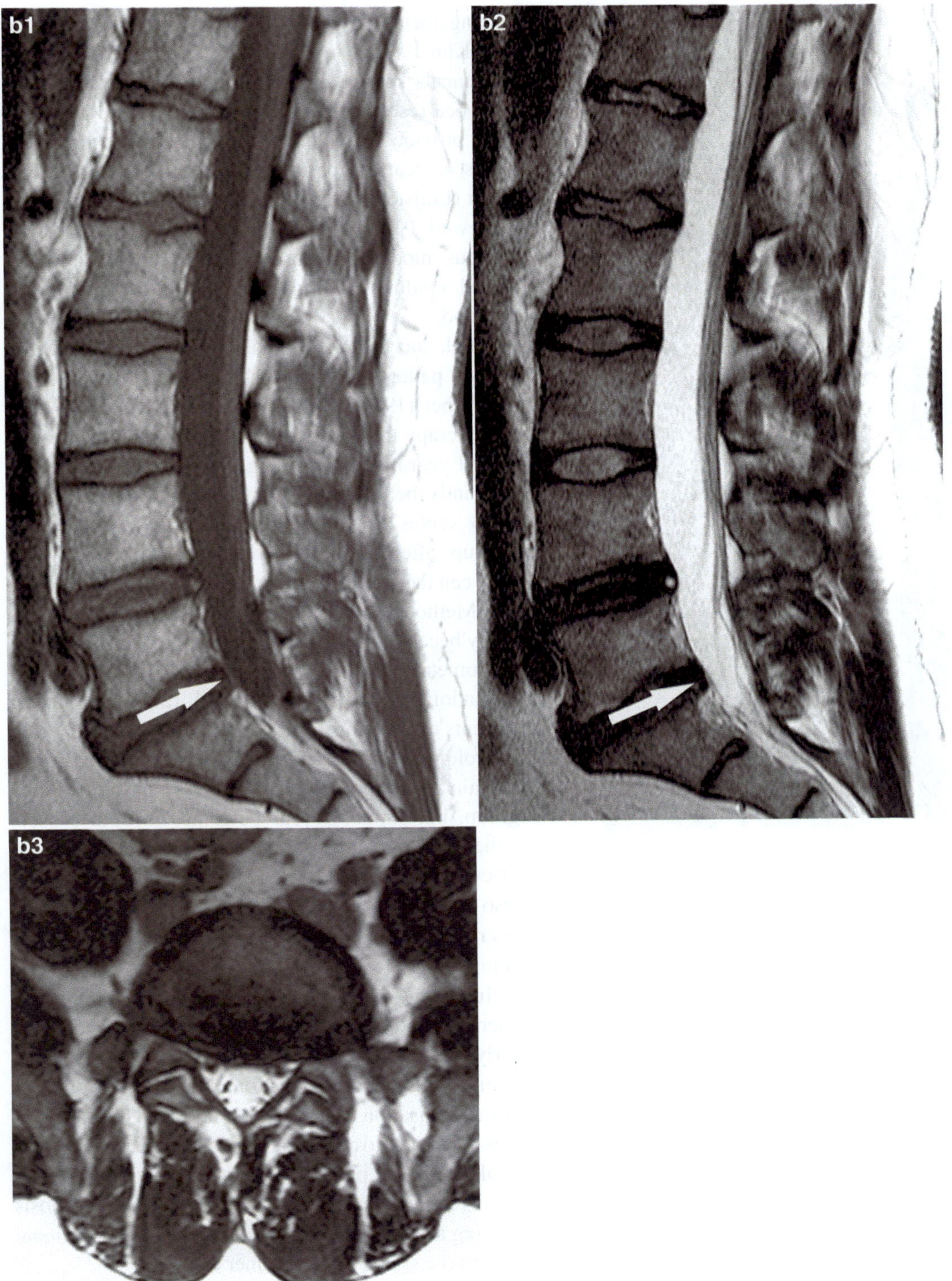

Fig. 5.5 Follow-up MRI study was ordered because of recurrence of sciatica 18 months later, which proved to be short-lived. At time of study the patient was experiencing only low back pain. *MRI*: (**b1–4**) shows marked reduction in size of herniation in sagittal images (**b1** and **b2**, *arrows*), now only a minor protrusion. Axial T2-weighted image (**b3**) shows left S1 root no longer compressed and MR myelogram (**b4**) reveals reduction in S1 root swelling and improved filling of distal root sleeve (*arrow*)

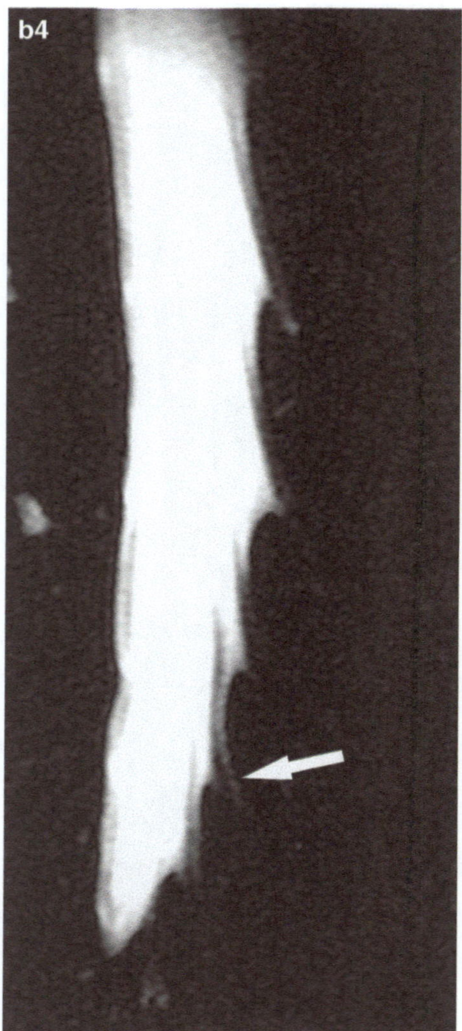

Fig. 5.5 (continued)

management at 1 year (Peul et al. 2008a, b; Carragee and Kim 1997)). A systematic review of conservative treatments such as injections, traction, physical therapy, bed rest, manipulation, medication and acupuncture, provided no evidence that one of these treatment types is clearly superior to the others, or to no treatment (Luijsterburg et al. 2007). Vroomen et al. (2000) reviewed 19 randomised controlled trials comparing various modes of conservative treatment and only found epidural steroid injection to be superior to placebo.

High success rates are also recorded in surgically treated patients (Davis 1994). In a randomised study by Weber (1983) comparing surgical and non-operative therapy in patients with radicular pain, the results after 1 year in the operated group of patients were significantly better than in those treated conservatively (90% versus 60% 'good' or 'fair' results). At later follow-up after 4 and 10 years, however, outcomes between the groups were no longer significantly different. Methodological criticism has been levelled at this study because of incomplete randomisation, subjective outcome measurements and inclusion bias (Saal 1996). A randomised study by Peul et al. (2007) comparing patients undergoing early surgery with those subjected to prolonged conservative therapy, showed a faster rate of pain relief and perceived recovery in the operated group, but similar 1-year outcomes in both groups. Other, non-randomised studies dealing with herniated discs (Atlas et al. 2005a; Weinstein et al. 2006) have also mentioned good results more frequently in the operated group, especially in those with severe complaints.

In patients with spinal stenosis, studies comparing operative and conservative therapy also showed better early results in the operative group, with benefits diminishing over time. Confounding factors were lack of randomisation (Atlas et al. 2005b) and high level of non-adherence to conservative management (Weinstein et al. 2008). In patients undergoing operation, better results were seen in cases with more severe stenosis causing a greater than 50% reduction in cross-sectional area of the spinal canal (Weiner et al. 2007).

In conclusion: surgical therapy appears to provide some benefits over conservative treatment especially in patients with intractable pain, as relief of symptoms is more rapid. In those with less severe complaints surgery offers little extra benefit. The long-term outcomes do not differ significantly between the two groups.

70% within 1 year (Weber et al. 1993) and that up to 70% of sciatica patients report improvement within 2 weeks, and 87% after 12 weeks, respectively (Vroomen et al. 1999). In the latter study there was no significant difference in outcome between a group treated with bed rest and a similar group followed by "watchful waiting".

Conversely, however, it then appears that in up to 30% of patients treated conservatively, significant complaints persist for a period of 1 year or longer. These are especially patients with higher initial scores for pain and disability, while female gender has also been mentioned as a predictor of slower rate of recovery and unsatisfactory outcome of conservative

Surgical therapy is not without downsides: beside a small risk of surgical or anesthesiological complications there is a risk of recurrence of symptoms. The latter risk is of course also present in conservative management. When several surgical interventions have failed to produce a satisfactory outcome this is sometimes referred to as the failed back surgery syndrome (FBSS, see Appendix 1).

Some clinical situations require urgent surgical intervention: an example is an acute cauda equina compression syndrome which is usually due to a large disc extrusion, and which features neurologic deficits such as paresis of the lower extremities, disorders of micturition and saddle anaesthesia. These deficits can be permanent, and early decompression within 48 h is recommended to optimise the prospect of recovery (Ahn et al. 2000; Shapiro 2000).

This has been disputed by some (Qureshi and Sell 2007; Gleave and Macfarlane 2002) who hold that severity of bladder function impairment at time of surgery rather than surgical delay is the most important determinant of outcome in these patients.

Other indications for early operation can be severe and incapacitating radicular pain not responding to conservative measures, which can sometimes be accompanied by signs of neurologic deficit such as paresis of flexor or extensor muscles of the foot, dermatomal sensory or loss of tendon reflexes.

Patients with indications for early or emergent surgery form a small minority. Given the fact that a high percentage of patients with a lumbar disc herniation will be cured spontaneously, early operation in all patients will constitute an unnecessary surgical procedure in many.

In the majority of cases conservative management will be attempted initially. If no sufficient improvement takes place, surgery becomes an option. A period of conservative management lasting 6–8 weeks before operation is regarded by most as appropriate.

In a minority of patients the radicular signs and symptoms will persist despite all non-surgical therapeutic measures. Beside involving a more lengthy period of sometimes incapacitating radicular pain, there are personal and public economic consequences when effective therapy is unnecessarily delayed.

It would be useful, therefore, to be able to predict the outcome of conservative management at onset. Severity of symptoms and gender have been mentioned above, and lists have been compiled setting out prognostic factors which favour positive outcome without operation. These range from psychosocial, educational and employment circumstances to findings at physical examination and evolution of symptoms in the first 6 weeks (Saal 1996).

Imaging features which have been reported to be associated with good or poor spontaneous early outcome of disc herniation and associated radicular symptoms, will now be described.

5.2.2.1 Shape and Size of the Herniation, Nerve Root Compression, Concomitant Pathology

Saal et al. (1990) in a follow-up MRI study of 11 non-operated patients with lumbar disc herniation, saw the greatest degree of resorption of the herniation in the largest extrusions, and the least resorption in contained protrusions. Similar findings were reported by others (Delauche-Cavallier 1992; Maigne 1992; Bush 1992), and Cowan (1992) stated that the classic disc herniation in a young patient is the most likely to show the greatest improvement at follow-up CT. Komori (1996) saw the greatest decrease in size in migrated disc fragments.

Saal and Saal (1989), however, saw rapid improvement in a group of patients undergoing aggressive conservative treatment, with no relationship between size of the extrusion and outcome.

Vroomen et al. (2002b) found a favourable outcome at 12 weeks best predicted by the following MRI features: annular rupture ($p < 0\ 0.02$) and nerve root compression ($p < 0.03$), followed by mediolateral location of the herniation ($p < 0.06$) and compression at the root sleeve ($p < 0.08$). It will be noted that these are the 'classical' imaging features of a radicular syndrome by a lumbar disc herniation. Unfavourable outcome was seen in cases with foraminal disc herniation ($p < 0.004$).

Saal (1996) mentioned the presence of concomitant spinal stenosis as a prognostic factor unfavourable for spontaneous symptom resolution. Carragee and Kim (1997) saw the best non-surgical outcomes in those with a small ratio of hernia size to canal size.

Epidural lipomatosis may also be associated with backache, radicular pain, neurogenic claudication and even cauda equina syndrome. The most common causes are endocrinologic. When morbid obesity is present, weight reduction therapy may be helpful (Robertson et al. 1997; Ishikawa et.al. 2006).

5.2.2.2 Gadolinium Enhancement of the Herniated Disc

Figure 5.6 provides a striking example of this. Gallucci et al. (1995) studied 15 patients undergoing conservative treatment for acute lumbar disc herniation, and found that gadolinium contrast enhancement around the extruded disc fragment seen in 11 patients predicted significant reduction in size of the herniation and good clinical outcome. In four patients without such enhancement the morphologic and clinical evolution was much less favourable. In a later study by the same group (Splendiani 2004) spontaneous regression of disc herniation was seen especially in cases with free fragments (100%), herniations with high T2 signal intensities (85%) and herniations with peripheral contrast enhancement (83%).

Komori et al. (1998) studied 48 patients with lumbar radiculopathy at least twice with gadolinium-enhanced MRI. In 22 patients with migrating disc herniations a rim of circular enhancement was seen around the herniation, which thickened in the course of time in 17 patients as the hernia diminished (see Fig. 5.6). In the other 5 patients no change in enhancement was seen, and little or no decrease in the size of the hernia. In 26 patients with disc extrusions without migration the rim enhancement, which was seen in 20 cases, was often poorer and occurred later. Decrease in size of the herniation took place in only those eight out of 15 cases where clear increase in enhancement in the course of time was present. In no case without any enhancement was a decrease in size of the hernia seen. It was hypothesised that the enhancement occurs in a rim of vascularised fibrous tissue containing macrophages which has been demonstrated in surgically removed disc samples (Haro et al. 1996) and represents an inflammatory reaction to the presence of foreign material in the epidural space.

5.2.3 Conclusion

When MRI reveals the presence of a disc herniation with characteristics favouring early spontaneous remission such as a mediolateral location, ruptured annulus fibrosus, and nerve root compression at the origin of the root sleeve, these are arguments in favour of pursuing a conservative course of management. Further arguments for such a policy are present when there is a large migrated extrusion with a high T2 signal and/or epidural rim enhancement in a young patient with 'classic' radiological findings as mentioned above.

The opposite is not necessarily true. When a patient with sciatica presents with an atypical clinical profile, and MRI shows a small non-enhancing protrusion within an intact annulus fibrosus resulting in a dural impression not involving the root or root sleeve, these findings appear not to favour an early operation but rather a critical review of the clinical diagnosis of a radicular compression syndrome. Early operation is instead indicated rather by clinical circumstances mentioned earlier: occurrence of a cauda equina syndrome or severe and incapacitating radicular pain. In the latter case the indication for operation may be reinforced by an MRI finding of a disc herniation located in the foramen, as spontaneous resolution is then statistically less likely.

5.3 Post-Operative Imaging

5.3.1 Introduction

When diagnostic imaging is performed in a patient who has previously undergone operation for a radicular syndrome, the reason is usually the persistence or recurrence of sciatic pain by a residual or recurrent herniation and/or spinal stenosis, except for those rare cases in which there is for instance a suspicion of a post-operative intraspinal hematoma, or post-operative spondylodiscitis.

In those cases where early post-operative pain relief is inadequate or temporary, the query will usually refer to possible incomplete removal or recurrence of the offending disc herniation. The problem here is that the MR image in this phase is degraded and obscured by the effects of the operation. In the following weeks to months these effects gradually clear, and the MR image can be interpreted with more confidence. Problems of interpretation remain, however, with epidural scar formation blurring the contours of the normal or herniated disc, and post-operative changes at the site of the operation frequently difficult to categorise as normal post-operative or abnormal findings. This picture may become even more confusing when a gadolinium contrast agent has been administered.

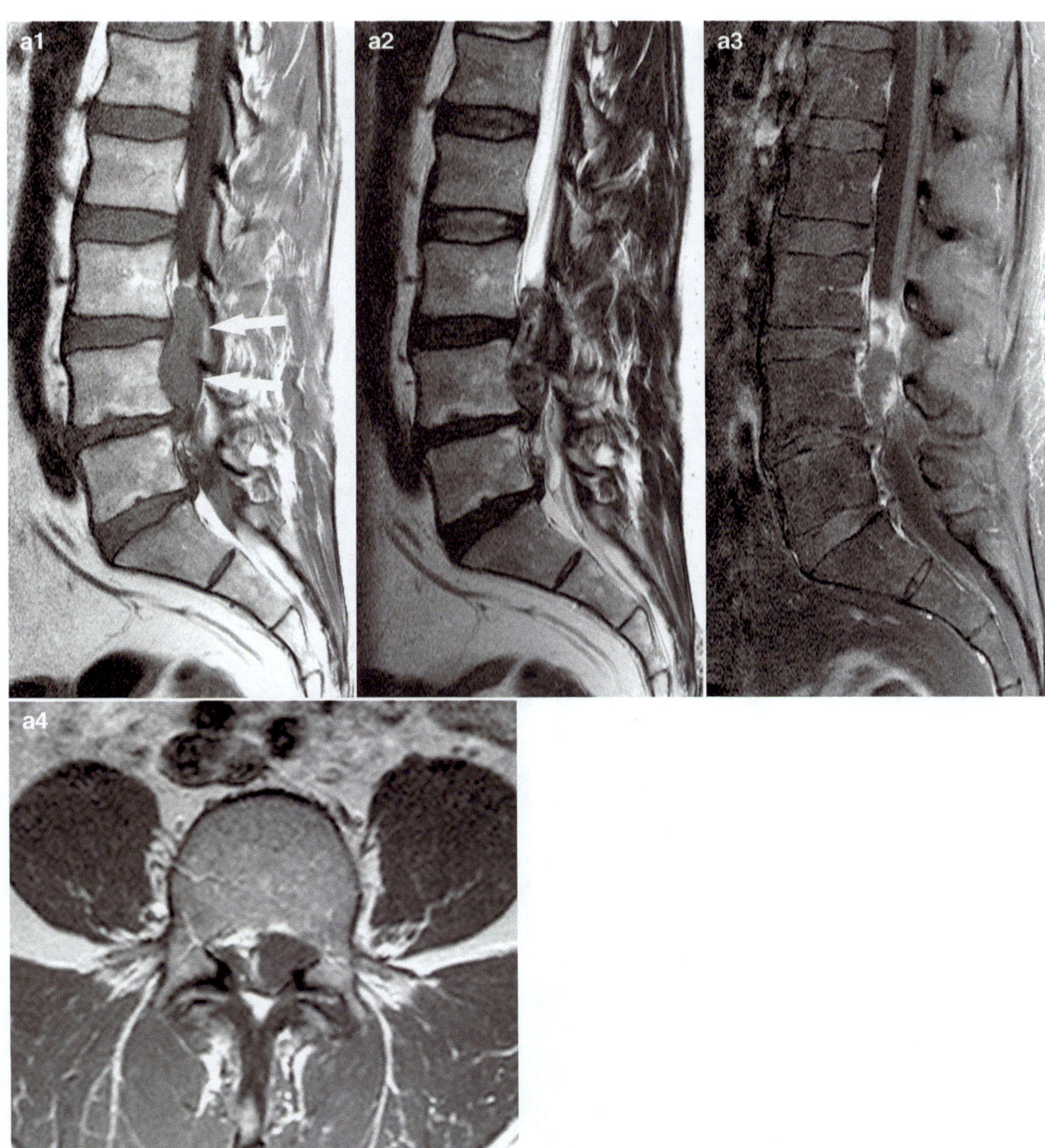

Fig. 5.6 Sequestrated extrusion with marked peripheral enhancement. *Presentation*: patient, male 54 years, presented with acute onset, during exertion, of low back pain irradiating to lateral aspect of left thigh and lower leg, numbness in left calf with left foot drop, absent left knee jerk and hypesthesia in lateral lower leg and entire foot. Testing revealed normal sensation, no limitation of straight-leg-raising. *MRI*: first study (**a1–4**) shows voluminous mass filling left half of spinal canal on sagittal T1- (**a1,** *arrows*) and T2-weighted images (**a2**). Post-gadolinium fat-suppressed T1-weighted images in sagittal (**a3**) and axial planes (**a4**) reveal this mass to be composed of peripheral enhancing tissue around central non-enhancing extrusion most likely originating from L4–5 disc.

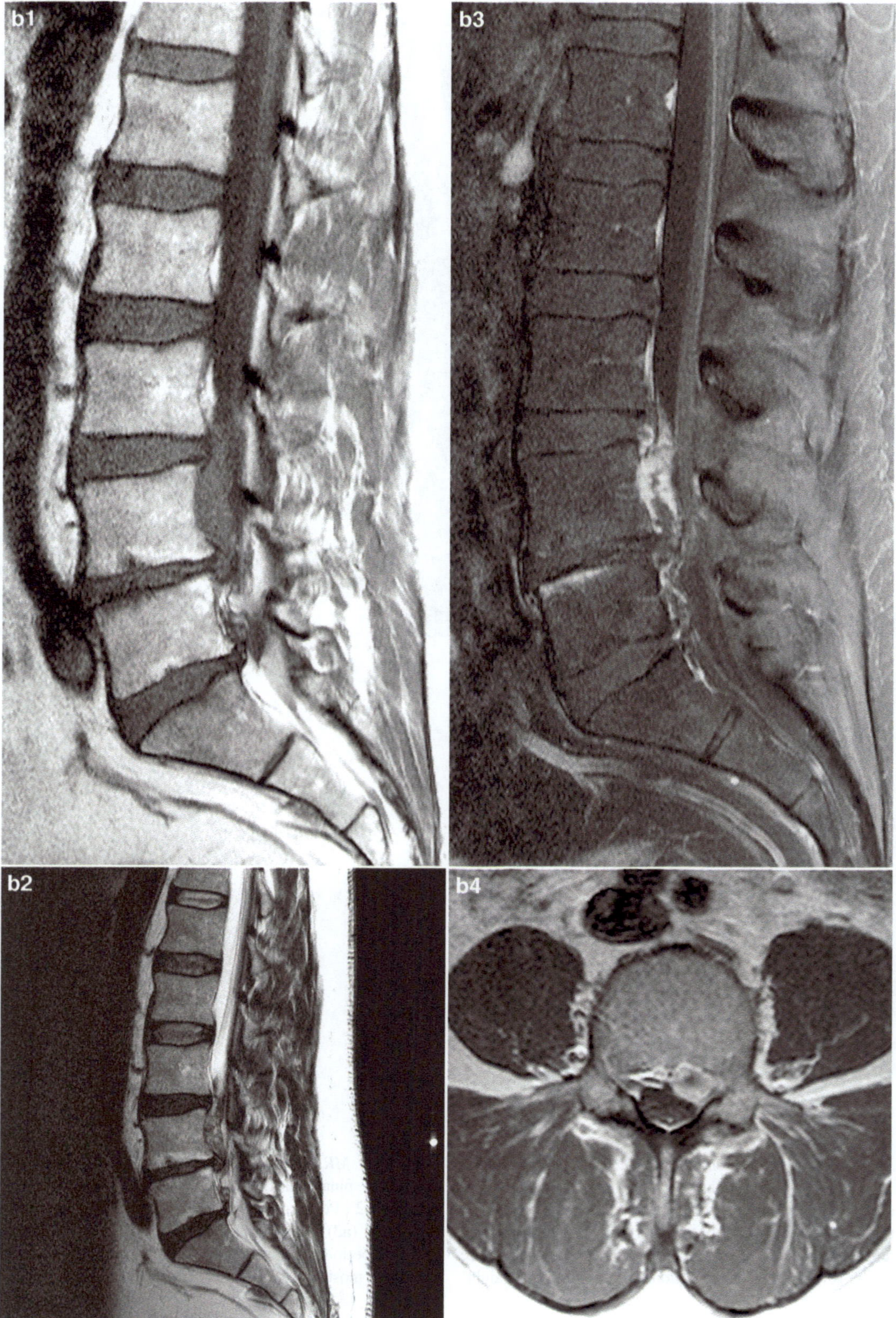

Fig. 5.6 *Follow-up MRI study* 2 months later (**b1–4**) shows substantial resorption of central non-enhancing portion of mass, with relative thickening of enhancing rim. At follow-up 2 months later foot drop was still present, pain and sensory symptoms had improved

5.3.2 Normal Post-Operative Findings

After a 'classical' wide laminectomy the laminar defect where the bone and the underlying flaval ligament have been removed, can usually be recognised without much difficulty. Where the lamina has been removed the dural sac often presents an outpouching or bulge into the operative defect, making it easier to recognise (see Fig. 5.1f). More lately microsurgical and endoscopic techniques have made it possible to gain access to the spinal canal via a partial laminectomy (laminotomy), or via the interlaminar ligaments without any bony resection at all. In addition, various percutaneous methods have been developed to reduce the volume of the herniated disc and relieve nerve root compression without the necessity of opening the spinal canal at all. These methods will not be discussed in detail here, nor will the use of various prostheses and instrumentation devices.

As mentioned, when the spinal canal has been opened to remove a herniated disc, MRI studies in the first 6–8 post-operative weeks can present a misleading picture. The images of the disc and the epidural structures are blurred and the anatomic contours hard to distinguish because of oedema and early post-operative scarring (Annertz 1995a). Frequently the herniation still appears to be present. The dural sac may be deformed over an area of up to 25% in asymptomatic post-operative patients (Van Goethem and Salgado 1997). After gadolinium contrast injection strong enhancement of subchondral vertebral bone marrow can occur which may mimic spondylodiscitis, and enhancement of epidural soft tissues also frequently occurs in asymptomatic post-operative patients (Dina et al. 1995). Enhancement of intradural nerve roots may persist up to 6 months after a successful operation with relief of symptoms (Boden 1992). Longer-lasting enhancement is usually associated with persistence of symptoms (Jinkins 1993).

5.3.3 Residual or Recurrent Disc Herniation and Epidural Scarring

Recurrence of radicular pain in a patient who has previously undergone surgical excision of a herniated disc may be due to a new herniation in another location; in this case the clinical presentation will be different if a different nerve root is compressed. When the presenting signs and symptoms are identical to those before surgery and imaging studies show a herniated disc in the same location as previously, this may be due to a true recurrence. On the other hand, complete disappearance of a herniation after operation is not routinely verified by imaging, so that it is always possible that the offending hernia was not (completely) removed. Whether due to recurrence or residue, the finding of a symptomatic post-operative disc herniation can be an indication for repeat surgery if the severity of the clinical presentation warrants it (Fig. 5.7).

It is important to bear in mind that disc herniations brought to light in patients who have previously undergone an operation can also be an incidental finding: in one study herniations were found in 16% of the disc levels in asymptomatic cases and in 38% of those with symptoms (Grane 1998).

Another possible MRI finding in post-operative patients is that of epidural scarring or fibrosis persisting after the early post-operative period mentioned above. It has been stated that patients with extensive scarring are 3.2 times more likely to experience recurrent pain (Ross et al. 1996). Unless there is severe deformation of the dural sac and root sleeves, however, fibrosis is considered by most to be a radiological finding which has no relationship to radicular signs and symptoms (Annertz et al. 1995b; Vogelsang et al. 1999; Van Goethem et al. 2002). Operative excision of epidural fibrosis is not considered useful.

The radiological problem caused by epidural fibrosis lies in the fact that the bright fat which normally outlines the epidural anatomy is replaced by fibrotic tissue which is much darker on a T1-weighted image, so that a post-operative disc herniation which is surrounded by fibrosis can be masked. An intravenous gadolinium contrast injection will usually cause bright and homogeneous enhancement of fibrotic scar tissue, which may even become iso-intense to epidural fat in a T1-weighted image (Fig. 5.8). With the obscuring effect of fibrosis thus eliminated, a post-operative disc herniation, which does not show enhancement, can be visualised much more clearly. Also, the effect of the herniation upon the dural sac or nerve root can now be assessed; it should be kept in mind that such disc herniations can also be asymptomatic. Post-operative disc herniations can show a rim of peripheral contrast enhancement in the same way that unoperated extrusions do.

The morphologic aspect of post-operative epidural fibrosis is different to that of a recurrent or residual disc

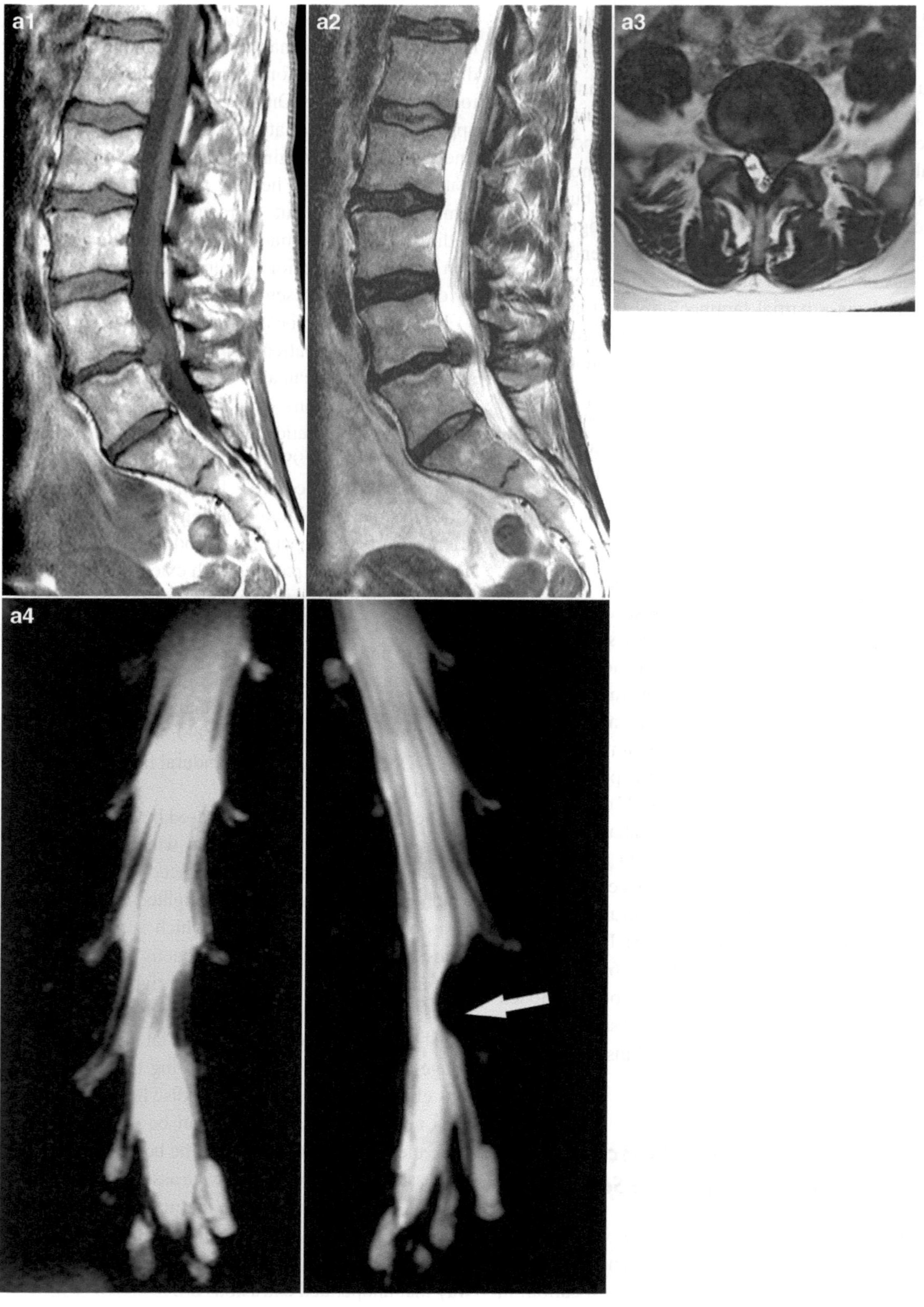

herniation: except in case of distant migration disc herniations are typically dome-shaped or mushroom-shaped and project into the spinal canal from the disc contour (see Chap. 4). There may be a rim of contrast enhancement around the herniation, but the herniation itself does not show enhancement unless there has been a delay (>10 min) between the contrast injection and the imaging sequence, which allows the contrast medium to permeate into the hernia itself (Ross 1991; Van Goethem 2002) This process is more rapid when a non-ionic MR contrast medium is used (Haughton et al. 2002).

Epidural fibrosis on the other hand may occur at some distance from the disc and tends to follow the contour of the dural sac; concave with respect to this structure, and shows homogeneous enhancement. Sometimes a small round defect is seen within the enhancing scar, this may represent either the emerging nerve root sleeve (see Fig. 5.8), or a small fragment of extruded disc. Comparison with the normal root sleeve on the opposite side will usually clarify this problem.

Beside causing enhancement of epidural fibrosis and rim enhancement of a disc herniation, intravenous injection of a gadolinium contrast agent also produces strong enhancement within epidural veins. This can create a misleading picture when a disc herniation displaces the dural sac, thus expanding the anterior epidural space and dilating the venous plexus (Fig. 5.9).

Post-gadolinium MR imaging is often performed routinely in patients who have undergone surgery for lumbar disc herniation, but this is not always necessary, even when non-contrasted T1-weighted images show epidural fibrosis obscuring a possible post-operative disc herniation.

In T1-weighted images epidural fibrosis is hypo-intense to epidural fat, practically iso-intense to herniated disc and dural sac, and hard to distinguish from these structures. Early reports (Ross 1991) indicated that T2-weighted images acquired with conventional spin-echo (CSE) technique did not provide a reliable distinction between epidural fibrosis and herniated disc, and stipulated T1-weighted pre- and post-gadolinium imaging in these cases. However, when fast spin-echo (FSE) technique is used to acquire T2-weighted images, fibrosis appears much brighter and usually more or less iso-intense to epidural fat. Therefore, T2-weighted FSE images usually present the same result as T1-weighted post-gadolinium images: a post-operative disc herniation is clearly outlined by the much brighter area of fibrosis (Fig. 5.10).

To recapitulate: The presence and extent of post-operative epidural fibrosis is best assessed in non-enhanced T1-weighted images as the dark gray scar tissue is then well-contrasted against the surrounding bright epidural fat. Demarcation of fibrosis against the normal or herniated disc or the dural sac is poor, however. Post-contrast T1-weighted and FSE T2-weighted images in effect make fibrosis almost invisible, and improve definition of the disc, and also of dural and epidural anatomy.

Remember that the objective in post-operative imaging is not primarily to demonstrate the presence of epidural fibrosis, which has little therapeutic significance, but rather to clearly outline a possible residual or recurrent disc herniation and to assess its effects on the nerve root. For the latter aim, sagittal and axial FSE T2-weighted images, complemented by MR myelography, are usually sufficient (Figs. 5.11 and 5.12). Post-gadolinium imaging can be reserved for the rare cases in which there remains room for doubt.

5.3.4 Spondylodiscitis

Post-operative discitis with adjacent spondylitis is a rare but severe complication of spinal surgery (Lindholm and Pylkkanen 1982; Bircher et al. 1988) with potentially serious consequences. Early diagnosis and prompt antibiotic treatment are important in shortening the course of the disease and limiting the consequences, but

Fig. 5.7 Recurrent/residual disc herniation. *Presentation*: patient, female 46 years, had long-standing low back pain, recently irradiating to left thigh, leg and lateral margin of left foot, sometimes to hallux. Examination revealed hypesthesia in L5 and possibly S1 dermatomes, absent left ankle jerk and limitation of straight-leg-raising to 30° at left. *MRI*: first study at presentation (**a1–4**) shows large left L4–5 extrusion on sagittal T1- (**a1**) and T2-weighted images (**a2**). Axial T2-weighted image (**a3**) and MR myelogram (**a4**) show severe compression of left half of dural sac and traversing L5 nerve root, with root swelling and non-filling L5 root sleeve (*arrow* in **a4**). Medial displacement of intradural S1 root. Patient underwent L4–5 laminectomy 2 months later. Initial results were good, but at 6 weeks post-operation patient reported persistence of left leg pain.

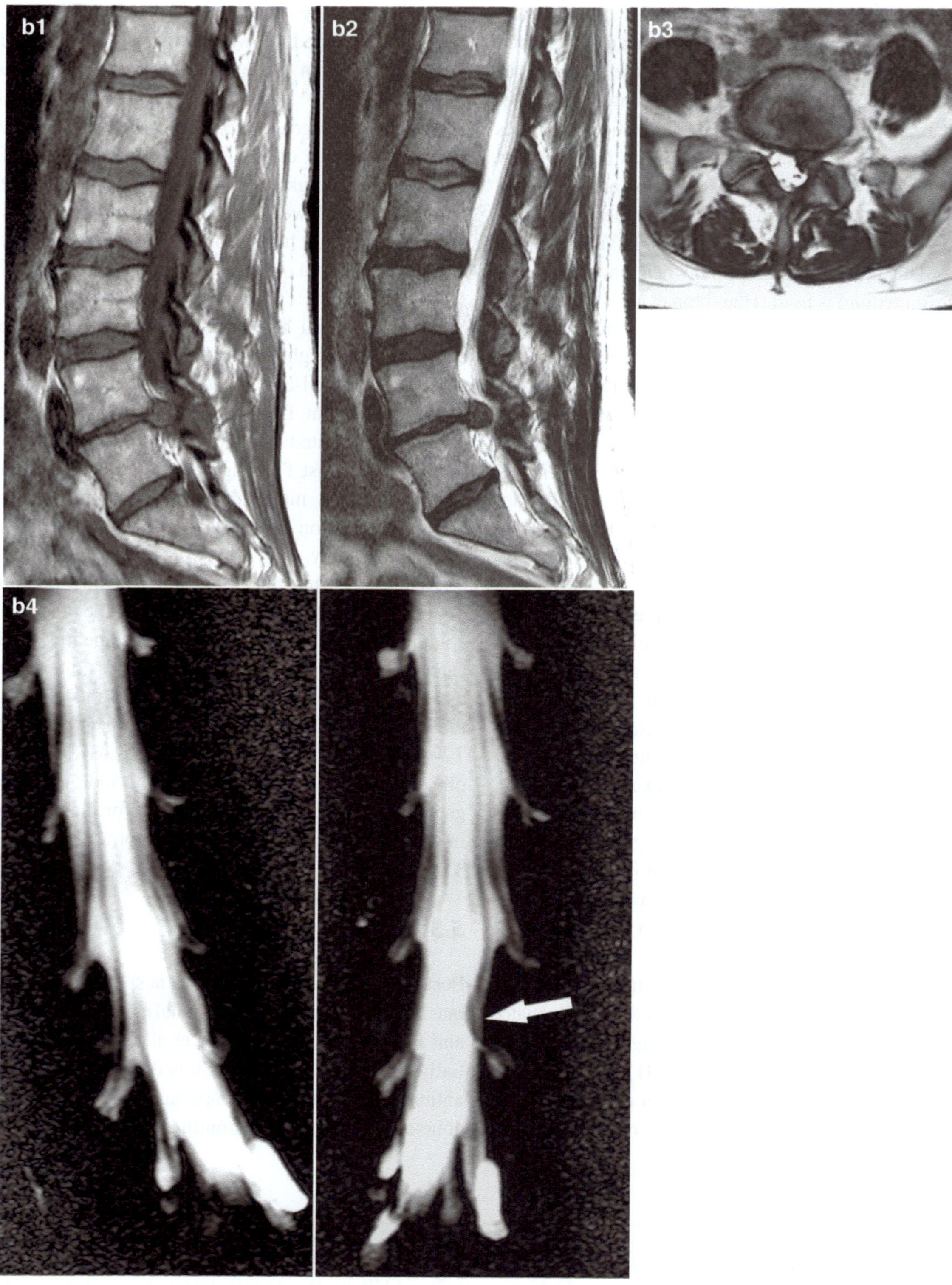

Fig. 5.7 *Follow-up MRI* study 3 months post-operation (**b1–4**) showed decrease in size of extrusion and less deformation of dural sac, with L5 root still displaced but now normal root sleeve filling (**b4**, *arrow*). Patient was re-operated several days later, again with initially good results. Three months post-operation there was recurrence of severe lumbago with pain irradiating to left leg and tingling sensation in left leg and sole of foot, with straight-leg-raising to 80° producing pain and tingling in sole of left foot.

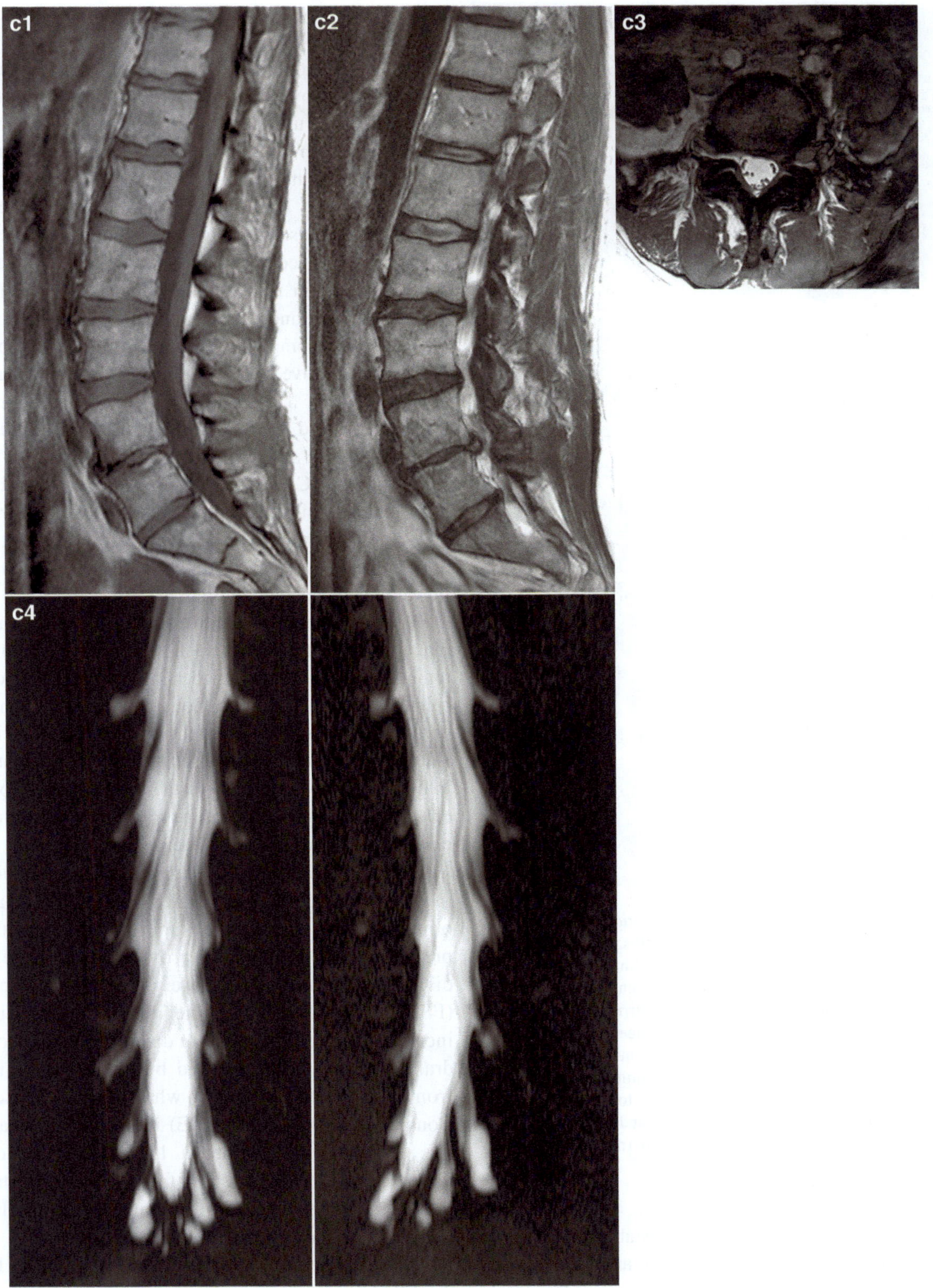

Fig. 5.7 *Follow-up MRI* 4 months after re-operation (**c1–4**) revealed a small left lateral L4–5 herniation without L5 root compression: normal aspect of intradural root and root sleeve on axial T2-weighted image (**c3**) and MR myelogram (**c4**). Note also smaller protrusions visible at other disc levels in sagittal T2-weighted image (**c2**), without signs of nerve root compression in MR myelogram (**c4**). No further operation undertaken

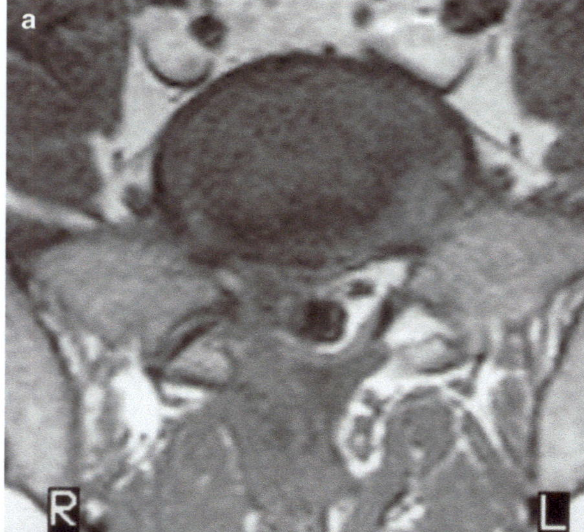

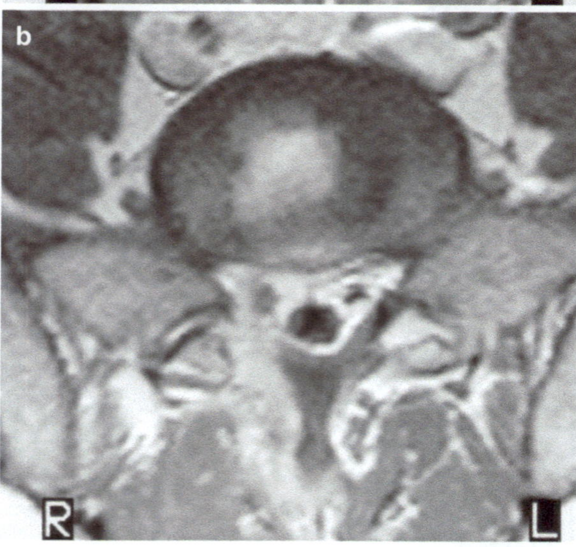

Fig. 5.8 Enhancing epidural scar. *Presentation*: patient, male 35 years, had undergone laminectomy 3 months previously, but suffered recurrence of sciatica. No further clinical data available. *MRI*: axial T1-weighted image (**a**) in patient after right L5-S1 laminectomy shows extensive epidural scarring which obscures right border of dural sac, right S1 root sleeve and L5-S1 disc contour. Recurrent herniation cannot be identified or excluded in this image. After IV injection of gadolinium contrast medium (**b**) scar tissue is seen to enhance almost to iso-intensity with normal epidural fat. Dural sac, S1 root and disc contour now clearly visible. No sign of recurrent disc herniation

the diagnosis is often difficult to establish. Presenting signs and symptoms can be aspecific and MRI findings in post-operative spondylodiscitis can quite closely resemble those seen in uncomplicated post-operative patients, while systemic signs of an infectious condition may be lacking.

Presumably in the majority of cases there is a direct contamination by micro-organisms of the surgically exposed disc, usually by *Staphylococcus aureus*. MRSA infection has been reported to be particularly devastating, with high mortality and morbidity (Al-Nammari et al. 2007). Inoculation with micro-organisms can also take place in diagnostic examinations such as discography or myelography. Typically severe local pain is reported in the operated spinal region, but not uncommonly there is also radicular pain. Onset of complaints is usually after a symptom-free post-operative period of 1–4 weeks; on average about 2 weeks. The erythrocyte sedimentation rate may be elevated over 50 mm and leukocyte counts increased, while subfebrile to febrile temperatures are regularly seen. C-reactive protein has been described as the most sensitive laboratory marker to assess presence of infection and response to therapy (Silber et al. 2002). Combinations of findings have greater diagnostic value than isolated findings.

Plain X-ray films have little or no value in the early diagnosis of post-operative spondylodiscitis. Computed tomography can be used for locating possible infectious spinal lesions when intravenous contrast injection is performed, but specificity in the post-operative period is low. CT- or ultrasound-guided aspiration of potential infectious lesions can help to establish the bacteriological diagnosis and guide antibiotic therapy when successful, but sometimes yields negative results.

MRI is presently the imaging technique of choice in spondylodiscitis. T1-weighted pre- and post-gadolinium MR images with fat suppression by spectral pre-saturation (SPIR, fatsat) provide the most useful diagnostic information. T2-weighted fast spin-echo (FSE) images are suitable for demonstrating increased intradiscal signal in discitis, but subchondral oedema is often masked by the bright signal from fatty bone marrow when FSE is used. Conventional spin-echo (CSE) images do not have this property, but require a lengthy acquisition. Suppression of bone marrow fat signal by spectral pre-saturation or short TI inversion recovery (STIR) is recommended (Fig. 5.13).

The following MRI features are of importance for the differential diagnosis between spondylodiscitis and aseptic post-operative changes:

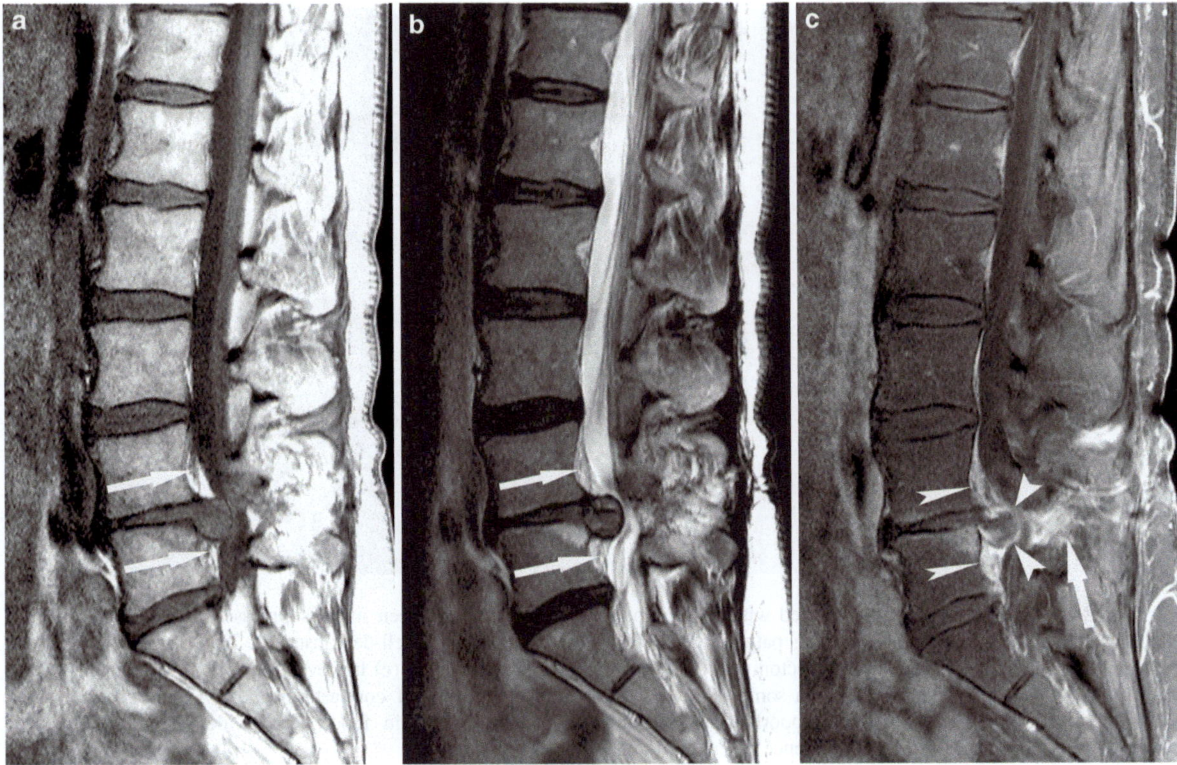

Fig. 5.9 Enhancing epidural scar and dilated veins. *Presentation*: patient, female 51 years, had been operated 10 months earlier for L4–5 lateral disc herniation with good initial results but recurrence of severe right sciatica 1 week previous to MRI study. *MRI*: L4–5 disc extrusion shown on sagittal T1- (**a**) and T2-weighted images (**b**) Post-gadolinium fat-suppressed T1-weighted image (**c**) shows interlaminar scar enhancement (*arrow*), also rim enhancement around extrusion (*arrowheads*). Normal enhancement of basivertebral and anterior epidural veins in upper lumbar region. Enhancement in anterior epidural space behind L4 and L5 vertebral bodies (*long arrowheads*) is not due to scar formation, which would also be visible in (**a**) but here is caused by expansion of epidural space by dorsal displacement of dural sac, with enhancement of dilated epidural veins. Veins can also be faintly seen in (**a**) and (**b**) (*long arrows*)

- Post-operative subchondral Modic type 1 bone marrow changes with decreased T1- and increased T2- signal have been described as rare in uncomplicated post-operative cases and said to favour the diagnosis of spondylodiscitis (Ross et al. 1987; Boden et al. 1992b). Others regard such changes to indicate bone marrow oedema, commonly seen in uncomplicated post-operative cases (Grane et al. 1998; Van Goethem and Salgado 2007). Enhancing end-plate regions can be seen in both conditions.
- Enhancement of the site of surgical incision in the posterior annulus fibrosus is commonly seen in uncomplicated post-operative cases. Intradiscal enhancement is a requisite for the diagnosis of spondylodiscitis, as is increased T2 signal within the disc (Boden et al. 1992a; Van Goethem and Salgado 2007).
- An enhancing paraspinal soft tissue mass favours the diagnosis of spondylodiscitis, but epidural enhancement is not a reliable indicator of this diagnosis.

Again, combinations of MRI findings are more reliable than isolated features: according to Dina et al. (1995) one or two of a triad of findings (Type I Modic bone marrow changes, bone marrow enhancement and increased T2 signal within the disc) were sometimes seen in asymptomatic patients, but only patients with spondylodiscitis simultaneously exhibited all three (see however Fig. 5.14).

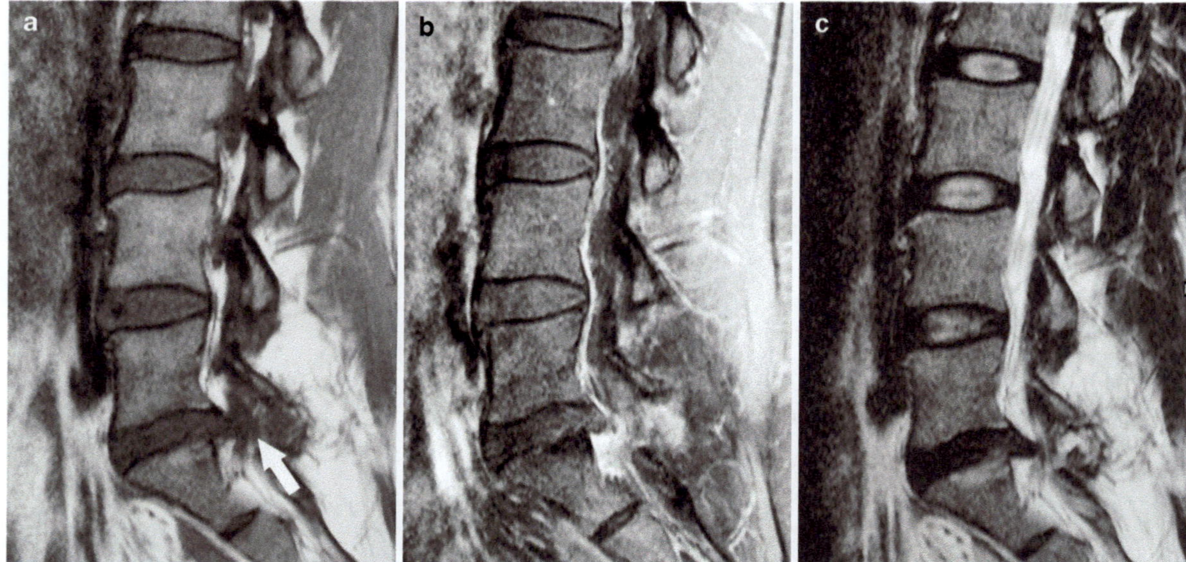

Fig. 5.10 Recurrent disc extrusion visualised with and without gadolinium contrast injection. *Presentation*: patient, female 34 years, had twice undergone previous laminectomy, but now suffered from persistent right S1 sciatica with some limitation of straight-leg-raising. *MRI*: L5-S1 extrusion poorly visualised on sagittal T1-weighted image (**a**) due to presence of epidural and interlaminar scarring (*arrow*). Scar enhancement after gadolinium contrast injection seen in fat-suppressed T1W image (**b**), and extrusion is now well-demonstrated. Note, however, that FSE T2-weighted image (**c**) however shows extrusion equally well, without necessity of contrast injection. A new operation was undertaken but again failed to provide significant relief of complaints

5.3.5 Hematoma, Pseudomeningocele

Bleeding can frequently be demonstrated at the site of operation in the immediate post-operative phase, and MRI will show the presence of blood products. Formation of a haematoma can cause a recurrence of radicular symptoms in the first hours to days after the operation, or increased neurologic deficit when the cauda equina is compressed, necessitating new surgery.

A post-operative pseudomeningocele is a CSF-filled cyst contiguous with the dural sac, not lined with an arachnoid membrane but with reactive fibrous tissue, occurring as a result of dural laceration during the operation (Bosacco et al. 2001) and is reported to occur at a rate of 3.5% in primary discectomy, 8.5% in surgery for spinal stenosis and 13% in revision disc surgery (Tafazal and Sell 2005) Such pseudocysts may be very extensive and extend craniocaudally and/or laterally in the paraspinal tissues. MRI is the best imaging technique in this condition, and clearly shows the fluid contents iso-intense to CSF on T1- and T2-weighted images, although the T2 fluid signals within the pseudocyst is typically brighter than that of the CSF within the dural sac, due to lack of cardiac-related pulsatile CSF movements which degrade the intradural CSF signal. Sometimes a communication with the contents of the dural sac can be identified. Intravenous gadolinium contrast injection occasionally gives rise to enhancement of the wall of the pseudomeningocele, making a differentiation from a post-operative abscess difficult without laboratory support (Fig. 5.15). The condition is commonly asymptomatic, but may give rise to aspecific low back

Fig. 5.11 Recurrent disc extrusion visualised without gadolinium contrast injection. *Presentation*: patient, female 49 years, suffered recurrence of backache and left gluteal pain without radicular signs after having been free of pain for about 10 months after a previous laminectomy. *MRI*: sagittal T1-weighted image (**a**) shows scarring at operative site L5-S1, impossible to assess recurrence of extrusion (*question mark*). T2-weighted images (**b-d**) clearly show disc extrusion (**b,** *arrow*) compressing right dural sac and S1 root (**c**), MR myelogram (**d,** *arrow*) shows dural impression and cut-off of S1 root sleeve filling (*arrow*). No gadolinium injection necessary in this case

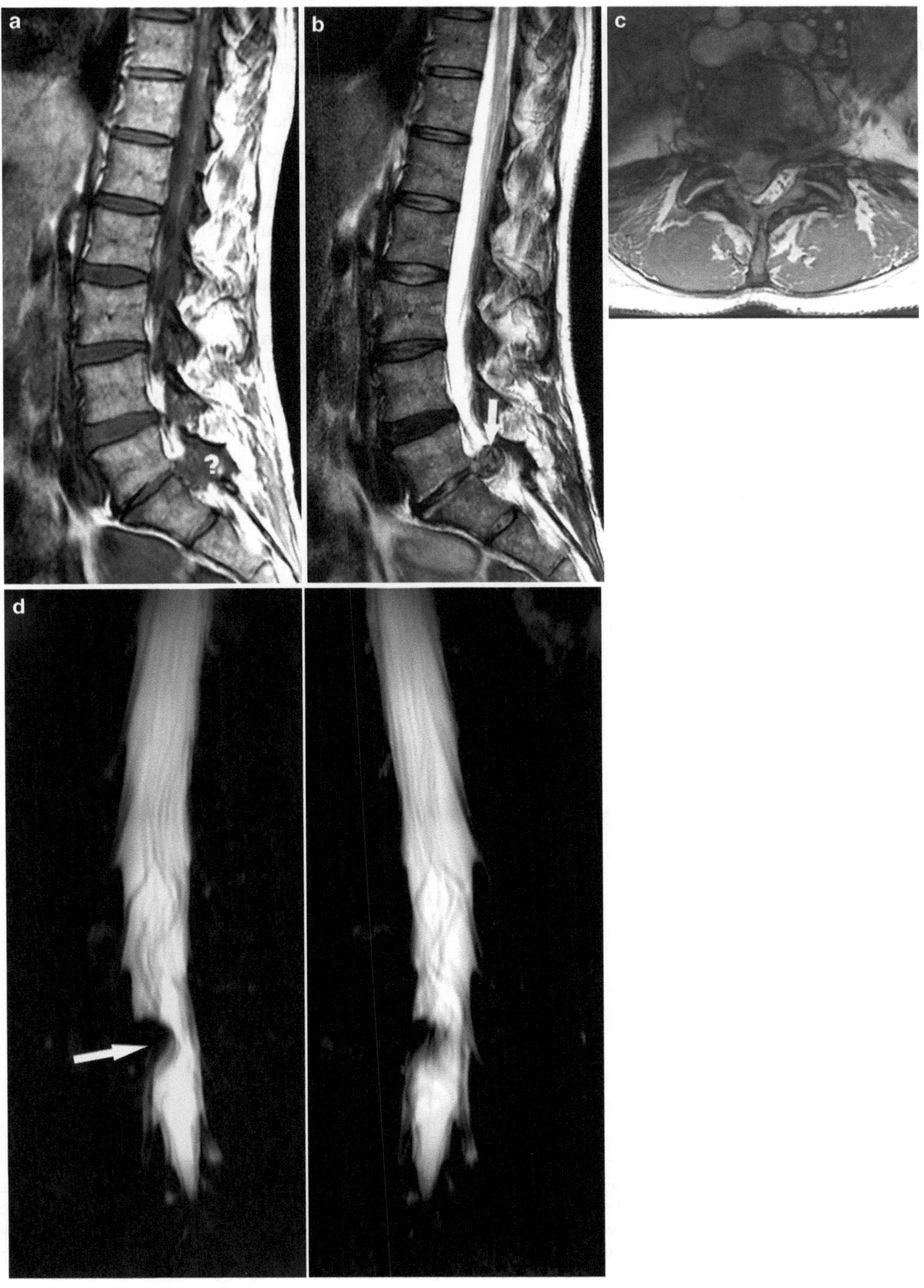

complaints, occasionally to headache caused by CSF hypotension, and rarely to nerve root compression.

5.3.6 Arachnoiditis

Adhesive arachnoiditis in low back patients is at present seen much less frequently than in the past, when oil-based or older high-osmolality water-soluble radiologic contrast media were injected into the dural sac to perform conventional myelography, Nowadays, intrathecal injection of anesthetics, corticosteroids or chemotherapeutic agents are a more common cause. Arachnoiditis may occur as a sequel to surgery, especially intradural procedures (Fitt and Stevens 1995; where residual blood in the dural sac may play a role, or after spondylodiscitis. Three morphologic groups can be distinguished (Delamarter et al. 1990). Group 1 is characterised by adhesion and 'clumping' of cauda equina fibres in the central region of the dural sac, while in Group 2 there is more peripheral adhesion of the roots to the dural walls, creating the appearance of an empty dural sac with thickened walls. In Group 3, there is a soft tissue mass replacing the sub-arachnoid space. Arachnoiditis is at present best demonstrated by T2-weighted MR imaging, including MR myelography (Fig. 5.16).

The matted nerve roots may sometimes show enhancement after injection of a gadolinium contrast medium (see Fig. 5.15), but frequently this is not the case (Sze 1990).

Fig. 5.12 Post-operative scarring visualised without gadolinium contrast injection. *Presentation*: patient, female 46 years, suffered from persistent lumbago and left sciatica after two surgical procedures for left L5-S1 disc herniation. *MRI*: sagittal T1-weighted image (**a**) shows post-operative situation at L5-S1; difficult to assess possible recurrence of herniation due to post-operative scarring (*question mark*). Sagittal T2-weighted image (**b**) shows annular defect at L5-S1 (*arrow*). Recurrent herniation appears unlikely, but epidural anatomy obscured. Axial T2-weighted image (**c**) clearly demonstrates normal left S1 root sleeve (*arrow*), surrounded by epidural scar but without compression by scar or recurrent herniation. MR myelogram (**d**) confirms normal filling of left S1 root sleeve (*arrow*). No gadolinium injection necessary in this case

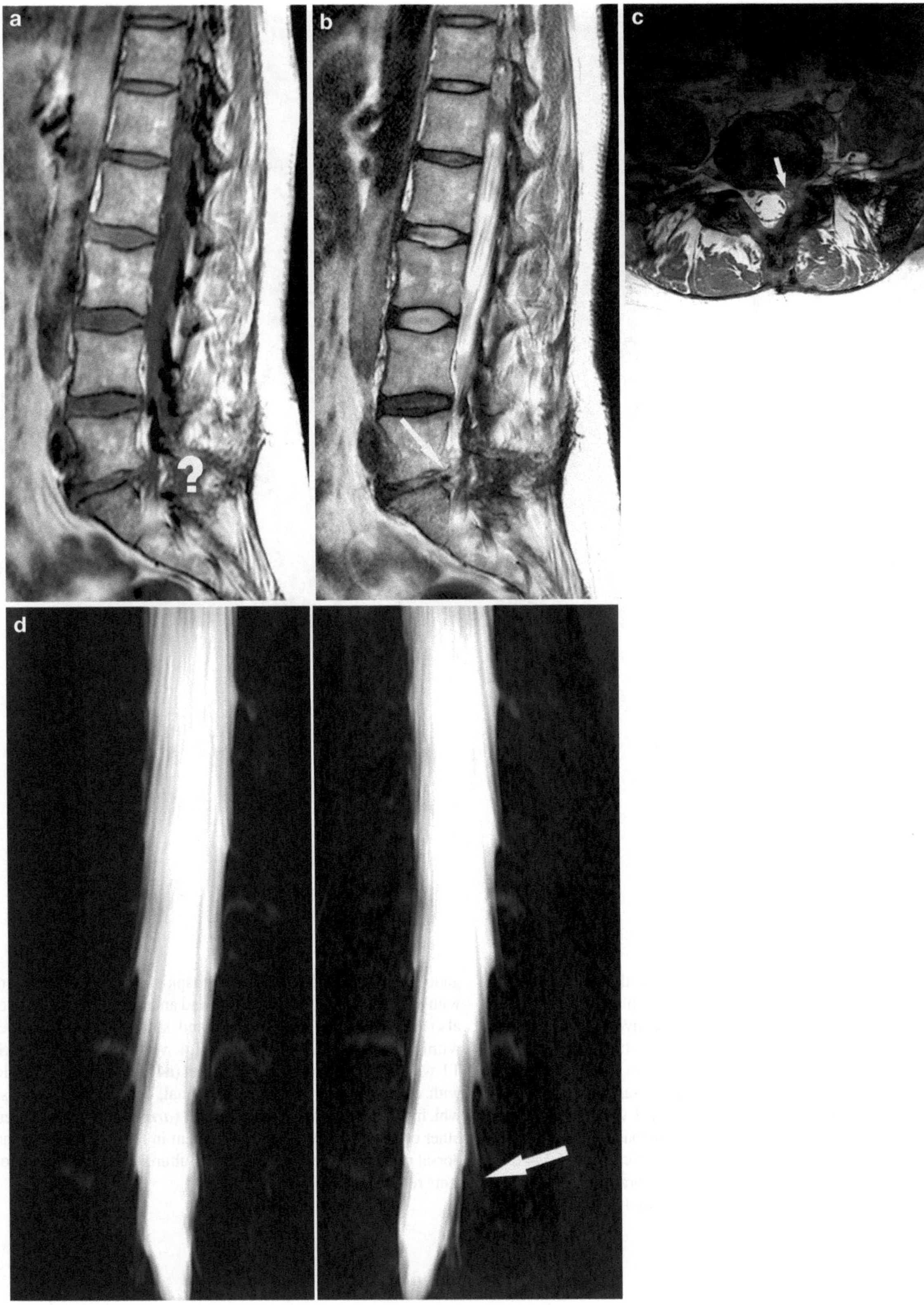

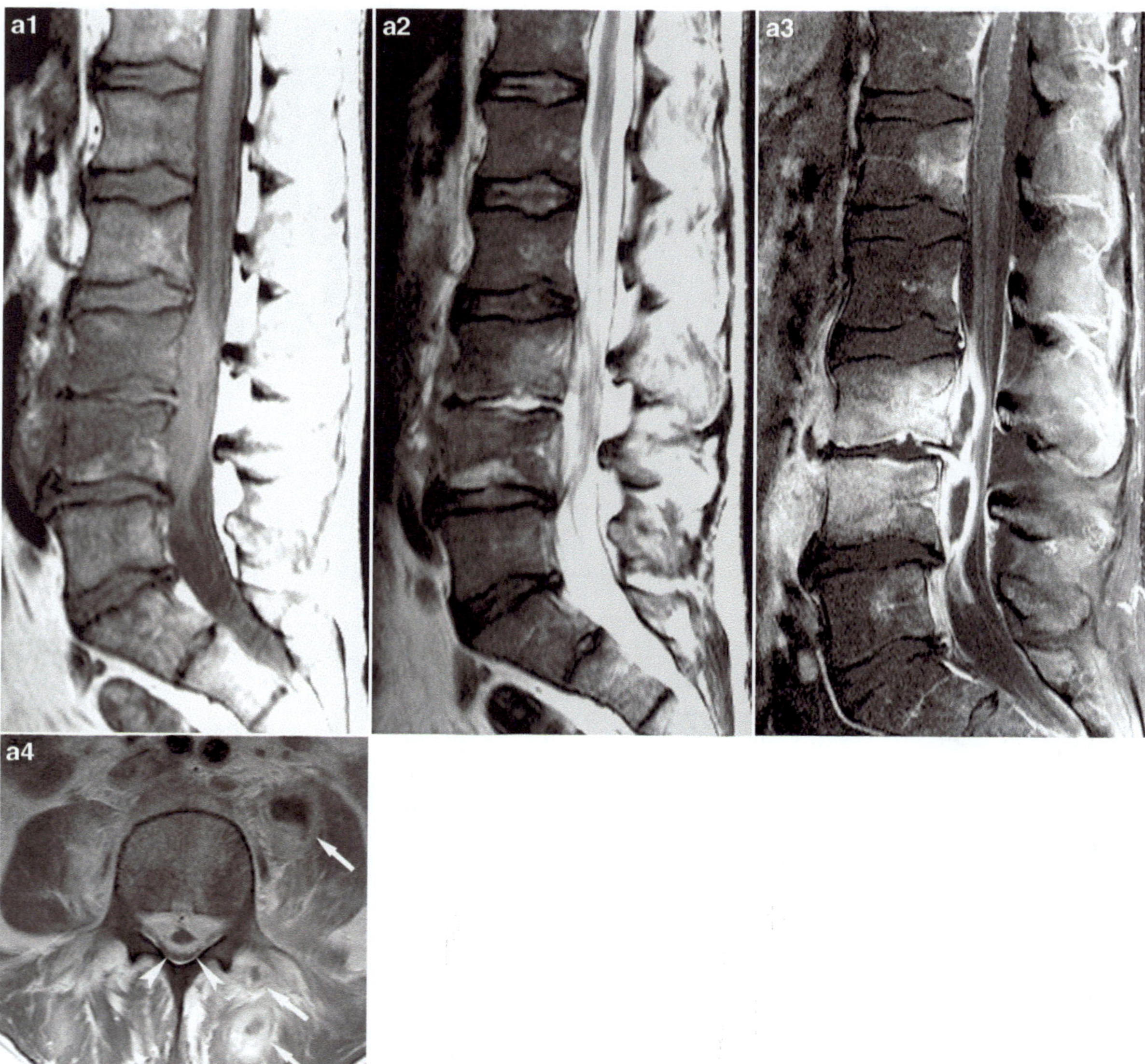

Fig. 5.13 MRI with follow-up in a case with spondylodiscitis. *Presentation*: patient, male 46 years, had been suffering from low back pain for several months, lately progressive and irradiating to both feet, with tingling and subjective loss of strength in both legs. Laboratory findings indicating infection, with leucocytosis, ESR 97 mm, CRP 127. *MRI*: at first presentation sagittal images show decreased bone marrow signal in L3 and L4 vertebral bodies on T1-weighted image (**a1**), also intraspinal mass hyperintense to CSF. T2-weighted image (**a2**) shows hyperintensity of L3–4 disc, with some signal increase in adjacent vertebral bodies; interruption of posterior L3–4 annulus. Fat-suppressed T1-weighted post-gadolinium image (**a3**) shows intraspinal pockets of empyema with also abscess formation within and anterior to L3–4 disc. Note also bone marrow enhancement and soft tissue enhancement within and anterior to L3 and L4 vertebral bodies. Axial T1-weighted post-gadolinium image (**a4**) shows pus collection with enhancing rim within spinal canal, compressing dural sac which is almost completely collapsed (*arrowheads*), also several other collections with rim enhancement in left psoas (*arrow*) and dorsal paraspinal muscles (*arrows*). Culture of dorsal abscess contents revealed staphylococcus aureus.

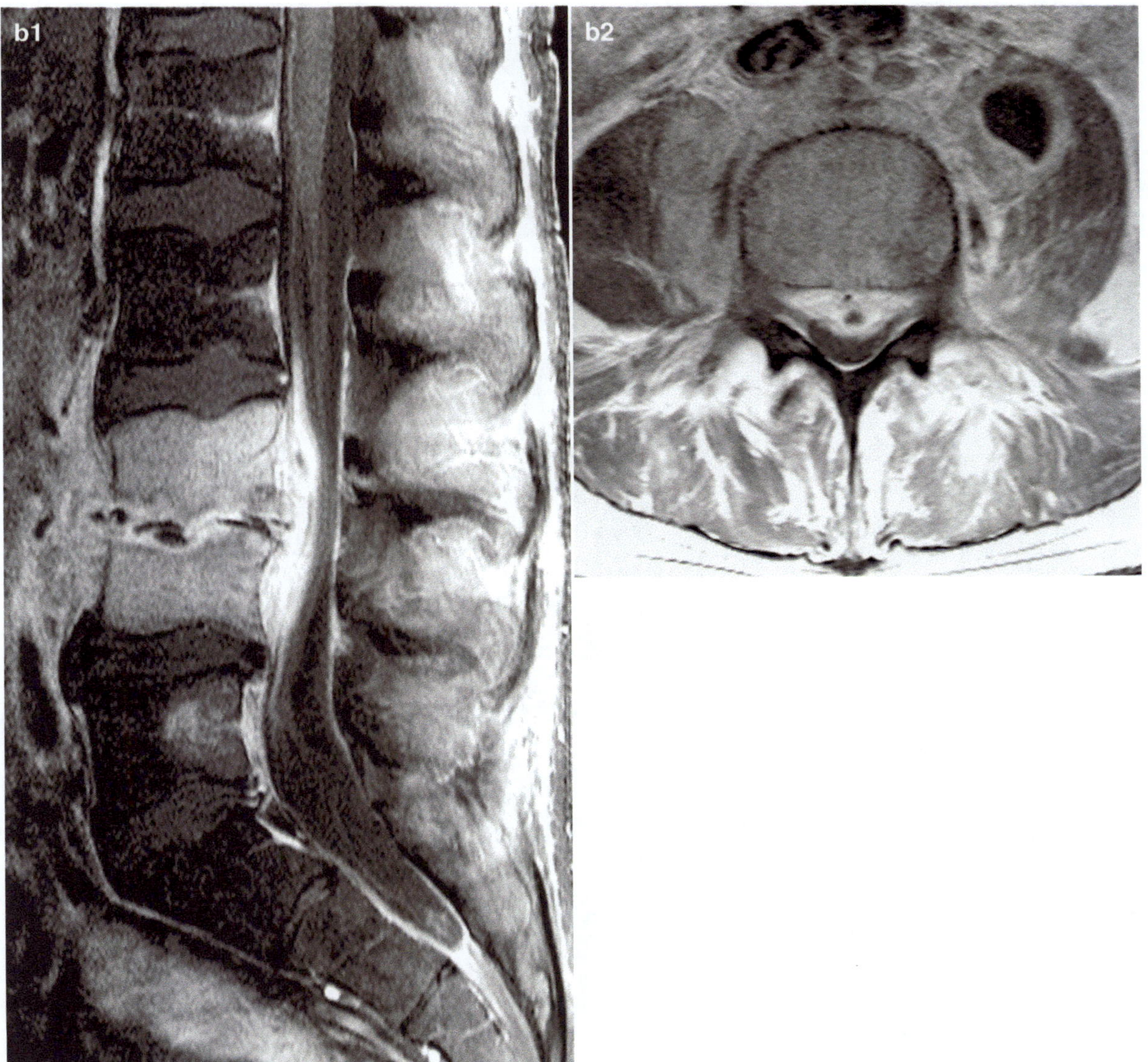

Fig. 5.13 *Follow-up MRI after 3 weeks* of antibiotic treatment: post-gadolinium sagittal (**b1**) and axial (**b2**) T1-weighted images revealed decrease in epidural mass effect, still strongly enhancing bone marrow and paraspinal soft tissues, unchanged left psoas abscess.

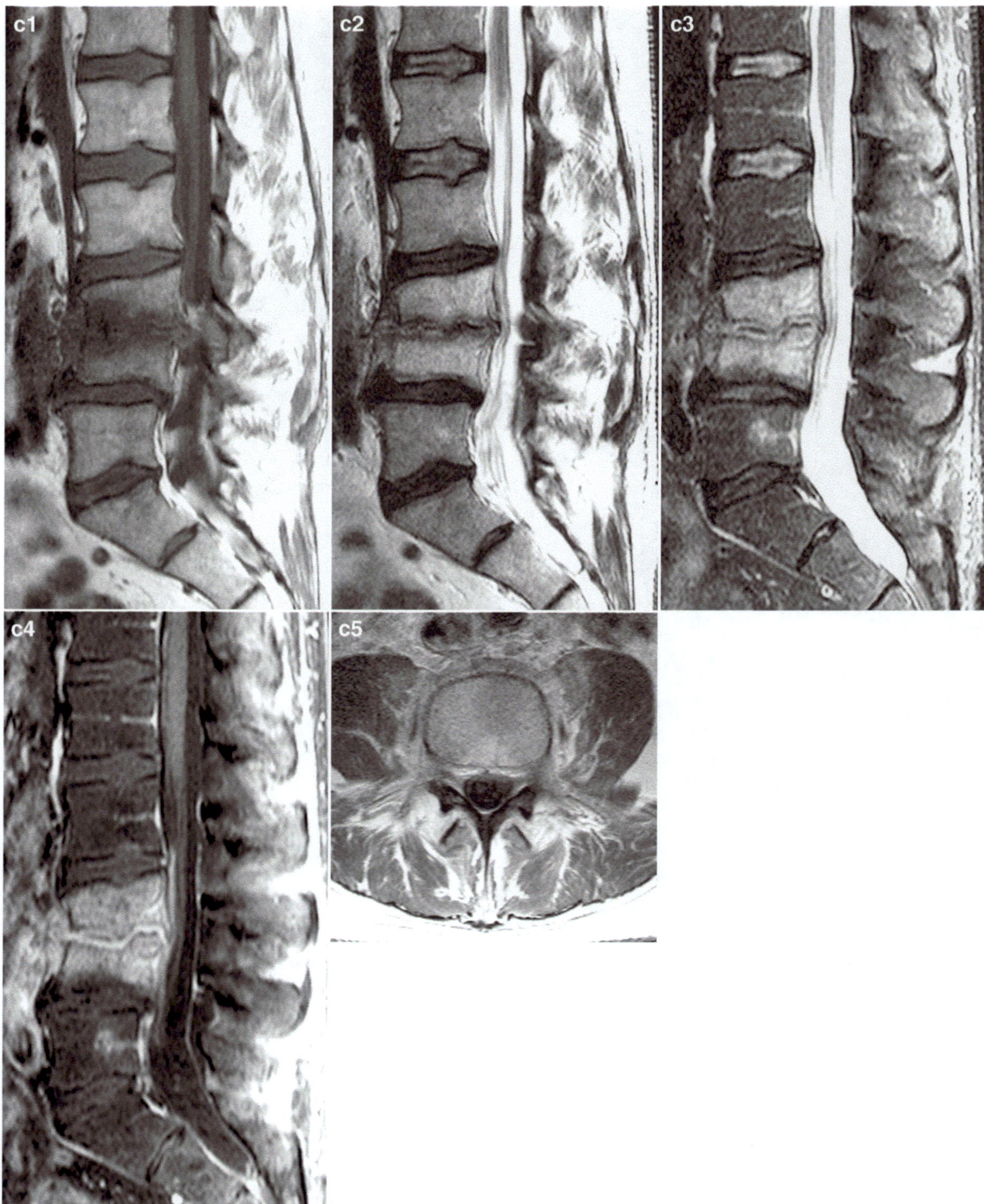

Fig. 5.13 *Follow-up MRI after 3 months*: sagittal T1- (**c1**); T2-weighted (**c2**) and fat-suppressed STIR images (**c3**) still show residual bone marrow signal changes with collapse of L3–4 disc space. Post-gadolinium fat-suppressed sagittal T1-weighted image (**c4**) shows enhancement of bone marrow, disc space and prevertebral region, and small linear area of epi-dural enhancement. Axial post-gadolinium T1-weighted image (**c5**) shows small left paravertebral enhancing pocket. Possible enhancement in dorsal paraspinal muscles, difficult to ascertain in this non-fat-suppressed image. Patient at this time free of pain, with normal laboratory findings

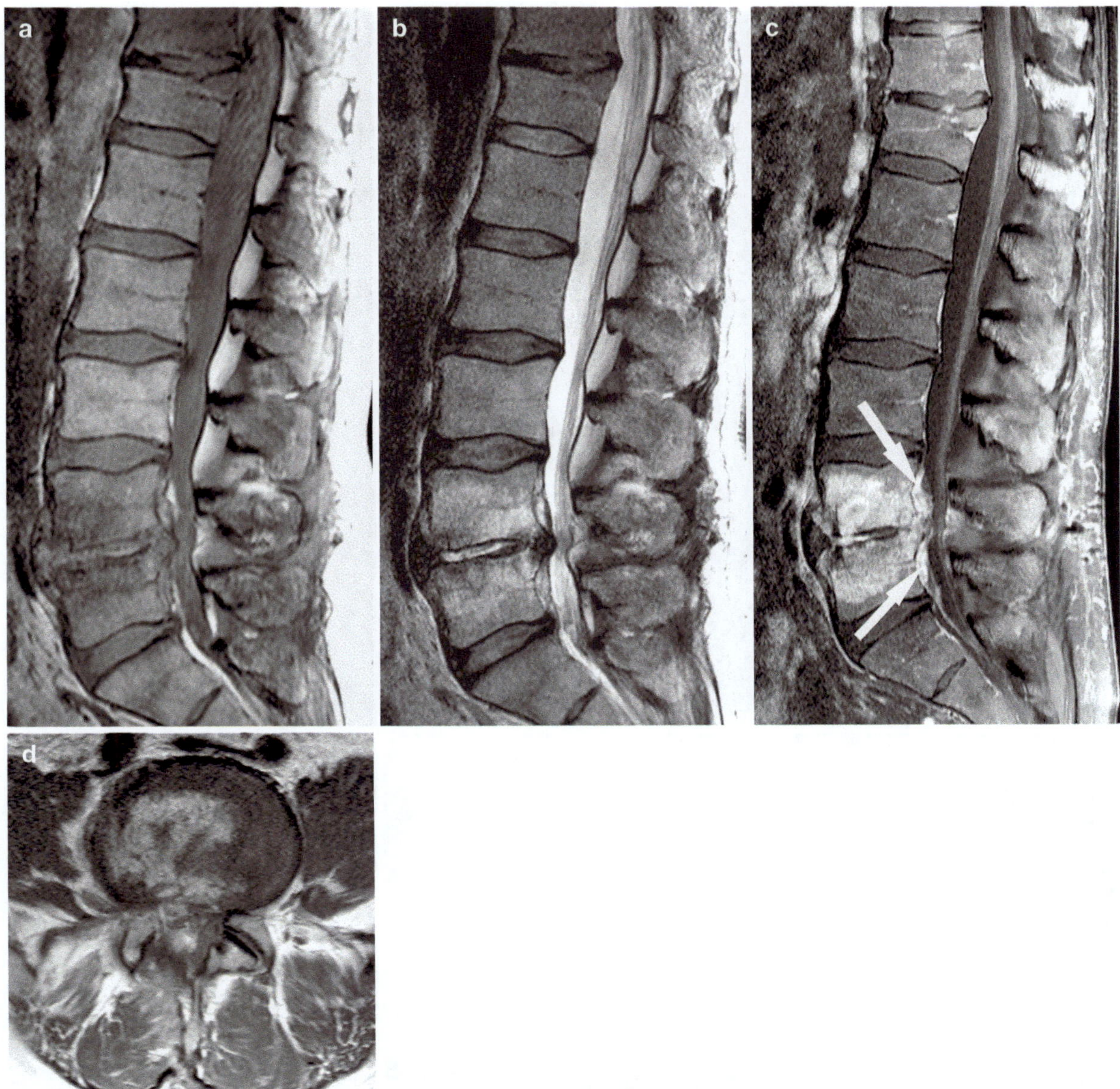

Fig. 5.14 Post-operative MRI changes without clinical or laboratory signs of spondylodiscitis. *Presentation*: patient, 55 years, underwent laminectomy for right L4–5 disc herniation, was initially free of pain after the operation, but suffered recurrence of pre-operative right L5 radicular pain after several weeks. *MRI*: eight months after operation sagittal T1- (**a**) and T2-weighted (**b**) images reveal L4 and L5 bone marrow changes: decrease of bone marrow fat signal in (**a**) and increase of fluid signal in (**b**), consistent with possible vertebral osteomyelitis but not specific for this diagnosis. Residual or recurrent herniation L4–5 with T2-hyperintense nucleus (**b**). Fat-suppressed post-gadolinium T1-W sagittal image (**c**) shows enhancing L4–5 disc and adjacent bone marrow, also epidural enhancement behind L4 and L5 vertebral bodies (*arrows*), probably due to expansion of anterior epidural space with dilated enhancing epidural veins (see also Fig. 5.9). Axial T1-weighted post-gadolinium image (**d**) shows disc enhancement, no clear paraspinal enhancement or abscess formation in this non fat-suppressed image. MRI was considered indicative of spondylodiscitis, but repeated clinical and laboratory assessments failed to support this diagnosis. The patient eventually underwent re-operation at L4–5, which resulted in partial relief of symptoms

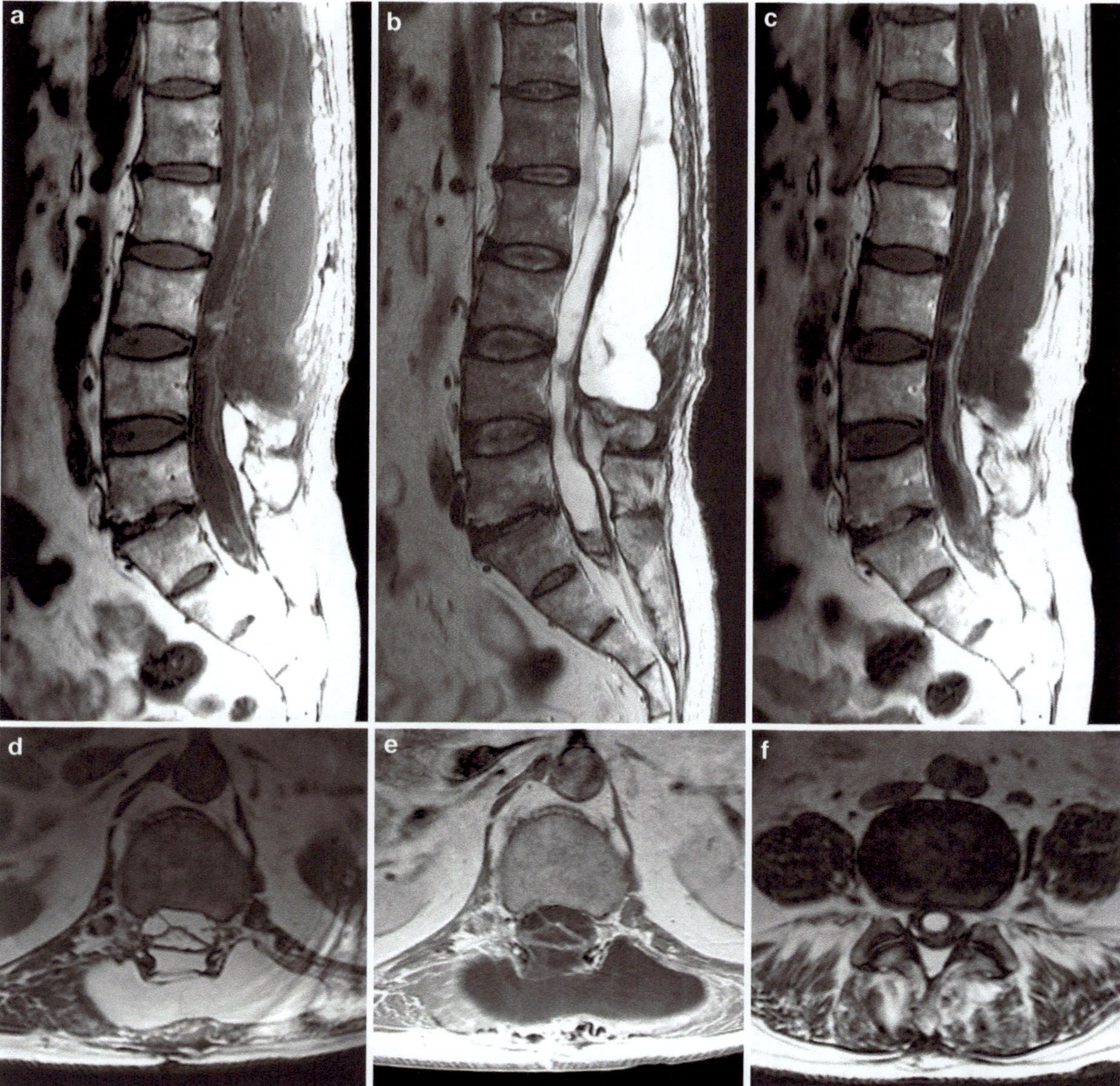

Fig. 5.15 Post-operative pseudomeningocele and arachnoiditis after excision of lumbar dermoid by laminectomy T10-L4. *Presentation*: patient, male 61 years, had undergone two previous untethering operations with dermoid excision, the first 38 years previously. Now recurrence of slowly progressive pain distally in both legs, with gradual loss of muscle strength. Patient underwent a third operation to remove the intraspinal mass which extended from T12 to L4. Post-operatively motor functions were unchanged, but there was disturbance of gait due to proprioceptive ataxia, which gradually improved in the course of the following months.

MRI: sagittal T1- (**a**) and T2-weighted (**b**) images show multi-level laminectomy with large CSF collection dorsal to spine, also irregular clumping and adhesions of cauda equina fibres sometimes forming septa, showing irregular contrast enhancement in post-gadolinium image (**c**). Axial T2-weighted and T1- weighted post-gadolinium images at L2 (**d, e**) and L4–5 (**f, g**) confirm adhesions of cauda equina fibres to one another and to dural sac at upper and lower lumbar levels, respectively. MR myelographic image (**h**) demonstrates point of connection of CSF collection with dural sac (*arrow*), and shows thickening of dural end-sac by arachnoiditis

Fig. 5.15 (continued)

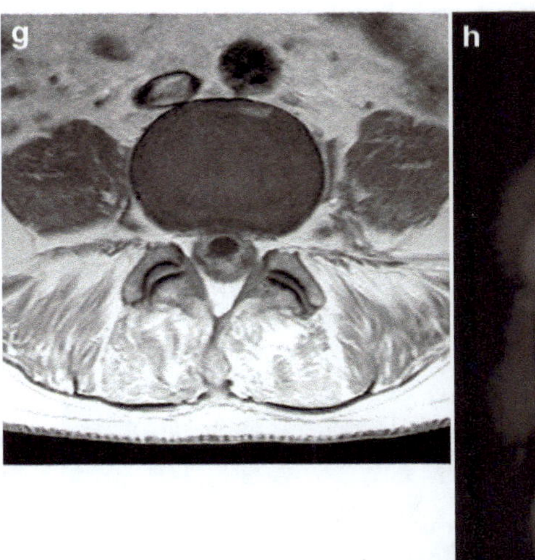

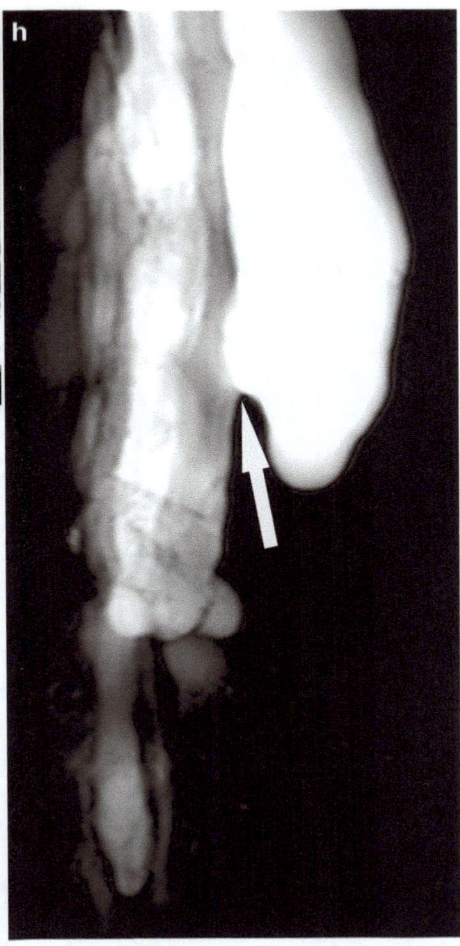

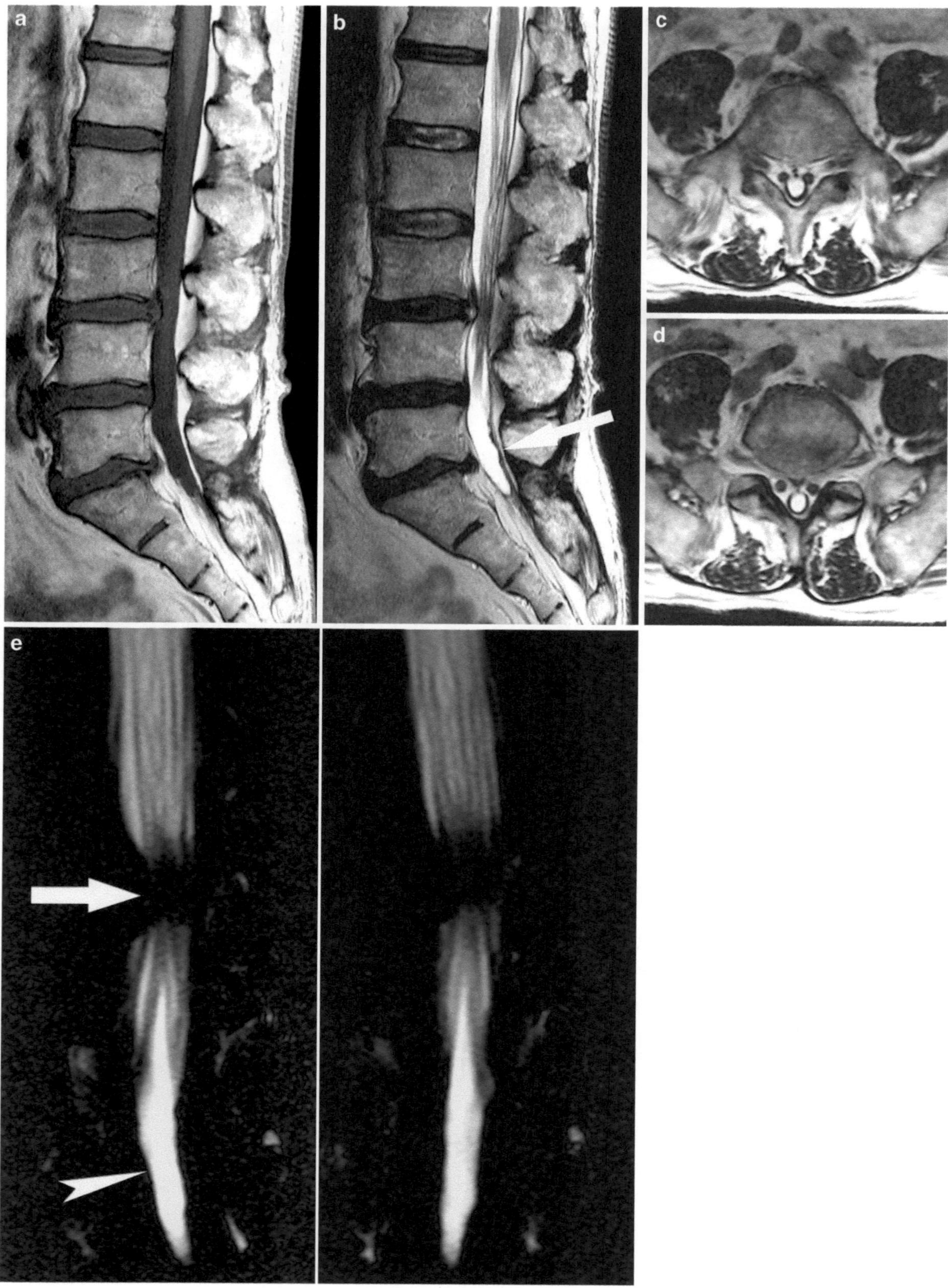

Fig. 5.16 Adhesive arachnoiditis after myelography incidentally found in patient referred for L4 radicular syndrome. *Presentation*: patient, male 72 years, underwent lumbar myelography many years previously, probably with an oil-based or high-osmolality ionic contrast medium. He suffered only from chronic aspecific low back pain until onset of an L4 radicular syndrome 4 months previous to MRI, with pain irradiating to medial aspect of right knee with loss of strength in iliopsoas and quadriceps muscles and decreased knee jerk at right. *MRI*: sagittal T1 (**a**) and T2-weighted (**b**) images show L3–4 protrusion, as well as classic aspect of empty dural sac caudal to L4–5 level (*arrow* in b). Axial T2-weighted images (**c, d**) confirm cauda equina fibres adherent to dural sac. This is also seen in MR myelographic images (**e**, *arrowhead*), which show empty dural sac, and also demonstrate L4 root compression by the L3–4 herniation (*arrow*). It is not clear whether the chronic low back pain could be attributed to the presence of arachnoiditis. Spontaneous remission of radicular complaints after 6 months

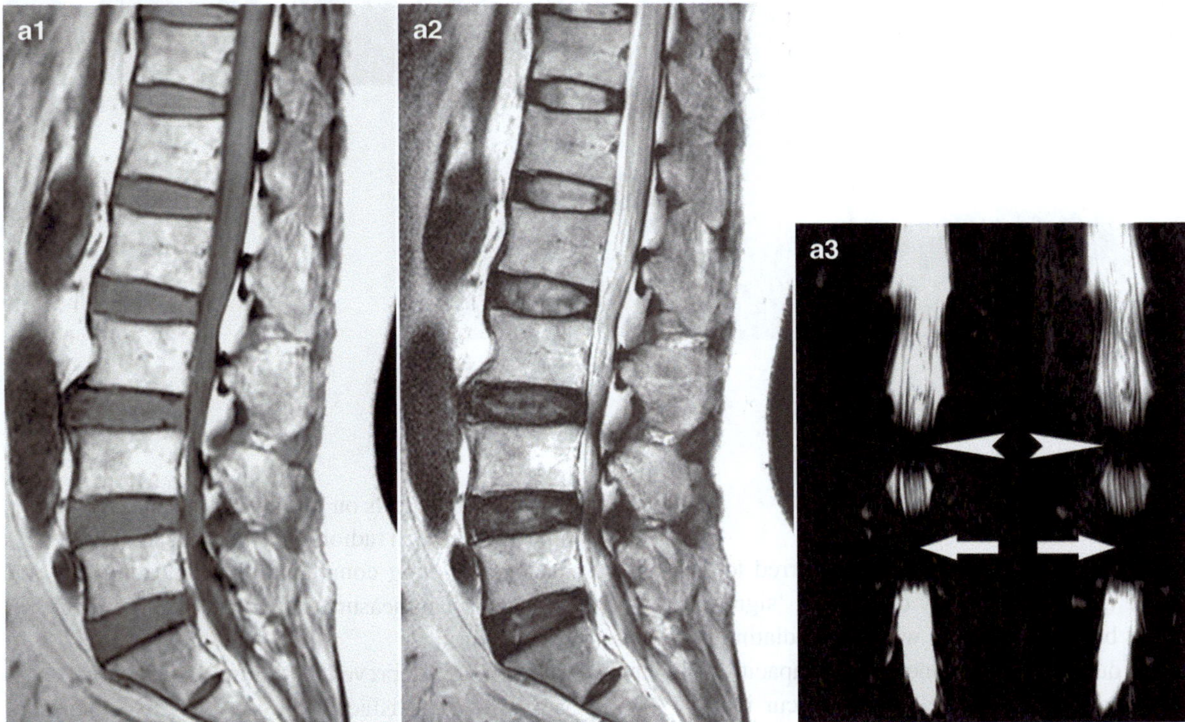

Fig. 5.17 Failed back surgery due to inappropriate level of operation. *Presentation*: patient, male 69 years, reported bilateral neurogenic claudication with numbness and cramping feelings in posterior thighs and calves after walking longer than 10 min, relieved by standing still. Examination revealed normal arterial pulsations in both legs and feet, no neurological deficits, normal straight-leg-raising on both sides. *MRI*: at first presentation sagittal T1 (**a1**) and T2-weighted (**a2**) images show multi-level lumbar spinal stenosis, with mid-sagittal bony diameters at L3 and L4 measuring 11 mm and 10 mm respectively. Further narrowing of canal by mild broad-based protrusion of L4–5 disc. Combination causing complete L4–5 CSF block on MR myelogram (*arrows* in **a3**). Note also less severe block at L3–4 (*arrowheads*), here apparently related to increase in retrodural fat rather than disc protrusion, in combination with developmental stenosis. Patient underwent decompressive laminectomy with initial good results. Three months later he reported relief of complaints of neurogenic claudication in the left leg, but persistence of these complaints at right. *Follow-up MRI* revealed that laminectomy had been performed at the L3 and L4 levels (**b1, 2**), but there was still compression of the dural sac at the L4–5 disc level, where the MR myelogram (**b3**) showed a complete CSF block (*arrow*). The L3–4 myelographic block present in the preoperative images, had been relieved. The patient underwent additional decompression at L4–5, with satisfactory results

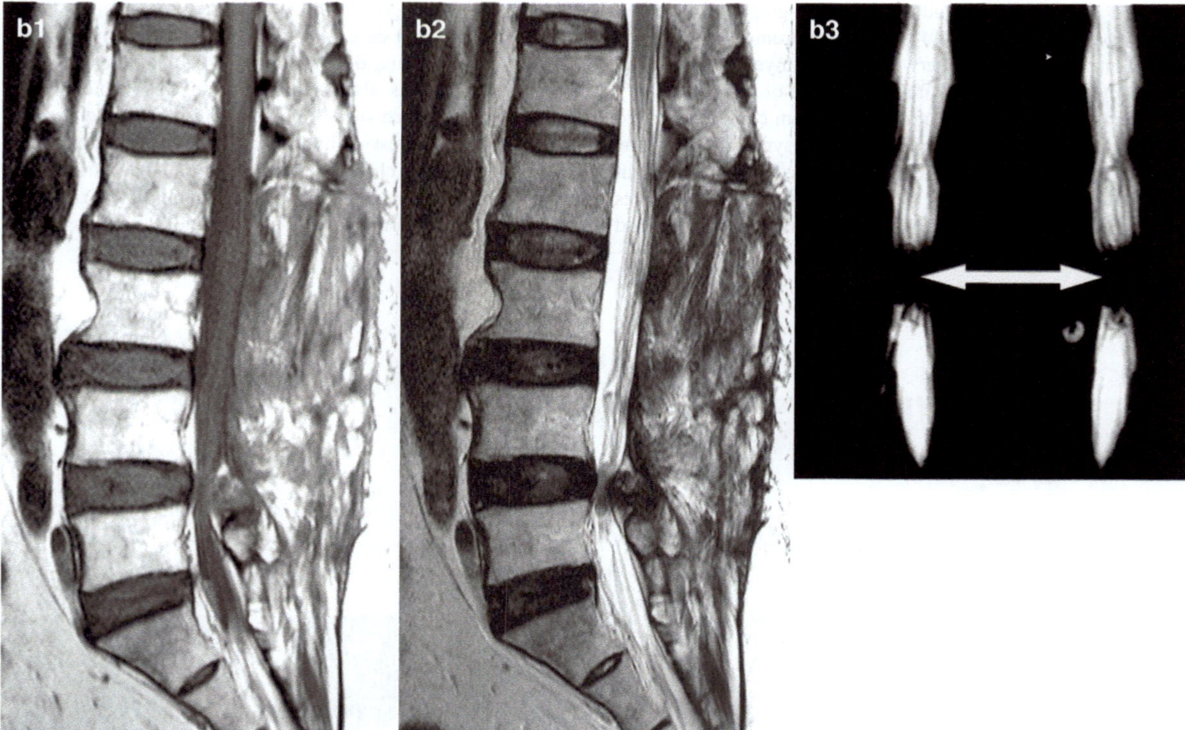

Fig. 5.17 (continued)

Appendix

Failed back surgery, sometimes referred to as a syndrome (FBSS), is loosely defined as: 'significant persistent back pain with or without irradiating pain and/or various degrees of functional incapacity following back surgery', and is believed to occur in 5–15% of patients who have undergone operation (Frymoyer 1988). Many causes have been named: surgical relief of nerve root compression by a herniated disc may be incomplete, or may even fail completely, for instance, when the wrong spinal level is operated, and/or in case of unrecognised concomitant stenosis (Fig. 5.17). The stability of the spine may have been compromised by the surgical procedure. A recurrent herniation of disc material may take place at the site of operation (see Fig. 5.7). When relief of pain is not achieved after one or more surgical interventions, and sometimes new radiological signs of post-operative epidural scar formation or intradural adhesive arachnoiditis occur, a therapeutic dead-end situation arises. Also because of concomitant psychosocial factors which are often mentioned in reports on this group, the causal relationship between such radiological findings and the persistent and crippling complaints is often not clear, and further surgical measures are considered ineffective in these conditions.

"The best way to prevent FBSS is to avoid surgery that leads to an unsatisfactory result" (Van Goethem and Salgado 2007). Other authors have also implicated inappropriate selection of patients for spinal surgery as a major cause of failure (Fager and Freidberg 1980; Frymoyer 1988). This can be best achieved by a careful selection of surgical candidates on the basis of selected clinical criteria supported by diagnostic imaging focused on key features and performed at the appropriate moment in the natural history. Diagnostic imaging should aim not only to depict in detail the myriad of degenerative spinal features which can be visualised with a high-resolution technique such as MRI, but should focus on separating the "wheat from the chaff", aiming to assess the relevance of imaging findings in relation to the clinical signs and symptoms.

References

Aejmelaeus R, Hiltunen H, Harkonen M et al (1984) Myelographic versus clinical diagnostics in lumbar disc disease. Arch Orthop Trauma Surg 103(1):18

Ahn UM, Ahn NU, Buchowski JM et al (2000) Cauda equina syndrome secondary to lumbar disc herniation: a meta-analysis of surgical outcomes. Spine 25(12):1515

Al-Nammari SS, Lucas JD, Lam KS (2007) Hematogenous methicillin-resistant *Staphylococcus aureus* spondylodiscitis. Spine 32(22):2480

Annertz M, Jonsson B, Stromqvist B et al (1995a) Serial MRI in the early postoperative period after lumbar discectomy. Neuroradiology 37(3):177

Annertz M, Jonsson B, Stromqvist B et al (1995b) No relationship between epidural fibrosis and sciatica in the lumbar postdiscectomy syndrome. A study with contrast-enhanced magnetic resonance imaging in symptomatic and asymptomatic patients. Spine 20(4):449

Atlas SJ, Keller RB, Wu YA et al (2005a) Long-term outcomes of surgical and nonsurgical management of sciatica secondary to a lumbar disc herniation: 10 year results from the maine lumbar spine study. Spine 30(8):927

Atlas SJ, Keller RB, Wu YA et al (2005b) Long-term outcomes of surgical and nonsurgical management of lumbar spinal stenosis: 8 to 10 year results from the maine lumbar spine study. Spine 30(8):936

Bartynski WS, Lin L (2003) Lumbar root compression in the lateral recess: MR imaging, conventional myelography, and CT myelography comparison with surgical confirmation. AJNR Am J Neuroradiol 24(3):348

Beattie PF, Meyers SP, Stratford P et al (2000) Associations between patient report of symptoms and anatomic impairment visible on lumbar magnetic resonance imaging. Spine 25(7):819

Bircher MD, Tasker T, Crawshaw C et al (1988) Discitis following lumbar surgery. Spine 13(1):98

Boden SD, Davis DO, Dina TS et al (1992a) Contrast-enhanced MR imaging performed after successful lumbar disk surgery: prospective study. Radiology 182(1):59

Boden SD, Davis DO, Dina TS et al (1990) Abnormal magnetic-resonance scans of the lumbar spine in asymptomatic subjects. A prospective investigation. J Bone Joint Surg Am 72(3):403

Boden SD, Davis DO, Dina TS et al (1992b) Postoperative diskitis: distinguishing early MR imaging findings from normal postoperative disk space changes. Radiology 184(3):765

Boos N, Rieder R, Schade V et al (1995) 1995 Volvo Award in clinical sciences. The diagnostic accuracy of magnetic resonance imaging, work perception, and psychosocial factors in identifying symptomatic disc herniations. Spine 20(24):2613

Borenstein DG, O'Mara JW Jr, Boden SD et al (2001) The value of magnetic resonance imaging of the lumbar spine to predict low-back pain in asymptomatic subjects: a seven-year follow-up study. J Bone Joint Surg Am 83-A(9):1306

Bosacco SJ, Gardner MJ, Guille JT (2001) Evaluation and treatment of dural tears in lumbar spine surgery: a review. Clin Orthop Relat Res (389):238

Bozzao A, Gallucci M, Masciocchi C et al (1992) Lumbar disk herniation: MR imaging assessment of natural history in patients treated without surgery. Radiology 185(1):135

Bush K, Cowan N, Katz DE et al (1992) The natural history of sciatica associated with disc pathology. A prospective study with clinical and independent radiologic follow-up. Spine 17(10):1205

Carlisle E, Luna M, Tsou PM et al (2005) Percent spinal canal compromise on MRI utilized for predicting the need for surgical treatment in single-level lumbar intervertebral disc herniation. Spine J 5(6):608

Carragee EJ, Kim DH (1997) A prospective analysis of magnetic resonance imaging findings in patients with sciatica and lumbar disc herniation. Correlation of outcomes with disc fragment and canal morphology. Spine 22(14):1650

Cowan NC, Bush K, Katz DE et al (1992) The natural history of sciatica: a prospective radiological study. Clin Radiol 46(1):7

Crisi G, Carpeggiani P, Trevisan C (1993) Gadolinium-enhanced nerve roots in lumbar disk herniation. AJNR Am J Neuroradiol 14(6):1379

Davis RA (1994) A long-term outcome analysis of 984 surgically treated herniated lumbar discs. J Neurosurg 80(3):415

Delamarter RB, Ross JS, Masaryk TJ et al (1990) Diagnosis of lumbar arachnoiditis by magnetic resonance imaging. Spine 15(4):304

Delauche-Cavallier MC, Budet C, Laredo JD et al (1992) Lumbar disc herniation. Computed tomography scan changes after conservative treatment of nerve root compression. Spine 17(8):927

Dina TS, Boden SD, Davis DO (1995) Lumbar spine after surgery for herniated disk: imaging findings in the early postoperative period. AJR Am J Roentgenol 164(3):665

Fager CA, Freidberg SR (1980) Analysis of failures and poor results of lumbar spine surgery. Spine 5(1):87

Fitt GJ, Stevens JM (1995) Postoperative arachnoiditis diagnosed by high resolution fast spin-echo MRI of the lumbar spine. Neuroradiology 37(2):139

Fries JW, Abodeely DA, Vijungco JG et al (1982) Computed tomography of herniated and extruded nucleus pulposus. J Comput Assist Tomogr 6(5):874

Frymoyer JW (1988) Back pain and sciatica. N Engl J Med 318 (5):291

Gallucci M, Bozzao A, Orlandi B et al (1995) Does postcontrast MR enhancement in lumbar disk herniation have prognostic value? J Comput Assist Tomogr 19(1):34

Gleave JR, Macfarlane R (2002) Cauda equina syndrome: what is the relationship between timing of surgery and outcome? Br J Neurosurg 16(4):325

Grane P (1998) The postoperative lumbar spine. A radiological investigation of the lumbar spine after discectomy using MR imaging and CT. Acta Radiol Suppl 414:1

Hakelius A (1970) Prognosis in sciatica. A clinical follow-up of surgical and non-surgical treatment. Acta Orthop Scand Suppl 129:1

Haro H, Shinomiya K, Komori H et al (1996) Upregulated expression of chemokines in herniated nucleus pulposus resorption. Spine 21(14):1647

Haughton V, Schreibman K, De Smet A (2002) Contrast between scar and recurrent herniated disk on contrast-enhanced MR images. AJNR Am J Neuroradiol 23(10):1652

Hitselberger WE, Witten RM (1968) Abnormal myelograms in asymptomatic patients. J Neurosurg 28(3):204

Hofman PA, Wilmink JT (1996) Optimising the image of the intradural nerve root: the value of MR radiculography. Neuroradiology 38(7):654

Ishikawa Y, Shimada Y, Miyakoshi N et al (2006) Decompression of idiopathic lumbar epidural lipomatosis: diagnostic magnetic resonance imaging evaluation and review of the literature. J Neurosurg Spine 4(1):24

Ito T, Takano Y, Yuasa N (2001) Types of lumbar herniated disc and clinical course. Spine 26(6):648

Jensen MC, Brant-Zawadzki MN, Obuchowski N et al (1994) Magnetic resonance imaging of the lumbar spine in people without back pain. N Engl J Med 331(2):69

Jensen TS, Albert HB, Soerensen JS et al (2006) Natural course of disc morphology in patients with sciatica: an MRI study using a standardized qualitative classification system. Spine 31(14):1605

Jinkins JR (1993) MR of enhancing nerve roots in the unoperated lumbosacral spine. AJNR Am J Neuroradiol 14(1):193

Karppinen J, Malmivaara A, Tervonen O et al (2001) Severity of symptoms and signs in relation to magnetic resonance imaging findings among sciatic patients. Spine 26(7):E149

Komori H, Okawa A, Haro H et al (1998) Contrast-enhanced magnetic resonance imaging in conservative management of lumbar disc herniation. Spine 23(1):67

Komori H, Shinomiya K, Nakai O et al (1996) The natural history of herniated nucleus pulposus with radiculopathy. Spine 21(2):225

Krudy AG (1992) MR myelography using heavily T2-weighted fast spin-echo pulse sequences with fat presaturation. AJR Am J Roentgenol 159(6):1315

Kuroki H, Tajima N, Hirakawa S et al (1998) Comparative study of MR myelography and conventional myelography in the diagnosis of lumbar spinal diseases. J Spinal Disord 11(6):487

Lane JI, Koeller KK, Atkinson JD (1996) MR imaging of the lumbar spine: enhancement of the radicular veins. AJR Am J Roentgenol 166(1):181

Lindholm TS, Pylkkanen P (1982) Discitis following removal of intervertebral disc. Spine 7(6):618

Luijsterburg PA, Verhagen AP, Ostelo RW et al (2007) Effectiveness of conservative treatments for the lumbosacral radicular syndrome: a systematic review. Eur Spine J 16(7):881

Maigne JY, Rime B, Deligne B (1992) Computed tomographic follow-up study of forty-eight cases of nonoperatively treated lumbar intervertebral disc herniation. Spine 17(9):1071

Modic MT, Obuchowski NA, Ross JS et al (2005) Acute low back pain and radiculopathy: MR imaging findings and their prognostic role and effect on outcome. Radiology 237(2):597

Modic MT, Ross JS, Obuchowski NA et al (1995) Contrast-enhanced MR imaging in acute lumbar radiculopathy: a pilot study of the natural history. Radiology 195(2):429

O'Connell MJ, Ryan M, Powell T et al (2003) The value of routine MR myelography at MRI of the lumbar spine. Acta Radiol 44(6):665

Peul WC, Brand R, Thomeer RT et al (2008a) Influence of gender and other prognostic factors on outcome of sciatica. Pain 138(1):180

Peul WC, Brand R, Thomeer RT et al (2008b) Improving prediction of "inevitable" surgery during non-surgical treatment of sciatica. Pain 138(3):571

Peul WC, van Houwelingen HC, van den Hout WB et al (2007) Surgery versus prolonged conservative treatment for sciatica. N Engl J Med 356(22):2245

Porchet F, Wietlisbach V, Burnand B et al (2002) Relationship between severity of lumbar disc disease and disability scores in sciatica patients. Neurosurgery 50(6):1253

Qureshi A, Sell P (2007) Cauda equina syndrome treated by surgical decompression: the influence of timing on surgical outcome. Eur Spine J 16(12):2143

Robertson SC, Traynelis VC, Follett KA et al (1997) Idiopathic spinal epidural lipomatosis. Neurosurgery 41(1):68

Ross J (1991) Imaging of the spine. WB Saunders, Philadelphia

Ross JS, Masaryk TJ, Modic MT et al (1987) Lumbar spine: postoperative assessment with surface-coil MR imaging. Radiology 164(3):851

Ross JS, Robertson JT, Frederickson RC et al (1996) Association between peridural scar and recurrent radicular pain after lumbar discectomy: magnetic resonance evaluation. ADCON-L European Study Group. Neurosurgery 38(4):855

Saal JA (1996) Natural history and nonoperative treatment of lumbar disc herniation. Spine 21(24 Suppl):2S

Saal JA, Saal JS (1989) Nonoperative treatment of herniated lumbar intervertebral disc with radiculopathy. An outcome study. Spine 14(4):431

Saal JA, Saal JS, Herzog RJ (1990) The natural history of lumbar intervertebral disc extrusions treated nonoperatively. Spine 15(7):683

Shapiro S (2000) Medical realities of cauda equina syndrome secondary to lumbar disc herniation. Spine 25(3):348

Silber JS, Anderson DG, Vaccaro AR et al (2002) Management of postprocedural discitis. Spine J 2(4):279

Splendiani A, Puglielli E, De Amicis R et al (2004) Spontaneous resolution of lumbar disk herniation: predictive signs for prognostic evaluation. Neuroradiology 46(11):916

Sze G (1990) New applications of MR contrast agents in neuroradiology. Neuroradiology 32(5):421

Tafazal SI, Sell PJ (2005) Incidental durotomy in lumbar spine surgery: incidence and management. Eur Spine J 14(3):287

Taneichi H, Abumi K, Kaneda K et al (1994) Significance of Gd-DTPA-enhanced magnetic resonance imaging for lumbar disc herniation: the relationship between nerve root enhancement and clinical manifestations. J Spinal Disord 7(2):153

Thelander U, Fagerlund M, Friberg S et al (1994) Describing the size of lumbar disc herniations using computed tomography. A comparison of different size index calculations and their relation to sciatica. Spine 19(17):1979

Toyone T, Takahashi K, Kitahara H et al (1993) Visualisation of symptomatic nerve roots. Prospective study of contrast-enhanced MRI in patients with lumbar disc herniation. J Bone Joint Surg Br 75(4):529

Van Goethem J, Salgado R (2007) Spinal imaging: diagnostic imaging of the spine and spinal cord. Springer, Berlin

Van Goethem JW, Parizel PM, Jinkins JR (2002) Review article: MRI of the postoperative lumbar spine. Neuroradiology 44(9):723

Vogelsang JP, Finkenstaedt M, Vogelsang M et al (1999) Recurrent pain after lumbar discectomy: the diagnostic value of peridural scar on MRI. Eur Spine J 8(6):475

Vroomen PC, de Krom MC, Slofstra PD et al (2000) Conservative treatment of sciatica: a systematic review. J Spinal Disord 13(6):463

Vroomen PC, de Krom MC, Wilmink JT et al (1999) Lack of effectiveness of bed rest for sciatica. N Engl J Med 340(6):418

Vroomen PC, de Krom MC, Wilmink JT et al (2002a) Diagnostic value of history and physical examination in patients suspected of lumbosacral nerve root compression. J Neurol Neurosurg Psychiatry 72(5):630

Vroomen PC, Van Hapert SJ, Van Acker RE et al (1998) The clinical significance of gadolinium enhancement of lumbar disc herniations and nerve roots on preoperative MRI. Neuroradiology 40(12):800

Vroomen PC, Wilmink JT, de KM (2002b) Prognostic value of MRI findings in sciatica. Neuroradiology 44(1):59

Weber H (1983) Lumbar disc herniation. A controlled, prospective study with ten years of observation. Spine 8(2):131

Weber H, Holme I, Amlie E (1993) The natural course of acute sciatica with nerve root symptoms in a double-blind placebo-controlled trial evaluating the effect of piroxicam. Spine 18(11):1433

Weiner BK, Patel NM, Walker MA (2007) Outcomes of decompression for lumbar spinal canal stenosis based upon preoperative radiographic severity. J Orthop Surg 2:3

Weinstein JN, Lurie JD, Tosteson TD et al (2006) Surgical vs nonoperative treatment for lumbar disk herniation: the Spine Patient Outcomes Research Trial (SPORT) observational cohort. JAMA 296(20):2451

Weinstein JN, Tosteson TD, Lurie JD et al (2008) Surgical versus nonsurgical therapy for lumbar spinal stenosis. N Engl J Med 358(8):794

Weishaupt D, Zanetti M, Hodler J et al (1998) MR imaging of the lumbar spine: prevalence of intervertebral disk extrusion and sequestration, nerve root compression, end plate abnormalities, and osteoarthritis of the facet joints in asymptomatic volunteers. Radiology 209(3):661

Wiesel SW, Tsourmas N, Feffer HL et al (1984) A study of computer-assisted tomography. I. The incidence of positive CAT scans in an asymptomatic group of patients. Spine 9(6):549

Index

MIX
Papier aus verantwortungsvollen Quellen
Paper from responsible sources
FSC® C105338

If you have any concerns about our products,
you can contact us on
ProductSafety@springernature.com

In case Publisher is established outside the EU,
the EU authorized representative is:
Springer Nature Customer Service Center GmbH
Europaplatz 3, 69115 Heidelberg, Germany

Printed by Libri Plureos GmbH
in Hamburg, Germany